Advances in Research on Neurodegeneration, Volume II

Etiopathogenesis

Advances in Research on Neurodegeneration

Advances in Research on Neurodegeneration, Volume II

Etiopathogenesis

Y. Mizuno
D. B. Calne
R. Horowski
Editors

Birkhäuser
Boston • Basel • Berlin

Yoshikuni Mizuno
Department of Neurology
Juntendo University School of Medicine
Hongo, Bunkyo, Tokyo 113
Japan

R. Horowski
Schering AG Berlin
Clinical Research
Special Research Projects
Müllerstraße 170–178
D-1000 Berlin 65
Germany

Donald B. Calne
The University of British Columbia
Director, Neurodegenerative Disorders Center
Purdy Pavillion
The Vancouver Hospital, Health Sciences Center
2211 Wesbrook Mall
Vancouver, B.C.
Canada V6T 1W5

Printed on acid-free paper.

© 1994 Birkhäuser Boston

Birkhäuser

Softcover reprint of the hardcover 1st edition 1994

ISBN 978-1-4684-9205-7   ISBN 978-1-4684-9203-3 (eBook)
DOI 10.1007/978-1-4684-9203-3

Typeset by Alden Multimedia, Northampton, England.

Contents

Preface

In 1991, a small annual meeting named "International Winter Conference on Neurodegeneration (IWCN)" was established; the aim of this meeting is to review the neurodegenerative disorders and to attempt to explore how progress might be made in this field, as the neurodegenerative disorders have been emerging to be one of the major causes of morbidity and mortality in modern societies. The first meeting took place in Seefeld, Austria, in February 1992; the topics for the first IWCN were chosen to provide a broad foundation of clinical science, which included the problem of aging, classification of neurodegenerative disorders and natural history, pathology, and clinical neurology of Alzheimer's disease, Parkinson's disease, and amyotrophic lateral sclerosis.

The fundamental pathology underlying these neurodegenerative disorders is neuronal cell death. For the understanding of pathophysiology and the development of neuroprotective treatment for these disorders, elucidation of the mechanism of neuronal cell death at the cellular and molecular level is essential. With this concept in mind, the second IWCN was held in Whistler Village in Canada in January 1993. Funding was generously provided by Schering AG, Berlin, and for the excellent organization we have to thank Ms. Ingeborg Runge.

In the second meeting, discussion was largely focused on the mechanism of neuronal death in the neurodegenerative disorders, as the subtitle of the meeting, "Etiopathogenesis," indicates. Papers were presented on genetic factors, trophic factors, metal ions (manganese, iron, and calcium), free radicals, mitochondrial metabolism, proteases, neurotoxins, and slow viruses in the neurodegenerative disorders. Much time was spent in the discussion; in particular, molecular events that appear to be taking place in the process of neuronal cell death were discussed from various aspects. Although we still do not know the primary events that initiate the cascade of cellular reactions which lead to neuronal death in different diseases, it is the hope of the organizers of the second IWCN that this second volume will give, to a wider group of investigators, ideas about what should be done to find the primary causes of these disorders and at what levels of the pathogenetic cascade new therapies might act.

Y. Mizuno
D.B. Calne
R. Horowski

List of Contributors

M. Flint Beal, Warren 408, Harvard Medical School, Massachusetts General Hospital, Fruit Street, Boston, Massachusetts 02114, USA

Dorit Ben-Shachar, Department of Pharmacology, TECHNION, Faculty of Medicine, Israel Institute of Technology, P.O. Box 9649, Haifa 31 096, Israel

Donald B. Calne, Neurodegenerative Disorders Centre, Purdy Pavillion, The Vancouver Hospital and Health Sciences Centre, 2211 Wesbrook Mall, Vancouver V6T 2B6, British Columbia, Canada

N.S. Chu, Department of Neurology, Chang Chung Medical College, Chang Gung Memorial Hospital, 199 Tung Awa North Road, Taipei 5a1, Taiwan

D. Carleton Gajdusek, Laboratory of Central Nervous System Studies, NINDS, Building 36, Room 5B-21, National Institutes of Health, Bethesda, Maryland 20892, USA

P.H. St. George-Hyslop, Center for Research in Neurodegenerative Diseases, Tanz Neuroscience Building, University of Toronto, 6 Queen's Park Cr. West, Toronto M5S 1A8, Ontario, Canada

Franz Hefti, Andrus Center, University of Southern California, University Park 0191, Los Angeles, California 90089, USA

John B. Hibbs, Jr., Department of Veterans Affairs Medical Center and, Division of Infectious Diseases, University of Utah School of Medicine, 500 Foothill Drive, Salt Lake City, Utah 84148, USA

Chrysanthy Ikonomidou, Department of Pediatric Neurology, St. Louis Children's Hospital, Washington University School of Medicine, One Children's Place, St. Louis, Missouri 63110, USA

Bernd Janetzky, Department of Neurology, University of Würzburg, Josef-Schneider Str. 11, 97080 Würzburg, Germany

William C. Koller, Department of Neurology, University of Kansas Medical Center, 3901 Rainbow Boulevard, Kansas City, Kansas 66160-7314, USA

Andreas Kupsch, Department of Neurology, Klinikum Grosshadern, Ludwig-Maximilians-Universität München, Marchioninistraße 15, 81377 München, Germany

Patrick L. McGeer, Kinsmen Laboratory of Neurological Research, University of British Columbia, 2255 Wesbrook Mall, Vancouver, B.C., Canada V6T 1W5

Edith G. McGeer, Kinsmen Laboratory of Neurological Research, University of British Columbia, 2255 Wesbrook Mall, Vancouver, B.C., Canada V6T 1W5

Yoshikuni Mizuno, Department of Neurology, Juntendo University School of Medicine, Hongo, Bunkyo, Tokyo 113, Japan

Toshiharu Nagatsu, Institute for Comprehensive Medical Science, Fujita Health University School of Medicine, Toyoake, Aichi 470-11, Japan

Makoto Naoi, Department of Biosciences, Nagoya Institute of Technology, Nagoya 466, Japan

Pierluigi Nicotera, Institute of Environmental Medicine, Division of Toxicology, Karolinska Institutet, Box 210, S-171 77, Stockholm, Sweden

Toskhimitsu Niwa, Department of Internal Medicine, Nagoya University Branch Hospital, Nagoya 461, Japan

Wolfgang H. Oertel, Department of Neurology, Klinikum Grosshadern, Ludwig-Maximilians-Universität München, Marchioninistraße 15, 81377 München, Germany

C. Warren Olanow, Department of Neurology, Mount Sinai Medical Center, One Gustave Levy Place, Box 1137, New York, New York, 10029, USA

Sten Orrenius, Institute of Environmental Medicine, Division of Toxicology, Karolinska Institutet, Box 210, S-171 77, Stockholm, Sweden

Daniel P. Perl, Neuropathology Division, Mount Sinai School of Medicine, One Gustave L. Levy Place, Box 1134, New York, New York 10029-6574, USA

Werner H. Poewe, Neurologische Abteilung, Universitätsklinikum Rudolf Virchow, Augustenburger Platz 1, D-13353 Berlin, Germany

Heinz Reichmann, Department of Neurology, University of Würzburg, Josef-Schneider Str. 11, 97080 Würzburg, Germany

Peter Riederer, Clinical Neurochemistry, Department of Psychiatry, University of Würzburg, Füchsleinstr. 15, 97080 Würzburg, Germany

Jill M. Roberts-Lewis, Cephalon, Inc., 145 Brandywine Parkway, West Chester, Pennsylvania 19380, USA

Mary J. Savage, Cephalon, Inc., 145 Brandywine Parkway, West Chester, Pennsylvania 19380, USA

Robert Siman, Cephalon, Inc., 145 Brandywine Parkway, West Chester, Pennsylvania 19380, USA

Lechoslaw Turski, Research Laboratories of Schering AG, Müllerstraße 178, 13342 Berlin, Germany

Mitsuo Yoshida, Department of Neurology, Jichi Medical School, Tochigi 329-04, Japan

Moussa B.H. Youdim, Department of Pharmacology, Bruce Rappaport Faculty of Medicine, TECHNION, Israel Institute of Technology, P.O. Box 9649, Haifa 31 096, Israel

Part I

GENETIC, GROWTH, AND ENVIRONMENTAL FACTORS

1

Genetic Evidence for a Novel Familial Alzheimer's Disease Locus on Chromosome 14: Analysis of Candidate Genes

P.H. St. George-Hyslop

Alzheimer disease (AD) is a common, fatal, degenerative disease of the adult human central nervous system associated with distinctive neuro-pathological features and with progressive cognitive and intellectual decline during mid- to late adult life (Kätzman, 1986). In some families AD is inherited as an autosomal dominant trait (St. George-Hyslop et al., 1989), subsequent studies have revealed that the disorder is genetically heterogeneous (St. George-Hyslop et al., 1991). Thus, a small proportion of FAD cases are associated with mutations in the amyloid precursor protein (*APP*) gene on chromosome 21 (Goate et al., 1991; Karlinsky et al., 1992; Murrell et al., 1991), while some pedigrees segregating senile onset FAD show linkage or association with genetic markers on chromosome 19 (Pericak-Vance et al., 1991). Many FAD pedigrees however have not shown strong evidence for linkage to either chromosome, suggesting the existence of additional FAD genes on other chromosomes. We report here the discovery of a novel FAD locus on chromosome 14 and the analysis of three candidate genes from this chromosome, and we provide preliminary results concerning the clinical application of molecular genetic data.

To identify the chromosomal locations of other FAD genes, we investigated the segregation of highly polymorphic simple sequence repeat (SSR) markers from chromosomes other than chromosomes 19 and 21 in a series of 21 FAD pedigrees (Table 1). Although these other FAD genes could be on any of the other autosomal chromosomes, we reasoned that we could efficiently identify these genes using clues gained from analysis of the biology of this disease to reduce the complexity of a genome search as much as possible. The discovery by this and other groups that the FAD phenotype in some pedigrees

ADVANCES IN RESEARCH ON NEURODEGENERATION, II
Y. Mizuno et al., Editors
© 1994 Birkhäuser Boston

Table 1. Phenotypes of FAD Pedigrees

Symbol	Mean Age of Onset (years)	Ethnic Origin	Neuropathological Confirmation[a]
FAD1	53	Canadian	+
FAD4	43	Italian	+
FAD2	48	German	+
FAD3	48	Jewish	+
M9	75	Jewish	
M2	67	American	+
M3	60	American	+
M4	60	American	
NIH2	48	Jewish	+
M8	61	American	
FLO2	61	Italian	+
TOR1	62	Canadian	
M11	70	American	
R1	70	Russian	
Mex1	45	Mexican	
FL1	74	Hispanic	
Tor1.1	43	Italian	+
M13	84	Jewish	+
TFL10	61	Italian	+
JPN1	42	Japanese	+
603	47	American	+

[a] Postmortem histopathological confirmation of AD has been possible in at least one instance in

was associated with mutations in the APP gene on chromosome 21 lent considerable support to an existing hypothesis that the primary event in the pathogenesis of AD is the extracellular deposition of the β/A4 fragment of *APP* (Joachim and Selkoe, 1992). Although most pedigrees do not segregate mutations in the APP gene, it is conceivable that the sequence of events that lead to the extracellular deposition of the β/A4 fragment of APP might more commonly arise from mutations in other genes involved in the metabolism of *APP* or in other aspects of the neuropathology of AD. This hypothesis argues that a search for additional FAD loci should be focused on those areas of the genome known to contain proteases, protease inhibitors, molecular chapterones, and genes coding for other components of the senile plaques or neurofibrillary tangles.

Several such candidate genes have been mapped to chromosome 14. Thus, it is possible that mutations in either the α-1-anti-chymotrypsin (*AACT*) gene (a serine protease inhibitor and a component of the extracellular senile plaque in AD brain), or in a member of the serine protease gene cluster (including cathepsin G) might lead to aberrant intracellular proteolytic cleavage of *APP*. Similarly, mutations in the *FBJ* osteosarcoma viral oncogene homolog (*cFOS*) gene, which is known to be abberantly expressed in AD hippocampus and which is a transacting transcriptional regulator of *APP* gene expression (in preparation) might cause dysregulation of *APP* gene expression (Pollwein et al., 1991; Zhong et al., 1992). Finally, mutations in the heat shock protein *HSP70*, which is also known to be abnormally expressed in AD brain tissue (Hamos et al., 1991) could theoretically cause defective processing of *APP* because heat shock proteins are thought to be molecular chaperones involved in intracellular trafficking of transmembrane proteins such as *APP*. Further evidence to support the proposition that chromosome 14 might harbor a putative FAD locus is provided by a report of AD associated with a familial Robertsonian translocation involving chromosomes 14 and 21. To determine whether the known candidate genes or other as yet unidentified genes on chromosome 14 might be the site of an FAD mutation in our pedigrees, we initially investigated the segregation of a series of eight SSR markers spanning the entire long arm of chromosome 14 (Wang et al., 1992; Weissenbach et al., 1992).

Methods

FAD Pedigrees

The diagnosis of living affected pedigree members was achieved according to NINCDS-ADRDA criteria (Khachaturian, 1985; McKhann et al., 1984) by a qualified specialist in neurology or psychiatry using institutionally approved protocols and the informed consent of the study participants. Diagnosis in deceased, affected pedigree members was achieved through review of medical and family records. Postmortem histopathological confirmation of AD has been possible in at least 1 instance in 13 pedigrees.

Pedigrees 1–19 inclusive have been reported in previous genetic linkage studies and in some phenotypic studies (St. George-Hyslop et al., 1991). Genetic studies of pedigree 603 have also been reported in detail elsewhere (Perlak-Vance et al., 1988; Schellenberg et al., 1991). None of these pedigrees have individually shown significant evidence of linkage to genetic markers on either chromosome 21 or on chromosome 19 (Pericak-Vance et al., 1988; St. George-Hyslop et al., 1989, 1991; and unpublished results). However, some of these pedigrees, when considered *cumulatively*, do provide evidence for linkage to chromosome 21 (*D21S1/S11-DS1S16*, multipoint Z = 4.25) (St. George-Hyslop et al., 1981). None of the pedigrees have missense mutations in the APP gene (Tanzi et al., 1992).

Genotyping Studies

Genomic DNA was obtained from informative living family members as described (St. George-Hyslop et al., 1989) and from formalin-fixed tissue using methods to be described elsewhere (Mortilla et al., in preparation). Genomic DNA, 100 ng from each individual, was amplified by polymerex chain reaction (PCR) using 10 pmol of the oligonucleotide primers in 10 µl of reaction buffer as described (Wang et al., 1992; Weissenbach et al., 1992) and cycled through 94×6 sec, 54×20 sec, 72×20 sec for 35 cycles. For *D14S43*, the primer sequences were 5'-TGGAACACTCAGGCGA-3' and 5'-ACTTTCTACTTTCCCT-CACT-3'. For *D14S51*, the annealing temperature was 60×20 sec. PCR productions were resolved according to size by denaturing polyacrylamide gel electrophoresis and visualized by autoradiography. Genotypes were determined relative to those of other pedigree members loaded on the same gel and relative to a sequencing standard. Alleles at each locus were scored in an identical way across all pedigrees.

Statistical Analyses

Lod (logarithm of the odds) scores were calculated with the LINKAGE programs using the same initial maximum likelihood parameters as previously described (St. George-Hyslop et al., 1991). A new mutation rate of 0.001 was used to force the analysis to consider all discordant individuals as obligate recombinants, thereby making it harder to detect linkage. Marker allele frequencies were deduced from spouses of members of these pedigrees and from one at-risk member of these pedigrees to ensure that the allele frequencies used accurately reflect the frequencies existent in the ethnic populations from which these pedigrees were drawn. No significant difference was observed between the observed allele frequencies and those previously reported for these markers. To allow inclusion of information on the segregation of FAD gene from currently asymptomatic pedigree members, we employed an age-of-onset correction as previously described. To ensure that errors in the empiric estimates of age-dependent risk were not misleading our analyses, we also analyzed the data by setting the penetrance of FAD to zero in the asymptomatic family members but retained their genotypes at the chromosome 14 marker loci.

For the *D14S43-D14S53* multipoint, the data were recoded to four allele systems using standard procedures to improve computational tractability. Maximum likelihood scores were then calculated assuming *D14S43* and *D14S53* to be at fixed map positions 3 cM apart, using the

LINKMAP program and the same maximum likelihood parameter sets described for the two-point analyses.

Direct Sequencing of Genomic DNA

DNA sequences of interest within the *cFOS* and *CTSNG* genes were amplified and purified by PCR from total genomic DNA (containing both chromosomes) from one affected member and one unaffected member (usually the married-in parent) from each FAD pedigree using the flanking primer pairs as described (Rogaev et al., in press; Wong et al., in press). PCR reactions were typically carried out in 50-μl volumes using 20 pmole of each primer, 100 ng of template genomic DNa, 10 mM Tris HCl (pH 9.0), 2.0 mM MgCl$_2$, 0.01% gelatin, 0.1% Triton X-100, 200 μM dNTPs, 50 mM KCl, 0.2 units Taq polymerase (Promega), and cycled through 30 cycles of 90×6 sec, 54×20 sec, and 72×20 sec, using an initial denaturation phase of 5 sec at 94 and a final elongation phase at 72 for 7 min. PCR products were gel purified and rendered single stranded by asymmetric PCR using a 100-fold excess of one primer, and then sequenced using either the original PCR primers or new internal primers and the protocols previously described by Vaula et al. (1992).

Restriction Mapping

The physical size and copy number of the *CTSNG* and *cFOS* genes was assessed using Southern blots of *Bam*HI restriction digests of genomic DNA from the same affected and unaffected pair of family members in each pedigree. These Southern blots were hybridized with ^{32}P-labeled PCR products containing exon 4 of *CTSNG* or *cFOS* gene. The resultant restriction pattern for FAD-affected pedigree members was then compared both to the restriction pattern observed in genomic DNA from unaffected relatives run in an adjacent lane, and to the restriction pattern predicted from the published nucleotide sequences for these genes (van Straaten et al., 1983; Yoshkai et al., 1981). Using suitable size standards on the ethidium bromide-stained gels we are able to clearly resolve differences of 300 bp at 3 kb (*CSTNG Bam*HI fragment) and of 500 bp at 6 kb (*cFOS*).

Single-Stranded Conformational Polymorphisms

Single-stranded conformational polymorphisms (SSCPs) were detected for exons 1, 2, and 3 of the *cFOS* gene, but reliable SSCPs could not be generated for exon 4 (Rogaev et al., in press). Internally labeled PCR product at $10\,\mu l$ was added to $40\,\mu l$ of a solution containing 95% formamide, 0.05% bromophenol blue, and 0.05% xylene cyanol. The samples were denatured by heating to 94 for 5 min, quenched in ice, and $4\,\mu l$ of the mixture was loaded onto a 6% nondenaturing polyacrylamide gel containing 5% glycerol and run at 4 for 5–8 hr at 20 W. Allele frequencies for the SSCP polymorphisms were established from the analysis of 57 unaffected spouses married into the FAD pedigrees, thereby providing a control group of similar ethnic origins. Mendelian inheritance was assessed by following segregation through a three-generation sibship constituting 20 meioses.

Results

Initial Genetic Linkage Studies

The genotype at each of the first eight chromosome 14 loci was determined for each pedigree member (Wang et al., 1992). Evidence for cosegregation of each marker locus with FAD was then sought by computing pedigree-specific lod scores using pairwise (disease versus a single locus) tests of linkage and the same maximum likelihood parameters as previously described by St. George-Hyslop et al., in 1991. Markers at the extreme telomeric (*D14S48, D14S51*) or extreme centromeric regions (*D14S50, D14S49, D14S52*) of chromosome 14q provided no strong evidence for cosegregation with FAD in either the overall data set (Table 2) or in individual FAD pedigrees (data not shown). However,

Table 2. Cumulative LOD Scores for Chromosome 14 Markers[a]

Locus ID No.	Recombination fraction						Z	θ
	0.00	0.05	0.10	0.20	0.30	0.40		
D14S50	$-\infty$	−8.07	−3.45	−1.34	−0.47	−0.19	–	–
D14S49	$-\infty$	−8.69	−4.13	−0.91	0.01	0.15	0.15	0.40
D14S52	$-\infty$	−2.74	−1.48	−0.58	−0.24	0.07	0.07	0.40
D14S43	$-\infty$	20.47	18.47	13.52	8.20	3.28	20.50	0.04
D14S53	$-\infty$	11.64	11.69	9.24	5.83	2.48	12.10	0.07
D14S55	$-\infty$	6.94	6.76	5.50	3.75	1.76	7.10	0.07
D14S48	$-\infty$	−3.11	−0.49	1.13	1.21	0.62	1.25	0.25
D14S51	$-\infty$	−9.82	−5.35	−2.61	−0.62	−0.14	–	–

[a] Cumulative two point lod scores for tests of linkage between FAD and each seven polymorphic DNA marker loci from chromosome 14. These markers have been arranged in the followed genetic map cen-*D14S50*-(23 cM)-*D14S49*-(24 cM)-*D14S52*-(25 cM)-*D14S43*-(3 cM)-*D14S53*-(9 cM)-*D14S55*-(2 cM)-*D14S48*-(18 cM)-*D14S51*-TEL (Figure 1) (Roses et al., 1992). Individual pedigree-specific lod scores for markers yielding significant overall lod scores are displayed in Table 3. Genotype data for these loci are available on request.

three markers spanning a 12-cM region in the center of the long arm of chromosome 14 (*D14S43*, *D14S53*, *D14S55*) gave highly significant two-point lod scores in the overall data set (Tables 2 and 3). More impressively, six independent pedigrees provided statistically significant lod scores for at least one of these markers (Table 3).

Multipoint analyses of the *D14S53* and *D14S43* data using LINK-AGE (Lathrop et al., 1985) confirmed these findings, providing a peak lod score of 23.4 at 5 cM distal to *D14S53*. This analysis did not permit definitive placement of FAD relative to these two markers because a similar lod score (23.17) was generated at 5 cM proximal to *D14S43* (the odds ratio favoring the former is 2:1). Typing of additional markers was therefore necessary (see following).

To ensure that these positive results did not arise from errors in the estimated statistical parameters necessary for the maximum likelihood calculations (i.e., marker allele frequencies and age-dependent penetrance functions) we analyzed the data using three different parameters sets as follows: *Set 1*, marker allele frequencies estimated from 66 spouses of affected individuals and one at-risk per family (these observed allele frequencies did not differ from those previously published, and did not differ substantially across ethnic groups although the sample sizes for some ethnic groups were small; results from these analyses are shown in Tables 2 and 3); *Set 2*, equal marker allele frequencies (data not shown); and *Set 3*, zero penetrance for the FAD trait in currently asymptomatic pedigree members (data not shown). We observed a 10%–50% increase in lod scores with *Set 2*, suggesting that the reported lod scores did not result from segregation of rare alleles, an observation that was confirmed by direct inspection of the genotype data. We observed a 10%–20% reduction in lod scores but still overwhelming evidence for linkage with *Set 3*. This minor reduction in lod scores probably reflects the loss of a small amount of information provided by consideration of age-adjusted risk for FAD in asymptomatic members in the initial analysis.

Cumulatively, therefore, we have provided robust evidence for the existence of a novel FAD susceptibility locus on chromosome 14q (FAD_{14}) near the marker *D14S43*.

Analysis of Genetic Heterogeneity and More Complex Models of Inheritance

A few pedigrees provided negative lod scores for the *D14S43*, *D14S53*, or *D14S55* loci (see Table 3). To determine whether these negative results reflected additional nonallelic heterogeneity, we investigated the

Table 3. Pedigree-Specific LOD Scores[a]
Table 3A: *D14S43* versus FAD

Family	Recombination Fraction						
	0.00	0.05	0.10	0.15	0.20	0.30	0.40
FAD4	2.17	1.87	1.57	1.30	1.05	0.60	0.23
FAD2	3.65	3.16	2.67	2.17	1.68	0.75	0.11
FAD3	6.99	6.45	5.86	5.23	4.55	3.05	1.40
M9	−0.22	−0.15	−0.10	−0.07	−0.04	−0.02	0.00
M2	0.27	0.24	0.20	0.17	0.14	0.08	0.03
M3	0.14	0.12	0.09	0.07	0.06	0.03	0.01
M4	0.31	0.25	0.18	0.13	0.09	0.03	0.00
NIH2	−∞	−0.75	−0.41	−0.23	−0.13	−0.03	−0.01
M8	−0.08	−0.10	−0.10	−0.09	−0.07	−0.04	−0.01
FLO2	0.64	0.54	0.44	0.35	0.26	0.12	0.04
TOR1	−0.13	−0.10	−0.08	−0.06	−0.04	−0.02	0.00
M11	0.26	0.22	0.18	0.14	0.11	0.05	0.01
R1	0.08	0.07	0.05	0.04	0.03	0.01	0.00
MEX1	−∞	1.79	1.85	1.75	1.56	1.05	0.48
FL1	0.05	0.00	−0.03	−0.05	−0.05	−0.03	−0.01
TOR1.1	1.72	1.52	1.30	1.09	0.87	0.48	0.17
M13	−0.51	−0.41	−0.32	−0.24	−0.17	−0.07	−0.02
FLO10	−0.26	−0.19	−0.15	−0.11	−0.08	−0.03	−0.01
JPN1	0.75	0.67	0.58	0.49	0.40	0.22	0.06
603	1.94	1.75	1.55	1.34	1.11	0.66	0.27
Total	−∞	20.47	18.47	16.09	13.52	8.20	3.28

Table 3B: *D14S53* versus FAD

Family	Recombination Fraction						
	0.00	0.05	0.10	0.15	0.20	0.30	0.40
FAD1	−∞	2.46	2.27	1.96	1.61	0.91	0.34
FAD4	2.52	2.21	1.90	1.59	1.30	0.76	0.32
FAD2	0.72	0.58	0.44	0.30	0.18	0.02	−0.03
FAD3	−∞	0.66	0.84	0.86	0.81	0.56	0.26
M9	−∞	−0.57	−0.32	−0.19	−0.12	−0.04	−0.01
M2	0.25	0.21	0.17	0.13	0.09	0.04	0.00
M3	−∞	−0.53	−0.28	−0.16	−0.09	−0.02	0.00
M4	0.26	0.21	0.16	0.11	0.07	0.02	0.00
NIH2	−∞	−0.30	−0.02	0.10	0.15	0.13	0.05
M8	−0.14	−0.16	−0.15	−0.12	−0.09	−0.04	−0.01
FLO2	−0.03	−0.02	−0.01	−0.01	−0.01	0.00	0.00
TOR1	0.07	0.06	0.05	0.04	0.03	0.01	0.00
M11	0.00	0.00	0.00	0.00	0.00	0.00	0.00
R1	0.00	0.00	0.00	0.00	0.00	0.00	0.00
MEX1	0.94	0.84	0.74	0.63	0.53	0.33	0.16
FL1	−∞	−1.44	−0.89	−0.58	−0.39	−0.15	−0.04
TOR1.1	5.38	4.93	4.45	3.95	3.41	2.26	1.04
M13	−∞	−0.79	−0.52	−0.36	−0.25	−0.11	−0.03
FLO10	0.14	0.11	0.09	0.07	0.05	0.02	0.01
JPN1	0.46	0.40	0.33	0.27	0.21	0.10	0.03
603	3.13	2.79	2.45	2.09	1.73	1.02	0.39
Total	−∞	11.64	11.69	10.68	9.24	5.83	2.48

Table 3C: *D14S55* versus FAD

Family	Recombination Fraction						
	0.00	0.05	0.10	0.15	0.20	0.30	0.40
FAD1	0.35	0.24	0.16	0.10	0.06	0.02	0.00
FAD4	$-\infty$	5.21	4.92	4.46	3.91	2.63	1.22
FAD2	−0.74	−0.62	−0.49	−0.36	−0.25	−0.10	−0.03
FAD3	0.68	0.56	0.46	0.37	0.29	0.15	0.06
M9	−0.06	−0.05	−0.04	−0.03	−0.02	−0.01	0.00
M2	$-\infty$	−0.72	−0.44	−0.29	−0.19	−0.08	−0.02
M3	0.00	0.00	0.00	0.00	0.00	0.00	0.00
M4	0.08	0.06	0.05	0.04	0.03	0.01	0.00
NIH2	0.07	0.06	0.05	0.04	0.03	0.01	0.00
M8	−0.21	−0.22	−0.20	−0.17	−0.14	−0.06	−0.02
FLO2	−0.19	−0.13	−0.09	−0.06	−0.04	−0.02	−0.01
TOR1	0.00	0.00	0.00	0.00	0.00	0.00	0.00
M11	0.08	0.06	0.05	0.04	0.03	0.01	0.00
R1	0.00	0.00	0.00	0.00	0.00	0.00	0.00
MEX1	1.82	2.30	2.23	2.04	1.79	1.18	0.53
FL1	−0.15	−0.17	−0.16	−0.14	−0.02	−0.06	−0.01
TOR1.1	0.36	0.29	0.23	0.18	0.13	0.06	0.02
M13	−0.25	−0.21	−0.16	−0.12	−0.09	−0.04	−0.01
FLO10	0.08	0.06	0.05	0.04	0.03	0.01	0.00
JPN1	0.28	0.21	0.15	0.10	0.06	0.02	0.00
603	0.00	0.00	0.00	0.00	0.00	0.00	0.00
Total:	$-\infty$	6.94	6.76	6.21	5.50	3.75	1.76

[a] Initially calculated as described for Table 2.

pedigree-specific lod scores for the three loci showing linkage and the *D14S43-D14S53* multipoint analysis using the admixture test. Although these tests of nonallelic heterogeneity were not significant when either two-point or multipoint data were used (odds against homogeneity were less than 10:1 in all analyses), it is apparent that most of the evidence for linkage arose from pedigrees with a presenile onset (< 65 years). The few pedigrees with a later onset cumulatively provided negative scores. It seems likely therefore that this region contains a gene that plays a major role in the susceptibility to FAD in at least a significant proportion to early-onset FAD pedigrees.

As noted earlier, several of the pedigrees showing robust evidence for linkage to chromosome 14 in this study (especially pedigrees FAD4 and 603) also provide noticeably positive lod scores ($0.75 > Z < 3.0$) for markers on chromosome 21 (Pericak-Vance et al., 1988; St. George-Hyslop et al., 1991). The interpretation of the chromosome 21 results in this and other data sets has been the subject of much speculation but remains problematic (Haines, 1991). The pedigree-specific lod scores for the current chromosome 14 loci far exceed those previously achieved for chromosome 21. However, while these new results now suggest that a major gene effect is unlikely on chromosome 21, they do not negate the possibility that important epistatic or modifier loci may exist in these pedigrees on chromosomes 21. Unequivocal evidence for the existence of modifier loci in early-onset FAD is provided by the observation of phenotypic heterogeneity between and within FAD pedigrees with identical APP mutations ($APP_{717val \rightarrow ile}$ and $APP_{692ala \rightarrow gly}$, respectively) (Hendricks et al., 1992; Roses et al., 1992). Thus, while it is still conceivable that the previous results for chromosome 21 *may* simply represent chance cosegregation of chromosome 21 markers through parts of these pedigrees, two other explanations need to be considered. First, the observed cosegregation may reflect nonrandom cosegregation between two acrocentric chromosomes (chromosomes 14 and 21). No evidence for this has been produced from other genetic linkage studies and can thus be discarded on intuitive grounds. The second and more appealing possibility is that the positive lod scores for chromosome 21 markers in these families reflect the cosegregation of certain alleles at one or more chromosome 21 loci (including perhaps APP) through parts of these pedigrees, and that these alleles may play a role in generating or modifying the AD phenotype in *some* of our early-onset pedigrees. This hypothesis predicts that in some of our pedigrees a two-locus model of inheritance of FAD may exist in which the FAD_{14} gene confers the vast bulk of the susceptibility while the chromosome 21 locus would modify that phenotype or add minor components to the risk. A strong but epistatic role for one or more chromosome 21 loci would be in keeping with three other observations. First, some of the putatively pathogenic mutations in APP (including APP_{717}) also do not segregate perfectly with the AD phenotype (Hendricks et al., 1992; Roses et al., 1991). Second, weakly positive pedigree-specific lod scores and highly significant sib pair and affected pedigree member results have been reported for the same chromosome 21 markers in at least two other FAD data sets (Heston et al., 1991; Pericak-Vance et al., 1988), an observation more in keeping with a modifier locus than the major pathogenic locus. Third, independent epidemiologic studies investigating the transmission of AD in families which are multiply affected suggest that although there is a major gene effect (with an estimated population frequency of 0.038), it accounts for only about 24% of the variance in risk for AD, thus implying that other minor genetic (such as those proposed here) and nongenetic factors play a role (Farrer et al., 1991). Although identification of these putative modifier loci on chromosome 21 may eventually provide useful insights into biochemical pathways that might be used therapeutically to modify or delay the symptoms of AD, we reasoned that this task might be more easily addressed once the major FAD susceptibility locus on chromosome 14 had been identified.

Analysis of Candidate Genes on Chromosome 14

As an initial step toward identification of the FAD_{14} gene, we investigated three of the four known candidate genes that have already been cloned using both genetic linkage and direct DNA sequencing strategies.

α-1-ANTICHYMOTRYPSIN (*AACT*)

The segregation of *AACT* in our FAD pedigrees was tested using the published Taq1 restriction fragment length polymorphism (RFLP) detected by the probe *PACE3.4*. Although this polymorphism is not particularly informative (PIC = 0.33), we did detect obligate recombinants between affected members of FAD3 and FAD4 (in each pedigree there being one affected subject with genotype AA and another with genotype BB). This result indicates that *AACT* does not segregate with FAD in these pedigrees, an observation in keeping with the fact that the *AACT* gene maps telomeric to *D14S48* in a region that can be excluded as the site of the FAD_{14} locus (see Fig. 1).

CATHEPSIN G (*CTSNG*)

To investigate *CTSNG*, we directly sequenced the entire open reading frame (protein coding sequence) of the *CTSNG* gene by using PCR to amplify each exon together with at least 20 bp of intronic sequence beyond the 5' and 3' intron-exon splice sites. No mutations were observed in affected members of any of the five pedigrees clearly linked to chr 14 (pedigree 603 is not part of the University of Toronto collection) (Wong et al., in press). Further, during the course of our analyses, the *CTSNG* gene was precisely mapped to a genetic position between the anonymous markers *D14S50* and *D14S49* (see Fig. 1) (NIH/CEPH, 1992), a region that again can be excluded as the site of the FAD_{14} locus.

FBJ OSTEOSARCOMA PROTO-ONCOGENE (*cFOS*)

The candidacy of the *cFOS* gene was also investigated by direct sequencing of PCR fragments isolated from the genomic DNA of affected subjects in the FAD pedigrees definitively linked to chromosome 14. A substitution mutation of T by C, which creates a Dsa1 restriction site, was discovered at position 1893 in the genomic sequence of the *cFOS* gene in all affected members of FAD1, FAD4, and Tor1.1 pedigrees (Rogaev et al., in press). Although this mutation cosegregates with the disease in these families, three other observations indicate that it is unlikely to be pathogenic. First, the mutation is a conservative third-position mutation in codon 84 of exon 2, which does not change the encoded amino acid (serine). Second, the normal sequence in the mouse genome contains a T rather than C at this position, yet mice are not known to develop AD or even *APP* deposition. Third, the same mutation was observed in two elderly unaffected control subjects.

However, the fact that the sequence polymorphism in codon 84 cosegregated with FAD in three of our pedigrees urged us to investigate the segregation of the *CFOS* gene in all our pedigrees. To do this, we developed a novel, moderately informative (PIC = 0.57) PCR-based SSCP. The segregation of the *cFOS* SSCP, which derives from the insertion or deletion of a G nucleotide at nucleotide position 2611 in the intronic sequence between exons 3 and 4 of the *cFOS* gene, was tested in all 19 pedigrees in our data set with early-onset FAD. No obligate recombination events were discovered, indicating that *cFOS* is closely linked to the FAD_{14} locus. Further, the *cFOS* gene appears to map within the obligate FAD_{14} region between *D14S63* and *D14S53* (see Fig. 1) (unpublished observations). However, in addition to the absence of missense mutations in the coding sequence of *cFOS*, two other results suggest that the *cFOS* gene is not the FAD_{14} locus. First, two of our pedigrees (FAD4 and Tor1.1) are thought to share a common remote ancestor, yet the segregating allele in each pedigree differed (FAD4: "A" allele; Tor1.1: "B" allele). Second, there is no evidence for association or disequilibrium between presenile-onset FAD and particular alleles of the *cFOS* SSCP in our data set. Although these observations cumulatively argue strongly against *cFOS*, it is still remotely possible that pathogenic mutations might exist in noncoding regulatory regions of the *cFOS* gene. Theoretically at least, such mutations might cause dysregulation of *cFOS* expression and thus dysregulation of transcription of *APP*.

Attempts to Define Flanking Markers for the FAD Locus

In light of the negative results obtained from the analysis of three of the four known candidate genes, we have begun to more precisely define the location of the FAD_{14} gene between close flanking markers as a prelude to attempting to isolate the FAD_{14} gene by positional cloning strategies (Collins, 1992). Several new markers (*D14S63*, *D14S77*, *D14S71*, and *D14S61*) have been mapped to 14q24 near the *D14S43* locus (see Fig. 1) (Weisenbach et al., 1992). Preliminary analyses with these markers in the five University of Toronto pedigrees definitively linked to chromosome 14 suggest that identical recombination events are detected by *D14S55*, *D14S53*, and *D14S61*, implying that *D14S61* represents a close telomeric flanking marker (see Fig. 1). Similarly, *D14S63* and *D14S52* detect similar recombination events, suggesting that *D14S63* represents a centromeric boundary. *D14S77*, *D14S71*, and *D14S43* revealed no recombinants in affected individuals, indicating that these markers, which span approximately 4 cM, are very close to the FAD_{14} locus.

Discussion

We have provided compelling evidence for the existence of a novel locus conferring major susceptibility to early-onset FAD. It seems unlikely that the FAD_{14} mutation resides in the *CTSNG*, *AACT*, or *cFOS* genes. We cannot yet exclude the possibility that the FAD_{14} mutation may exist in the as yet uncharacterized *HSP70* gene tentatively mapped to chromosome 14q24 by *in situ* hybridization using probes derived from the chromosome 6 *HSP70* gene. Nevertheless, preliminary and still incomplete analyses with additional markers from this region provide evidence that the FAD_{14} locus maps somewhere between *D14S63* and *D14S61*. Further refining of this genetic location will thus serve as a basis for attempts to clone the FAD_{14} locus by a positional cloning strategy. However, we have shown that the molecular genetic data can be applied to clinical problems, albeit under fairly stringent restrictions. Paramount among these restrictions is that application of these genetic markers be confined to pedigrees with stringent evidence for a chromosome 14 etiology of their AD (i.e., a family-specific lod score with one or more chromosome 14 markers $> +3.00$). In addition, unlike other neurodegenerative diseases (e.g., Huntington-disease), absence of the FAD_{14} gene in at-risk members of these pedigrees provides no protection from the acquisition of other forms of AD, including the probably more common sporadic forms.

From a more fundamental point of view, two observations indicate that identification of the FAD_{14} gene will be of significance for clinical medicine at least. First, it is apparent that the FAD_{14} locus accounts for the vast majority of cases with early-onset FAD (in contrast to *APP* mutations, which account for less than 3% of all early-onset FAD cases). Second, whether the FAD_{14} mutation resides in the putative *HSP7-*homolog or in another as yet unidentified gene on chromosome 14q24, it is almost certain that this gene will be a hitherto unsuspected player in the pathogenesis of AD. In contrast, discovery of mutations in the *APP* gene by this and other groups was disappointing because it was already apparent that *APP* plays some role in the pathogenesis of AD. Uncovering the identity and function of the FAD_{14} gene, which may in fact have no direct relationship to *APP*, will likely provide powerful new insights into the pathogenesis of AD. Ultimately, a more complete knowledge of the biochemical pathogenesis of the AD phenotype should in turn assist attempts to discover rational therapeutic and diagnostic tools to combat all forms of the disease. Identification of this FAD gene may have application beyond the problem of Alzheimer's disease because many of the neuropathological features of AD (e.g., neuronal loss, senile plaques, and neurofibrillary tangles) are also features of normal aging.

Acknowledgments

This work was supported by grants from the Medical Research Council of Canada, the Alzheimer Association of Ontario, the Alzheimer Society of Canada, the Alzheimer and Related Disorders Association, the American Health Assistance Foundation, and the National Institute of Neurologic Disease and Stroke. The author thanks G. Galway, Q. Fong, and L. Jiang for technical assistance, and postdoctoral fellows Dr. E. Rogaev, G. Vaula, and M. Mortilla.

References

Collins FS (1992): Positional cloning: let's not call it reverse anymore. *Nat Genet* 1:3–6
Farrer L, Myers R, Connor L, Cupples LA, Growden J (1991): Segregation analysis reveals evidence for a major gene for Alzheimer's disease. *Am J Hum Genet* 48:1026–1033
Goate A, Haynes AR, Owen MJ, Farrall M, James LA, Lai LY, Mullan M, Rossor M, JH (1989): Predisposing locus for Alzheimer disease on chr 21. *Lancet* 1:352–355
Goate AM, Chartier-Harlin M-C, Mullan M, Brown J, Crawford F, Fidani L, Guiffra L, Laynes A, Hardy JA (1991): Segregation of a missense mutation in the amyloid precursor protein gene with familial Alzheimer disease. *Nature* 349:704–706
Haines JL (1991): The genetics of Alzheimer disease: a teasing problem. *Am J Hum Genet* 48:1021–1025
Hamos JE, Oblas B, Pulaski-Salo D, Welch WJ, Bole DG, Drachman DA (1991): Expression of heat shock proteins in Alzheimer's disease. *Neurology* 41(3):345–350
Hendricks M., et al. (1992): Presenile dementia and cerebral hemorrhage linked to a mutation at codon 692 of the B-amyloid precursor protein gene. *Nat Genet* 1:218–221
Heston LL, Orr HT, Rich SS, White JA (1991): Linkage of Alzheimer disease susceptibility locus to markers on human chromosome 21. *Am J Hum Genet* 40:449–453
Joachim CL, Selkoe DJ (1992): The seminal role of beta amyloid in the pathogenesis of Alzheimer disease. *Alzheimer Dis Assoc Disord* 6(1):7–34
Karlinsky H, Vaula G, Haines JL, Mortilla M, Crapper-MacLachlan DR, St. George-Hyslop P (1992): Molecular and prospective phenotypic characterization of a pedigree with familial Alzheimer disease and a dissense mutation in codon 717 of the B-amyloid precursor protein (APP) gene. *Neurology* 42:1445–1453

Katzman R (1986): Alzheimer's disease. *N Engl J Med* 314(15):964–973

Khachaturian ZS (1985): Diagnosis of Alzheimer disease. *Arch Neurol* 42:1097–1105

Lathrop GM, Lalouel JM, Julier C, Ott J (1985): Multi-locus linkage analysis in humans: detection of linkage and estimation of recombination. *Am J Hum Genet* 37(3):482–498

McKhann G, Drachman D, Folstein M, Katzman R, Price D, Stadlan EM (1984): Clinical diagnosis of Alzheimer disease: Report of the NINCDS-ADRDA Work Group under the auspices of the Dept. of Health and Human Services task force on Alzheimer disease. *Neurology* 34:939–944

Murrell J, Farlow M, Ghetti B, Benson MD (1991): A mutation in the amyloid precursor protein associated with hereditary Alzheimer's disease. *Science* 254:97–99

NIH/CEPH Collaborative Mapping Group (1992): A comprehensive genetic linkage map of the human genome. *Science* 258:67–86

Pericak-Vance MA, Bedout JL, Gaskell PC, Roses AD (1991): Linkage studies in familial Alzheimer disease – evidence for chromosome 19 linkage. *Am J Hum Genet* 48:1034–1050

Pericak-Vance MA, Yamoaka LH, Haynes CS (1988): Genetic linkage studies in Alzheimer's disease families. *Exp Neurol* 102:271–279

Pollwein P, Masters CL, Beyreuther K (1991): The expression of the amyloid precursor protein (APP) is regulated by two GC-elements in the promoter. *Nucleic Acids Res* 20:63–68

Rogaev EI, Lukiw WJ, Vaula G, Haines JL Rogaeva EA, Tsuda T, Alexandrova N, Liang Y, Mortilla M, Craper-McLachlan DR, St. George-Hyslop PH: Analysis of the *cFOS* gene on chr 14 and its relationship to the 5′ promoter of the amyloid precursor protein (*APP*) gene on chr 21 in familial Alzheimer disease. *Neurology* (in press)

Roses AD, Pericak-Vance M, Alberts M, Saunders A, Taylor H, Gilbert J, Schwartzbach C, Peacock M, Bhasin R, Goldgaber D (1992): Locus heterogeneity in Alzheimer disease. In: *Heterogeneity in Alzheimer Disease*, Boeller F, et al., eds. Berlin: Springer-Verlag (in press)

Schellenberg GD, Pericak-Vance MA, Wijsman EM, Moore DK, Gaskell PC, Yamaoka LA, Bedout JL, Bird T, Roses AD (1991): Linkage analysis of familial Alzheimer disease using chromosome 21 markers. *Am J Hum Genet* 48:563–583

St. George-Hyslop PH, Haines JL, Farrer LA, van Broeckhoven C, Goate AM, Crapper-McLachlan DR (1991): Genetic linkage studies suggest that Alzheimer's disease is not a single homogeneous disorder. *Nature* 347:194–197

St. George-Hyslop PH, Myers RH, Haines JL, Farrer LA, Tanzi RE, Abe K, James MF, Conneally PM, Polinsky RJ, Gusella JF (1989): Familial Alzheimer's disease: progress and problems. *Neurobiol Aging* 10:417–425

St. George-Hyslop PH, Tanzi RE, Polinsky RJ, Haines JL, Nee L, Watkins PC, Myers RH, Conneally PM, JF G (1987): The genetic defect causing familial Alzheimer disease maps on chromosome 21. *Science* 235:885–889

Tanzi RE, Vaula G, Romano D, Mortilla M, Huang T, Tupler R, Wasco W, St. George-Hyslop P (1992): Assessment of amyloid B protein gene mutations in a large set of familial and sporadic Alzheimer disease cases. *Am J Hum Genet* 51:273–282

van Straaten F, Mueller R, Curran T, Van Beveren C, Verma IM (1983): Complete nucleotide sequence of a human c-onc gene: deduced amino acid sequence of the human c-fos protein. *Proc Natl Acad Sci USA* 80:3183–3187

Vaula G, Mortilla M, Tupler R, Lukiw W, Tanzi RE, Polinsky R, Foncin J-F, Bruni AC, Montesi MP, Sorbi S, St. George-Hyslop PH (1992): A novel but non-pathogenic mutation in exon 4 of the human amyloid precursor protein (APP) gene. *Neurosci Lett* 144:46–48

Wang Z, Weber JL (1992): Continuous linkage map of human chromosome 14 short tandem repeat polymorphisms. *Genomics* 13:532–536

Weissenbach J, Gyapay G, Dib C, Vignal A, Morisette J, Millasseau PGV, Lathrop M (1992): A second generation linkage map of the human genome. *Nature* 359:794–798

Wong L, Liang Y, Tsuda T, Fong Q, Galway G, Alexandrova N, Rogeava E, Likiw W, Smith J, Rogaev E, Crapper-MacLachlan D, St. George-Hyslop P: Mutation of the gene for the human lysosomal serine protease Cathepsin G is not the cause of aberrant APP processing in familial Alzheimer disease. *Neurosci Lett* (in press)

Yoshkai S, Sasaki H, Doh-ura K, Furuya H, Sakaki Y (1991): Genomic organization of the human amyloid beta protein precursor gene. *Gene* 102:291–292

Zhang P, Hirsch EC, Danier P, Duyckaerts C, Javoy-Agid F (1992): c-FOS protein-like immunoreactivity: distribution in the human brain and over-expression in the hippocampus of patients with Alzheimer disease. *Neuroscience* 46:9–21

2

Growth Factors in Parkinson's Disease

PATRICK L. MCGEER AND EDITH G. MCGEER

There is currently intense interest in the possible role of neurotrophic factors in neurodegenerative diseases, because deficiencies may play an etiological role and administration may have therapeutic effects (Hefti et al., 1989, 1990). Particular attention has been focused on Alzheimer's disease (AD) and Parkinson's disease (PD), the former because of the importance of nerve growth factor (NGF) in maintaining basal forebrain cholinergic neurons. With regard to PD, the possibility that transplants may be helpful because of the stimulation of neurotrophic activity has been mooted, and NGF has even been tried clinically as a method of promoting the survival of adrenal medulla cells grafted into the basal ganglia (Olson et al., 1991; Silani et al., 1990). In more basic work, a number of identified factors have been shown to promote survival of dopamine neurons in culture or to protect such cultured neurons against neurotoxins such as 6-hydroxydopamine (6-OHDA) or MPP$^+$, the active principle of MPTP.

A very limited amount of *in vivo* work has also been done. Table 1 lists some of the neurotrophic factors studied either in culture or *in vivo*. A number of semipopular articles (Snyder, 1991; Weiss, 1993) have suggested the possible use of two of these, glial-derived neurotrophic factor (GDNF) and brain-derived growth factor (BDNF), in PD. GDNF seems to be amazingly selective toward dopaminergic neurons and will certainly be explored further. There have been some controversial reports about BDNF. This member of the neutrophin family [which also includes NGF and neurotrophin-3 (NT-3)] has generally been found protective to dopaminergic neurons in culture (Table 1). However, intranigral infusions of BDNF in rats actually down-regulate dopaminergic parameters (Lapchak et al., 1993). BDNF also apparently fails to protect dopamine neurons against axotomy-induced degeneration (Knüsel et al., 1992; Lapchak et al., 1993), but this probably represents an extremely severe insult to the system.

ADVANCES IN RESEARCH ON NEURODEGENERATION, II
Y. Mizuno et al.
© 1994 Birkhäuser Boston

Table 1. Brief Summary of Some of the Literature on the Effects of Various Neurotrophic Factors on Dopaminergic Neurons or Dopaminergic Parameters[a]

Factor	References Reporting Effects on Dopaminergic Neurons	
	In Culture	*In Vivo*
Platelet-derived growth factor (PDGF)	14 (No effect; 3)	
Epidermal growth factor (EGF)[b]	2, 6#, 16#	6#
Basic fibroblast growth factor (bFGF)	3, 4 10, 16#	15#
Acidic fibroblast growth factor (aFGF)	3	
Insulin-like growth factors (IGF-I and -II)	9	
Nerve growth factor (NGF)	(No effect; 11, 18)	5#
Brain-derived growth factor (BDNF)[c]	7#, 11, 17#, 19#	(No effect, 1; 8##, 12##)
Glial-derived neurotrophic factor (GDNF)	13	
Ciliary neurotrophic factor (CNTF)		21##
Neurotrophin-3 (NT-3)[b]	(No effect; 18)	
Interleukin-1	(No effect; 3)	

[a]Symbols against reference numbers are used to indicate that study involved use of a neurotoxin (#) or axotomy (##). Negative reports are in parentheses. Reference numbers: 1, Altar et al., 1992; 2, Caspar et al., 1991; 3, Engele and Bohn, 1991; 4, Ferrari et al., 1989; 5, Garcia et al., 1992; 6, Hadjiconstantinou et al., 1991; 7, Hyman et al., 1991; 8, Knüsel et al., 1992; 9, Knüsel and Hefti, 1991; 10, Knüsel et al., 1990; 11, Knüsel et al., 1991; 12, Lapchak et al., 1993; 13, Lin et al., 1993; 14, Nikkhah et al., 1993; 15, Otto and Unsicker, 1990; 16, Park and Mytilineou, 1992; 17, Skaper et al., 1993; 18, Snyder, 1991; 19, Spina et al., 1992; 20, Steinbusch et al., 1990; 21, Hagg and Varon, 1993.
[b]The mRNAs for both EGF and NT-3 are found in the substantia nigra and ventral tegmental area of rats (Gall et al., 1992).
[c]High concentrations of BDNF are reported in pallidal areas (Fallon et al., 1984), and the amount in striatum is increased after dopamine denervation (Okazawa et al., 1992).

Our own work has been focused on basic fibroblast growth factor (bFGF). bFGF is a pluripotential peptide with angiogenic, mitogenic and growth-promoting properties. It appears in several molecular weight forms, all of which appear to be derived from a single gene. In general, bFGFs of less than 20 kDa are referred to as low molecular weight forms, while those of more than 20 kDa are referred to as high molecular weight forms. The fundamental structures of rat, bovine, and human bFGF have been determined by cDNA sequencing. It has been speculated that differences in molecular weight may be the result of alternative initiation sites of transcription, and that these differences might result in modified physiological activity (for reviews, see Baird and Böhlen, 1990; Gospodarowicz, 1987; Rifkin and Moscatelli, 1989; Thomas, 1987).

BFGF is richly distributed in brain, where it is known to have neurotrophic properties. It has been reported to be present in midbrain dopaminergic neurons of human (Bean et al., 1991), monkey (Bean et al., 1991), and rat (Bean et al., 1991; Cintra et al., 1991). It promotes the survival of these neurons *in vitro* (Fallon et al., 1984; Knusel et al., 1990) and protects them from the neurotoxic actions of MPTP *in vivo* (Otto and Unsicker, 1990). In our studies (Tooyama et al., 1992) on the localization of bFGF in rat brain, we used three antibodies: R917, a rabbit antiserum raised against purified bovine bFGF; Fn, a rabbit polyclonal antibody raised against a synthetic peptide with the sequence 1–24 of bFGF (generously given by Dr. T. Pearson) (Kardami et al., 1990), and MAB78, a monoclonal antibody raised against human recombinant bFGF that recognizes an epitope within the 1–9 amino terminal region (generously given by Dr. J. Kakinuma) (Seno et al., 1989). When Western blots of recombinant bFGF were probed with these antibodies, all three recognized the classical 18-kDa band of bFGF as well as a fainter band of about 36 kDa, which is probably a dimer of bFGF. In similar analyses of rat midbrain extracts, all antibodies recognized a single band of about 27–28 kDa, but no 18-kDa band was detectable in crude brain homogenates with any of the antibodies.

R917 proved to be the best antibody for immunohistochemical work on rat brain. It gave intense neuronal staining in a ventromedial subpopulation of dopaminergic neurons in the midbrain tegmentum and in the paraventricular nucleus of the hypothalamus. In addition, faint staining of a very few neurons was seen in the supraoptic nucleus. Nonneuronal structures were also observed, but these were confined to radial glia and tanycytes in ventral parts of the third ventricle centered in the infundibulum. No other circumventricular organs contained positive cells or fibers. Positive staining was abolished by preincubation of the serum with either 20 µg/ml of recombinant bFGF, the original bFGF product, or a heparin-bound rat extract.

Positive fibers were observed in the midbrain tegmentum, and could be traced rostrally through the medial forebrain bundle. Fine terminals were distributed in specific brain regions, including striosomes and the dorsolateral rim of the striatum, the anterodorsal portion of the nucleus accumbens shell, the infralimbic cortex, and the medial prefrontal cortex. Scattered punctate staining was seen in some forebrain areas such as the olfactory tubercle; such staining was reduced in the cingulate cortex and was absent in the sulcal cortex surrounding the olfactory sulcus.

The interesting point was the apparent concentration of high molecular weight bFGF-like proteins in the ventral dopaminergic neurons, which may be particularly vulnerable in PD (Gibb, 1991). The dorsally located calbindin-positive dopaminergic neurons, which project to the neostriatal matrix (Gerfen et al., 1987) and seem to be relatively spared (Yamada et al., 1990) in PD, did not show bFGF-like immunoreactivity with this antibody. These data suggest that trophic specialization may occur within the dopaminergic system, and it therefore seemed well worth examining bFGF immunoreactivity in normal and parkinsonian human brain.

Human Studies

The substantia nigras from six cases of PD and six age-matched neurologically normal controls were compared (Tooyama et al., 1993). Each PD case was diagnosed clinically premortem, with the diagnosis being confirmed at autopsy by a decrease of pigmented neurons in the substantia nigra (SN), the existence of significant numbers of Lewy bodies in the residual SN neurons, and an absence of pathological evidence of other disorders, such as progressive supranuclear palsy, that result in SN degeneration. In these studies, we used the monoclonal antibody MAB78 (see earlier).

On Western blot examination of the cytosolic extract of control human SN, the bFGF antibody recognized three bands with molecular weights of 18, 27 and 29 kDa. These correspond to the 18-kDa classical bFGF and two high molecular weight forms of bFGF, respectively (Baird and Böhlen, 1990). Further proof of specificity was that no positive staining was obtained in control or PD brain using the antibody preincubated with human recombinant bFGF.

All six parkinsonian cases showed the expected depletion of pigmented neurons (Gibb, 1991; McGeer et al., 1977; Yamada et al., 1990; Zarow and Chui, 1991), especially in the mid- and lateral divisions of the SN. At the level of the oculomotor nucleus, the mean number of remaining neurons was 30.3% of the control mean (Table 2). In addition, there were many extraneuronal deposits of melanin as well as fragmentation of cells and gliosis.

The depletion of bFGF-immunopositive cells in PD was much more drastic than the depletion of pigmented cells. In control cases, 93.7% of pigmented cells were bFGF positive and 88.4% of bFGF-immunopositive cells were pigmented (Table 2). This finding, that most pigmented neurons of the SN are immunopositive for bFGF in normal control cases, is in accord with previous reports (Bean et al., 1991; Cintra et al., 1991). In PD, on the other hand, only 8.2% of pigmented cells were immunopositive for bFGF, while 91.8% of these were immunonegative. Paradoxically, however, a proportion of the pigmented neurons in PD showed extremely strong bFGF immunoreactivity. Such neurons were observed in five of the parkinsonian cases but never in control cases. Overall, about 20% of the bFGF immunopositive neurons in PD showed this intense

Table 2. Numbers (±SEM) of Neurons Containing Melanin, bFGF, or Both in 30-μm Sections of the Substantia Nigra at the Level of the Oculomotor Nerve ($n = 6$ in each group)

Type of Neuron	Type of Case			
	Controls	Parkinsonians	Percent	p
bFGF, Total	1408 ± 45.2	66 ± 14.6	4.69	.0001
Pigmented total	1328 ± 76.6	403 ± 8.7	30.35	.0001
bFGF, Pigmented	1245 ± 70.4	33 ± 11.5	2.65	.0001
bFGF, Nonpigmented	163 ± 34.9	33 ± 7.8	20.25	.004
Pigmented, non-bFGF	83 ± 16.4	370 ± 18.0	445.8	.0001
bFGF, Pigmented/ Pigmented total	0.937	0.082		

immunoreactivity. Lewy bodies for bFGF were also occasionally stained for bFGF. This was observed in four of the parkinsonian cases, including the one that showed no intensely staining neurons.

The loss of bFGF in PD SN neurons might be interpreted as part of a common down-regulation of growth factors and other proteins as a preterminal event. However, it is clear that the loss of bFGF precedes any observable loss in tyrosine hydroxylase (TH), suggesting a dissociation of bFGF levels from neurotransmitter synthetic capacity. Moreover, it is difficult to explain the intensification of bFGF staining seen in some neurons in the PD cases on the basis of terminal down-regulation. Some dysfunction must exist that results in a down-regulation in most dopamine neurons but an up-regulation in some. Of course, these results, using a single antibody to an epitope on the amino terminal region, also do not prove whether the whole of bFGF-like molecules are down-regulated in PD or whether the amino terminal end is cleaved or somehow buried so that it is inaccessible to the antibody. Only further work can help to answer this question.

Another interesting question is whether the action of bFGF on dopaminergic neurons is direct or indirect. Some of the tissue culture work has suggested that the effect of factors such as bFGF, aFGF, and EGF on dopaminergic neurons may be indirect and depend on glia (Casper et al., 1991; Engele and Bohn, 1991; Park and Mytilineou, 1992). The reported high specificity of the glial-derived factor GDNF for dopaminergic neurons might support such indirect action. On the other hand, the presence of FGF receptor mRNA in SN neurons has been shown by *in situ* hybridization studies (Wanaka et al., 1990), as has an apparent anterograde transport of radioactive bFGF from the SN to the striatum in the rat (McGeer et al., 1992). Both reports suggest a possible direct action of the bFGF on dopaminergic neurons. In the transport studies, the amount transported was small (Table 3) and the identity of the transported material was not proven; nevertheless, the apparent

Table 3. Relative Amounts of Radioactivity in Injection Site and Target Area[a]

Injection Site	Target Area	Types of Lesion	n	Amount in Injection Site as Percentage of Injected	Amount in Target Area as Percentage of Injection Site
SN	CP	None	5	36 ± 6	0.428 ± 0.077^a
SN	CP	KA	3	43 ± 5	0.350 ± 0.051^a
SN	CP	6-OHDA	4	40 ± 11	0.080 ± 0.033^b
CP	SN	None	2	51 ± 8	0.009 ± 0.009^b

[a]Rats were sacrificed 5 hr after the stereotaxic injection of approximately 1 ng of $[I^{125}]$bFGF into rat substantia nigra. ANOVA analyses showed no significant difference between the groups in the percent of radioactivity remaining at the injection site ($p > 0.7$) but a significant difference in the percent of radioactivity in the target area (i.e., the place to which injected material might be transported) ($p < 0.01$). Data are given as mean $\pm$SEM. Those carrying a common superscript are not significantly different from one another but are significantly different from those with a different superscript. Abbreviations: SN, substantia nigra; CP, caudate/putamen; KA, kainic acid; 6-OHDA, 6-hydroxydopamine; n, number of experiments.

specificity with regard to the striatum as compared to the thalamus argues that the bFGF was probably not broken down with the radioactivity being reconstituted into a mixture of proteins.

Even if the bFGF acts directly on the dopaminergic neurons, it is not clear whether the action is paracrine or autocrine. Further insight into the mechanism could be obtained by *in situ* hybridization studies on the SN for the mRNA of bFGF itself.

An examination of the expression of FGF receptors in SN neurons of PD and control cases would also be of great interest. A normal or enhanced receptor activity on surviving neurons would suggest that a deficiency of bFGF may be linked to the disease process.

References

Altar CA, Boylan CB, Jackson C, Hershenson S, Miller J, Wiegand SJ, Lindsay RM, Hyman C (1992): Brain-derived neutrophic factor augments rotational behavior and nigrostriatal dopamine turnover in vivo. *Proc Natl Acad Sci USA* 89:11347–11351

Baird A, Böhlen P (1990):Fibroblast growth factors. In: *Peptide Growth Factors and Their Receptors*, Sporn MB, Roberts AB, eds, pp. 369–418. Berlin/Heidelberg: Springer-Verlag

Bean AJ, Elde R, Cao YH, Oellig C, Tamminga C, Goldstein M, Pettersson RF, Hökfelt T (1991): Expression of acidic and basic fibroblast growth factors in the substantia nigra of rat, monkey, and human. *Proc Natl Acad Sci USA* 88:10237–10241

Casper D, Mytilineou C, Blum M (1991): EGF enhances the survival of dopamine neurons in rat embryonic mesencephalon primary cell culture. *J Neurosci Res* 30:372–381

Cintra A, Cao YH, Oellig C, Tinner B, Bortolotti F, Goldstein M, Pettersson RF, Fuxe K (1991): Basic FGF is present in dopaminergic neurons of the ventral midbrain of the rat. *Neuroreport* 2:597–600

Engele J, Bohn MC (1991): The neurotrophic effects of fibroblast growth factors on dopaminergic neurons in vitro are mediated by mesencephalic glia. *J Neurosci* 11:3070–3078

Fallon JH, Seroogy KB, Loughlin SE, Morrison RS, Bradshaw RA, Knaver DJ, Cunningham DD (1984): Epidermal growth factor immunoreactive material in the central nervous system: location and development. *Science* 224:1107–1109

Ferrari G, Minozzi M-C, Toffano G, Leon A, Skaper SD (1989): Basic fibroblast growth factor promotes the survival and development of mesencephalic neurons in culture. *Dev Biol* 133:140–147

Gall CM, Gold SJ, Isackson PJ, Seroogy KB (1992): Brain-derived neurotrophic factor and neurotrophin-3 mRNAs are expressed in ventral midbrain regions containing dopaminergic neurons. *Mol Cell Neurosci* 3:56–61

Garcia E, Rios C, Sotelo J (1992): Ventricular injection of nerve growth factor increases dopamine content in the striata of MPTP-treated mice. *Neurochem Res* 17:979–982

Gerfen CR, Herkenham M, Thibault J (1987): The neostriatal mosaic: II. Patch- and matrix-directed mesostriatal dopaminergic and non-dopaminergic systems. *J Neurosci* 7:3915–3934

Gibb WRG (1991): Neuropathology of the substantia nigra. *Eur Neurol* 31 (Suppl 1): 48–59

Gospodarowicz D (1987): Isolation and characterization of acidic and basic fibroblast growth factor. *Methods Enzymol* 147:106–119

Hadjiconstantinou M, Fitkin JG, Dalia A, Neff NH (1991): Epidermal growth factor enhances striatal dopaminergic parameters in the 1-methyl-4-phenyl-1,2,3,6-tetrahydrophyridine-treated mouse. *J Neurochem* 57:479–482

Hagg T, Varon S (1993): Ciliary neurotrophic factor prevents degeneration of adult rat substantia nigra dopaminergic neurons in vivo. *Proc Natl Acad Sci USA* 90: 6315–6319

Hefti F, Hartikka J, Knusel B (1989): Function of neurotrophic factors in the adult and aging brain and their possible use in the treatment of neurodegenerative diseases. *Neurobiol Aging* 10:515–533

Hefti F, Michel PP, Knusel B (1990): Neurotrophic factors and Parkinson's disease. *Adv Neurol* 53: 123–127

Hyman C, Hofer M, Barde YA, Juhasz M, Yancopoulos GD, Squinto SP, Lindsay RM (1991): BDNF is a neurotrophic factor for dopaminergic neurons of the substantia nigra. *Nature* 350:230–232

Kardami E, Murphy LJ, Liu L, Padua RR, Fandrich RR (1990): Characterization of two preparations of antibodies to basic fibroblast growth factor which exhibit distinct patterns of immunolocalization. *Growth Factors* 4:69–80

Knüsel B, Hefti F (1991): Trophic actions of IGF-I, IFG-II and insulin on cholinergic and dopaminergic brain neurons. *Adv Exp Med Biol* 293:351–360

Knüsel B, Michel PP, Schwaber JS, Hefti F (1990): Selective and nonselective stimulation of central cholinergic and dopaminergic development in vitro by nerve growth factor, basic fibroblast growth factor, epidermal growth factor, insulin and the insulin-like growth factors I and II. *J Neurosci* 10:558–570

Knüsel B, Winslow JW, Rosenthal A, Burton LE, Seid DP, Nikolics K, Hefti F

(1991): Promotion of central cholinergic and dopaminergic neuron differentiation by brain-derived neurotrophic factor but not neurotrophin 3. *Proc Natl Acad Sci USA* 88:961–965

Knüsel B, Beck KD, Winslow JW, Rosenthal A, Burton LE, Widmer HR, Nikolics K, Hefti F (1992): Brain-derived neurotrophic factor administration protects basal forebrain cholinergic but not nigral dopaminergic neurons from degenerative changes after axotomy in the adult rat brain. *J Neurosci* 12:4391–4402

Lapchak PA, Beck KD, Araujo DM, Irwin I, Langston JW, Hefti F (1993): Chronic intranigral administration of brain-derived neurotrophic factor produces striatal dopaminergic hypofunction in unlesioned adult rats and fails to attenuate the decline of striatal dopaminergic function following medial forebrain bundle transection. *Neuroscience* 53:639–650

Lin L-FH, Doherty DH, Lile JD, Bektesh S, Collins F (1993): GDNF: a glial cell-derived neurotrophic factor for midbrain dopaminergic neurons. *Science* 260:1130–1132

McGreer EG, Singh EA, McGeer PL (1992): Apparent anterograde transport of basic fibroblast growth factor in the rat nigrostriatal dopamine system. *Neurosci Lett* 148:31–33

McGeer PL, McGeer EG, Suzuki JS (1977): Aging and extrapyramidal function. *Arch Neurol* 34:33–35

Nikkhah G, Odin P, Smits A, Tingstrom A, Othberg A, Brundin P, Funa K, Lindvall O (1993): Platelet-derived growth factor promotes survival of rat and human mesencephalic dopaminergic neurons in culture. *Exp Brain Res* 92:516–523

Okazawa H, Murata M, Watanabe M, Kamei M, Kanazawa I (1992): Dopaminergic stimulation up-regulates the in vivo expression of brain-derived neurotrophic factor (BDNF) in the striatum. *FEBS Lett* 313:138–142

Olson L, Backlund E-O, Ebendal T, Freedman R, Hamberger B, Hansson P, Hoffer B, Lindblom U, Meyerson B, Strömberg I, Sydow O, Seiger Å (1991): Intraputaminal infusion of nerve growth factor to support adrenal medullary autografts in Parkinson's disease. One-year follow-up of first clinical trial. *Arch Neurol* 48:373–381

Otto D, Unsicker K (1990): Basic FGF reverses chemical and morphological deficits in the nigrostriatal system of MPTP-treated mice. *J Neurosci* 10:1912–1921

Park TH, Mytilineou C (1992): Protection from 1-methyl-4-phenylpyridinium (MPP$^+$) toxicity and stimulation of regrowth of MPP($^+$)-damaged dopaminergic fibers by treatment of mesencephalic cultures with EGF and basic FGF. *Brain Res* 599:83–97

Rifkin DB, Moscatelli D (1989): Recent developments in the cell biology of basic fibroblast growth factor. *J Cell Biol* 109: 1–6

Seno M, Iwane M, Sasada R, Moriya N, Kurokawa T, Igarashi K (1989): Monoclonal antibodies against human basic fibroblast growth factor. *Hybridoma* 8:209–221

Silani V, Falini A, Strada O, Pizzuti A, Pezzoli G, Motti EFD, Vegeto A, Scarlato, G (1990): Effect of nerve growth factor in adrenal autografts in parkinsonism. *Ann Neurol* 27:341–342

Skaper SD, Negro A, Facci L, Dal Toso R (1993): Brain-derived neurotrophic factor selectively rescues mesencephalic dopaminergic neurons from 2,4,5-trihydroxypheynlalanine-induced injury. *J Neurosci Res* 34:478–487

Snyder SH (1991): Parkinson's disease. Fresh factors to consider. *Nature* 350:195

Spina MB, Squinto SP, Miller J, Lindsay RM, Hyman C (1992): Brain-derived neurotrophic factor protects dopamine neurons against 6-hydroxydopamine and N-methyl-4-phenylpyridinum ion toxicity: involvement of the glutathione system. *J Neurochem* 59:99–106

Steinbusch HWM, Vermeulen RJ, Tonnaer JADM (1990): Basic fibroblast growth factor enhances survival and sprouting of fetal dopaminergic cells implanted in the denervated rat caudate-putamen: preliminary observations. *Prog Brain Res* 82:81–86

Thomas KA (1987): Fibroblast growth factors. *FASEB J* 1:434–440

Tooyama I, Walker D, Yamada T, Hanai K, Kimura H, McGeer EG, McGeer PL (1992): High molecular weight basic fibroblast growth factor-like protein is localized to a subpopulation of mesencephalic dopaminergic neurons in the rat brain. *Brain Res* 593:274–280

Tooyama I, Kawamata T, Walker D, Yamada T, Hanai K, Kimura H, Iwane M, Igarashi K, McGeer EG, McGeer PL (1993): Loss of basic fibroblast growth factor in substantia nigra neurons in Parkinson's disease. *Neurology* 43:372–376

Wanaka A, Johnson EM Jr, Milbrandt J (1990): Localization of FGF receptor mRNA in the adult rat central nervous system by in situ hybridization. *Neuron* 5:267–281

Weiss R (1993): Promising protein for Parkinson's. *Science* 260: 1072–1073

Yamada T, McGeer PL, Baimbridge KG, McGeer EG (1990): Relative sparing in Parkinson's disease of substantia nigra dopamine neurons containing calbindin-D28K. *Brain Res* 526:303–307

Zarow C, Chui HC (1991): A simple method for assessing neuronal number in the human substantia nigra. *Soc Neurosci Abstr* 17:1450.

3

Contribution of Cell Culture to Understanding Neuronal Aging and Degeneration

Franz Hefti

Cell culture systems are frequently used to study molecular mechanisms, and they serve as models for developmental processes occurring *in vivo*. Further, in addition to this role as developmental models, the cultures are often used as predictors for responses occurring in the adult organism. For example, nerve growth factor (NFG) promotes differentiation of peripheral sympathetic, basal forebrain cholinergic but not mesencephalic, dopaminergic neurons and, in adult rodents, intracerebral NGF administration prevents lesion-induced degenerative changes of sympathetic neurons, forebrain cholinergic neurons but not mesencephalic dopaminergic neurons. These correlations support the notion that cultures can serve as models to predict pharmacological responses in adult rats. Cell cultures are particularly valuable because of their high capacity to test novel neuroactive molecules, in contrast to the low capacity of *in vivo* test systems. They can serve to identify most promising drugs or neurotrophic molecules for testing *in vivo*.

Culture systems available are primary cultures of dissociated cells, various types of explant cultures, and cultures of immortalized brain cells. The complexity of the brain makes it difficult to prepare homogenous cultures of dissociated cells belonging to specific populations. Dissection, plating, and growth techniques that improve the purity of the cultures, while retaining reasonable yields and viability, are constantly being developed. Some culture systems separate neurons from glial cells; other systems have been optimized to study actions on specific populations of neuronal cells. This chapter provides a brief summary of two examples of the use of primary neuronal cultures to predict effects of neurotrophic factors *in vivo*. These examples are followed by a brief assessment of the value of cell cultures to study processes of neurotoxicity and aging.

ADVANCES IN RESEARCH ON NEURODEGENERATION, II
Y. Mizuno et al.
© 1994 Birkhäuser Boston

Trophic Effect of NGF on Cholinergic Neurons in Culture
and NGF Prevention of Cholinergic Neurodegeneration in
Adult and Aging Animals: Basis for Clinical Trials in
Alzheimer's Disease

Various culture systems have been used to demonstrate that NGF plays
a role in the development of brain neurons. NGF increases the
expression of choline acetyltransferase (ChAT) in various culture
systems containing cholinergic neurons from the septum, nucleus
basalis, or striatum. Under specific culture conditions, NGF promotes
survival and fiber growth of septal cholinergic neurons. These trophic
effects are rather dramatic and are highly selective for forebrain
cholinergic neurons. The cholinergic neurons are one among a small
number of brain neuron populations expressing NGF receptors (see
Hefti et al., 1989; Lapchak et al., 1992, for reviews). The cell culture
findings led to many studies indicating that NGF administration is
effective in preventing cholinergic degeneration following experimental
injury or degeneration associated with normal aging.

In adult rats with transections of the cholinergic septohippocampal
pathways, NGF administration prevents degenerative changes in cholinergic cell bodies. When the transections are partial to produce a partial
cholinergic denervation of hippocampal tissue, NGF administration
increases the function of the surviving presynaptic cholinergic terminals, prevents postsynaptic cholinergic receptor supersensitivity, and
improves the behavioral performance of the experimental rats in a
radial maze (Lapchak et al., 1992b). In adult rats with nucleus basalis
lesions, NGF treatment increases presynaptic cholinergic function and
the behavioral performance of the rats in a water maze (Dekker et al.,
1991). NGF administration to a subpopulation of behaviorally impaired
rats increases cholinergic cell body size and behavioral performance
(Mandel et al., 1989). In select rat strains, NGF administration increases
the presynaptic cholinergic function (Williams, 1991). Some of the
findings obtained on rats have been extended to primates, where it was
shown that NGF treatment protects cholinergic cell bodies from axotomy-induced degeneration (Koliatsos et al., 1991).

Based on the loss of cholinergic neurons and the pronounced trophic
action of NGF on these cells, NGF has been proposed as a therapeutic
treatment for Alzheimer's disease (Hefti and Schneider, 1989). The
therapeutic use of NGF to counteract cholinergic neuron dysfunction
represents the best documented case for neurotrophic therapy of a
neurological disease. Based on the substantial body of evidence suggest-

ing beneficial actions of NGF on cholinergic neurons, limited clinical trials have been initiated and effects in a single Alzheimer's patient have been reported (Olson et al., 1992). The practical use of NGF in Alzheimer's disease will remain limited because of the necessity of intracranial infusion of the protein. However, alternative strategies are likely to result in practically useful treatments.

Neurotrophic Actions on Dopaminergic Neurons in Culture: Predictions for Prevention of Neurodegeneration in Adult Animals and Therapeutic Use in Parkinson's Disease

Degeneration of the dopaminergic neurons of the substantia nigra is responsible for the symptoms of Parkinson's disease, making this disease a very attractive target for neurotrophic factor therapy. Accordingly, the search for a molecule able to protect dopaminergic cell bodies in animals with experimental lesions, resembling the protective effects exerted by NGF on forebrain cholinergic neurons, is a major goal of many investigators. Cell culture studies have identified brain-derived neurotrophic factor (BDNF), epidermal growth factor (EGF), and basic fibroblast growth factor (bFGF) as factors that can promote differentiation of mesencephalic dopaminergic neurons (Hyman et al., 1991; Knüsel et al., 1990, 1991). BDNF seems particularly interesting given its ability to partially protect dopaminergic neurons from toxicity induced by MPP^+ (1-methyl-4-phenylpyridinium; Beck et al., 1992). Initial findings suggest that neuroprotection of dopaminergic neurons by trophic factors can be demonstrated in animal models. Intracerebral administration of bFGF or EGF to adult mice with MPTP, the metabolic precursor of MPP^+, promotes the recovery of dopaminergic parameters (Hadjiconstantinou et al., 1991; Otto and Unsicker, 1990). However, while effective in culture, BDNF failed to prevent the loss of dopaminergic cells after nigrostriatal transections (Knüsel et al., 1992), and so far no other factor has been reported to counteract the degenerative changes of dopaminergic neurons after axotomy. Available findings clearly are not sufficient evidence for the prediction that any of the known factors will be able to attenuate the dopaminergic cell degeneration in Parkinson's disease.

Use of Cultures to Study Toxicity-Induced Degeneration

Cell cultures seem particularly useful to study mechanisms and prevention of toxicity at the cellular and molecular level, as illustrated by several examples. Cultures of fetal rat mesencephalon have been used to demonstrate that BDNF treatment partially protects dopaminergic neurons from toxic actions of MPP^+, the active metabolite of MPTP (1-methyl-4-phenyl-1,2,3,6-tetrahydropyridine), which destroys dopaminergic neurons *in vivo* and results in a parkinsonian syndrome. BDNF pretreatment of such cultures resulted in a shift of the MPP^+ dose–response curve to higher concentrations (Beck et al., 1992). Cultures proved very useful in establishing the structure–activity relationship for the toxic effect of MPP^+ (Michel et al., 1989).

Primary cultures of cortical neurons have been used by several investigators to assess the toxicity of fragments of the amyloid precursor protein (APP), which are believed to be responsible for neuron loss in the vicinity of neuritic plaques. These studies provided conflicting results and suggest very complex relationships between the structure of the APP fragments and their toxicity (Pike et al., 1991).

The concept of excitotoxicity receives strong support from cell culture studies. A large number of excitatory amino acid analogs have been tested on primary cultures of rat brain neurons, and these studies illustrate the advantage of the high capacity of culture systems (Goldberg et al., 1987). Exposure of cultures to anoxia is experimentally easy and many findings related to neuroprotection have been obtained on such systems (Cheng and Mattson, 1991; Goldberg et al., 1987).

These examples demonstrate that cell cultures lend themselves to the study of acute toxicity induced by compounds added to the culture medium. While it is tempting to extrapolate such findings to toxicity generated by chronic low-level exposure, it cannot be overemphasized that mechanisms of acute, high-concentration toxicity may be very different from chronic exposure to a low concentration of the same agent. Thus, cell cultures are no viable substitute for chronic exposure of intact organisms to suspected chronic toxins.

Use of Cell Cultures as Models for Aging

Primary cultures are typically kept for several days, sometimes up to several weeks. While the terms "long term" and "aging in culture" are liberally used in the literature, the time spans of these studies are not comparable with aging of the species from which the cells were derived. Long-term cultures growing over several months are technically demanding. Optimization of culture conditions for long-term growth conditions requires long periods of time. Extreme care is required to avoid loss of cultures to contamination. Also, over long periods of growth, individual cultures tend to differentiate in individual directions; that is, specific neuronal or nonneuronal populations become predominant in individual culture dishes, making them increasingly dissimilar with progressing culture time. Taken together, these limitations make it necessary to start with a very large number of cultures for a meaningful long-term experiment. These limitations tend to erase the advantages of culture systems over living animals to study aging processes.

Primary cultures of adult nervous system cells could overcome many of the limitations of fetal cell cultures. Unfortunately, very limited progress has been made in the preparation of cultures from adult neurons. Cultures can be prepared from adult sensory neurons (Lindsay, 1988); however, most brain neurons can be dissociated but they do not survive or grow in cultures. In contrast, it is possible to generate cultures of nonneuronal cells from adult tissue. In such cultures, however, it is necessary to show that the cells indeed are representative of the population to be studied rather than being derived from a small minority of cells retaining fetal properties.

Conclusions

Cell cultures are easily prepared from fetal tissue and represent very useful systems to analyze the efficacy or toxicity of test compounds and growth factors. False-positives are possible when findings obtained on these developmental systems are extrapolated to the situation in a living adult organism. Cell cultures seem less suitable to study long-term toxicity or aging.

References

Beck KD, Knüsel B, Winslow JW, Rosenthal A, Burton LE, Nikolics K, Hefti F (1992): Pretreatment of dopaminergic neurons in culture with brain-derived neurotrophic factor attenuates toxicity of 1-methyl-4-pyridinium. *Neurodegeneration* 1:27–36

Cheng B, Mattson M (1991): NGF and bFGF protect rat hippocampel and human cortical neurons against hypoglycemic damage by stabilizing calcium homeostasis. *Neuron* 7:1031–1041

Dekker AJ, Langdon DJ, Gage FH, Thal LJ (1991): NGF increases cortical acetylcholine release in rats with lesions of the nucleus basalis. *Neuroreport* 2:577-580

Goldberg MP, Weiss JH, Pham PC, Choi DW (1987): N-methyl-D-aspartate receptors mediate hypoxic neuronal injury in cortical cultures. *J Pharmacol Exp Ther* 243:764–772

Hadjiconstantinou M, Fitkin JG, Dalia A, Neff NH (1991): Epidermal growth factor enhances striatal dopaminergic parameters in the 1-methyl-4-phenyl-1,2,3,6-tetrahydropyridine-treated mouse. *J Neurochem* 57:479–482

Hefti F, Schneider LS (1989): Rationale for the planned clinical trials with nerve growth factor in Alzheimer's disease. *Psychiatr Dev* 4:297–315

Hefti F, Hartikka J, Knüsel B (1989): Function of neurotrophic factors in the adult and aging brain and their possible use in the treatment of neurodegenerative diseases. *Neurobiol Aging* 10:515–533

Hyman C, Hofer M, Barde YA, Juhasz M, Yancopoulos GD, Squinto SP, Lindsay RM (1991): BDNF is a neurotrophic factor for dopaminergic neurons of the substantia nigra. *Nature* 350: 230–233

Knüsel B, Michel PP, Schwaber J, Hefti F (1990): Selective and nonselective stimulation of central cholinergic and dopaminergic development in vitro by nerve growth factor, basic fibroblast growth factor, epidermal growth factor, and the insulin-like growth factors. *J Neurosci* 10:558–570

Knüsel B, Winslow JW, Rosenthal A, Burton LE, Seid DP, Nikolics K, Hefti F (1991): Promotion of central cholinergic and dopaminergic neuron differentiation by brain-derived neurotrophic factor but not neurotrophin-3. *Proc Natl Acad Sci USA* 88: 961–965

Knüsel B, Beck KD, Winslow JW, Rosenthal A, Burton LE, Widmer HR, Nikolics K, Hefti F (1992): Brain-derived neurotrophic factor administration protects basal forebrain cholinergic but not nigral dopaminergic neurons from degenerative changes after axotomy in the adult rat brain. *J Neurosci* 12:4391–4402

Koliatsos VE, Clatterbuck RE, Nauta HJW, Knüsel B, Burton LE, Hefti F, Mobley WC, Price DL (1991): Human nerve growth factor prevents degeneration of basal forebrain cholinergic neurons in primates. *Ann Neurol* 30:831–840

Lapchak PA, Araujo DM, Hefti F (1992): Neurotrophins in the central nervous system. *Rev Neurosci* 3:1–23

Lapchak PA, Jenden DJ, Hefti F (1992): Pharmacological stimulation reveals recombinant human nerve growth factor-induced increases of in vivo hippocampal cholinergic function measured in rats with partial fimbrial transections. *Neuroscience* 50:847–856

Lindsay RM (1988): Nerve growth factors (NGF, BDNF) enhance axonal regeneration but are not required for survival of adult sensory neurons. *J Neurosci* 8:2394–2405

Mandel RJ, Gage FH, Thal LJ (1989): Spatial learning in rats: correlation with cortical choline acetyltransferase and improvement with NGF following NBM damage. *Exp Neurol* 104:208–217

Michel P, Dandapani BK, Sanchez-Ramoz J, Efange S, Pressman BC, Hefti F (1989): Toxic effects of potential environmental neurotoxins related to 1-methyl-4-phenylpyridinium (MPP$^+$) on cultured rat dopaminergic neurons. *J Pharmacol Exp Ther* 248:842–850

Olson L, Nordberg A, von Holst H, Backman L, Ebendahl T, Alafuzoff I, Amberla K, Hartvig P, Herlitz A, Lilja A, Lundquist H, Langstron B, Meyerson B, Persson A, Viitanen M, Winblad B, Seiger A (1992): Nerve growth factor affects ^{11}C-nicotine binding, blood flow, EEG and verbal episodic memory in an Alzheimer patient. *J Neurol Transm* [P-D Sect] 4:79–95

Otto D, Unsicker K (1990): Basic FGF reverses chemical and morphological deficits in the nigrostriatal system of MPTP-treated mice. *J Neurosci* 10:1912–1921

Pike CJ, Walencewicz AJ, Glabe CG, Cotman CW (1991): Aggregation-related toxicity of synthetic beta-amyloid protein in hippocampal cultures. *Eur J Pharmacol* 207:367–368

Williams LR (1991): Exogenous nerve growth factor stimulates choline acetyltransferase activity in aging Fischer-344 male rats. *Neurobiol Aging* 12:39–46

4

Neuroepidemiology of Parkinson's Disease: Environmental Influences

WILLIAM C. KOLLER

Descriptive epidemiology of Parkinson's disease (PD), by providing a profile of the disease, should be useful in the etiological investigation of PD. Etiological hypotheses need to be consistent with known epidemiologic factors, and descriptive epidemiologic observations may generate a new hypothesis. Analytic epidemiology seeks to identify risk factors that could lead to clues for causal associations with the disease.

The neuroepidemiology of PD could provide a novel etiologic hypothesis for PD. However, significant problems exist for the epidemiologic investigation of PD. Large populations of individuals need to be studied because of the relatively low frequency of PD. Another major difficulty is the accuracy of diagnosis, particularly by nonneurologists. For instance, essential tremor has been found to account for 10% to 40% of false-positive diagnoses of PD in community based studies (Marttila and Rinne, 1976; Snow et al., 1989). Recent studies suggest that approximately 20% of PD cases are misdiagnosed, even by neurologists, when the diagnosis is confirmed by neuropathological postmortem examination (Hughes et al., 1992).

Incidence studies are hampered not only by a low frequency of new cases but also with the problem of exact identification of when the disease began (Koller, 1992). Total case ascertainment is not possible because of the difficulty of identifying very mild cases and the fact that some PD features may be considered part of the normal aging process. Indeed, underestimation of PD has been reported to be 30% to 40% in both community and hospital-based studies (D'Alessandro et al., 1987; Morgante et al., 1992; Schoenberg et al., 1985).

ADVANCES IN RESEARCH ON NEURODEGENERATION, II
Y. Mizuno et al.
© 1994 Birkhäuser Boston

Prevalence

Prevalence studies were not performed until the 1950s. Since that time, many studies using diverse methods have attempted to define the prevalence of PD in various parts of the world (Ashok et al., 1986; Bademosi et al., 1991; Bharucha et al., 1988; Bodmer, 1973; Brewis et al., 1966; Broman, 1963; Casetta et al., 1990; Dupont, 1977; Gudmundsson, 1967; Harado et al., 1983; Ho et al., 1989; Jenkins, 1966; Kessler, 1972; Kurland, 1958; Li et al., 1985; Nobrega et al., 1969; Okada et al., 1990; Rajput et al., 1984b; Rosati et al., 1978; Schoenberg et al., 1988; Wang et al., 1991; Wender et al., 1989). For instance, some investigators have included all forms of parkinsonism such as drug-induced and post encephalitic types (Kurland, 1958; Nobrega et al., 1969; Rajput et al., 1984a, b). It is important to note that prevalence ratios are affected by the length of diagnostic delay, the incidence of the disease, and survival rates. Therefore, variations in the prevalence of PD in different countries may not necessarily reflect true differences. Wide variations in prevalence ratios have been reported. A range of 60 to 187/100,000 has been reported in Caucasians in Europe and North Americans. The lowest prevalence ratios have been reported in orientals (China and Japan) and in Africa (Nigeria and Libya) and in southern Europe (Sardinia). A study of blacks in Copiah County, (Mississippi, United States) found a much higher prevalence rate than for blacks in Nigeria (Schoenberg et al., 1988). Because of the limitations associated with all these studies, it is possible that the results are artifactual. On the other hand, these trends may be important as to different causation or risk factors for PD.

Age-Related Morbidity

Both the reported prevalence and incidence rates of PD increase with advancing age. Age-specific incidence rates are very low under 40 years of age and increase sharply to peak in the age group 70–79 years, decreasing at 80–85 years. However, case ascertainment in the very elderly may be poor because of patient inaccessibility, such as individuals in nursing homes.

Gender Differences

A slight male predominance of PD has been reported in most studies. The male/female ratios for prevalence range from 4.08 to 0.90. It can be concluded that there is no major difference in the pattern of the disease between the genders. An increase in males might have been expected if male-dominated occupations were associated with an increased risk of PD.

Time Trends

No substantial change occurred in age-adjusted incidence rates for PD in Rochester, Minnesota (United States) from 1945 to 1979 (Kurland, 1958; Nobrega et al., 1969; Rajput et al., 1984b). Incidence rates in Sardinia from 1961 to 1971 and in Iceland from 1954 to 1963 likewise showed no marked temporal fluctuations. These data suggest that at least in these locations PD has occurred at a relatively stable rate. If environmental toxins were recently introduced into these areas, an increasing prevalence would have been expected. However, if there is a long-latency toxin, a survey of longer time periods may be necessary.

Mortality Rates

Mortality data do not adequately reflect the frequency of PD. The death certificates of only 30% to 60% of patients dying of PD list this diagnosis. (Kessler, 1973). The proportion of death certificates that fail to mention PD as the underlying cause of death may be as high as 85% (Kessler, 1973; Marmot, 1981). Using death certificate data, a north–south gradient of PD mortality has been reported in the United States (Kurtzke and Murphy, 1990). However, this may not reflect a true difference.

Investigations in Young-Onset PD

Several investigations have studied young-onset PD in the hope that potential toxic exposure may have been more robust or more recent (Rajput et al., 1986; Terävälnen et al., 1986). Rajput and colleagues found that PD patients with onset of disease before age 40 were likely to have lived in a rural environment and to have drunk well water. No specific abnormalities were found in the well water. In another study using a clinic-based survey of 110 consecutive patients and a mail survey of a lay organization self-reported to have PD, it was also found that young-onset PD patients (onset before age 54 years) were more likely to live in a rural environment and to have drunk well-water (Tanner et al., 1987).

Analytic Epidemiology

Analytic studies using case-control or interventional methods seek to identify risk factors for PD. If PD has a long latency period, as has been suggested, this approach may yield valuable information. However, these data may be affected by recall bias or inaccurate recollection. Further, risk factors should not be equated with causal factors.

A number of case-control studies have attempted to assess the role of environmental risk factors in PD (Aquilonius and Hartvig, 1986; Barbeau and Roy, 1985; Ho et al., 1989; Jimenez-Jimenez et al., 1988; Koller et al., 1990; Semchuk et al., 1991; Tanner et al., 1987). The findings in these studies have not been consistent. However, an increased risk for PD for living in a rural environment and exposure to various chemicals has been found in many investigations.

The notion that the occurrence of PD is associated with rural living or farming dates to the mid 1980s (Barbeau et al., 1987; Rajput et al., 1984a, b, 1986). In the intervening years, the issue has been examined numerous times with most report corroborating but some refuting the association between PD and rural living (Granieri et al., 1991; Ho et al., 1989; Koller et al., 1990; Meador et al., 1987; Semchuk et al., 1991). The discrepancies in results may be attributable, in part, to differing study populations and methodology. Clearly, rural living is not the sole determinant of PD because many PD patients lack such a history. Assuming that rural living is a link to the cause of PD, distinguishing which feature of rural living serves as the actual risk factor for PD is difficult. Consideration has been given to well water consumption and its constituents, including chemicals and minerals (Rajput et al., 1987b). It is also possible that certain ethnic groups are overrepresented in some rural areas and thus a genetic component could contribute to the association between rural living and PD. Aging in itself is associated with rural living because one of four Americans over age 65 years reside in rural settings (Clifford et al., 1985).

Protective Agents

Some studies have suggested that certain environmental agents might protect against the development of PD. These include cigarette smoking (Baumann et al., 1980; Burch, 1981), childhood measles (Sasco and Paffenberger, 1985), alcoholic consumption (Koller, 1983), and cancer (Jannson and Jankovic, 1985). Other studies, however, have failed to demonstrate a protective effect for childhood measles (Tanner et al.,

1987), smoking (Rajput et al., 1987a; Tanner et al., 1987), and cancer (Rajput et al., 1987a). The inverse relationship between PD and smoking has been the most consistent. This observation could have a physiological (nicotine protects nigral neurons) or a psychological (part of premorbid PD personality) explanation. Dietary factors may also be important. Two reports suggest that a diet high in vitamin E, an anoxidant, might decrease the risk of PD (Golbe and Farrell, 1988; Tanner et al., 1988). However, retrospective dietary histories are often unreliable.

Environmental Toxin As a Cause of PD

The discovery that MPTP caused a clinical syndrome similar to PD and was a specific substantia nigra neurotoxin gave further strength to the notion that a chemical similar in structure to MPTP and having a similar mechanism of action might cause PD (Jenner and Marsden, 1988; Tetrud and Langston, 1987). The toxicity of MPTP results from its metabolism by monoamine oxidase B to MPP^+, which accumulates in dopamine neurons via the dopamine uptake system (Calne and Langston, 1983). MPP^+ is then actively taken up into mitochondria and there inhibits NADH Co Q reductase (complex I) of the mitochondrial respiratory chain body, causing a fall in ATP and eventually cell death. Structural analogs of MPTP can also cause parkinsonism and mitochondrial dysfunction (Langston et al., 1984a, b; Mitchell et al., 1985). MPTP appears to cause more restricted changes in the brain compared to the more diffuse changes seen in PD (Barbeau et al., 1981; Burns et al., 1983). It is also not clear if Lewy bodies are associated with MPTP-induced parkinsonism.

The cause of the epidemic of dementia-parkinsonism of the Western Pacific is unknown. It has been suggested that the condition may be environmentally induced by ingestion of the cycad plant (Spencer et al., 1991). This hypothesis is controversial. If a toxin in the cycad plant is shown to cause the neurodegenerative illness of the Western Pacific, the concept of an environmental toxin causing PD would be strengthened.

The putative environmental toxin that could cause PD could be either an uncommon or common toxin. The fact that a cluster or epidemic of true PD has never been documented makes it unlikely that a large exposure to an uncommon toxin in the environment is solely responsible for PD. Another possibility is that one or more environmental toxins exists that can induce PD in only selected individuals. These susceptible individuals could have impaired ability to detoxify a potentially damaging chemical. An impairment of enzymes metabolizing sulfur-containing

Table 1. Some necessary properties of environmental neurotoxins causing PD

Present for at least 150 years
Lack acute toxicity
Worldwide distribution
Demonstrate selectivity
Explain progressive nature of PD
Closely mimic clinical symptoms of PD
Closely mimic pathological changes of PD

compounds has been reported to occur in PD (Steventon et al., 1989; Waring et al., 1989). Such a defect would be consistent with this hypothesis.

Conclusion

It is concluded that there is evidence that an environmental toxin may be involved in the cause of PD. This environmental neurotoxin would need to possess various properties (Table 1). It would need to have been present at least 150 years longer if PD were present before then. This chemical would have to lack acute toxicity and not cause parkinsonism immediately as MPTP does. Because PD has a worldwide distribution, so much the chemical or chemicals that cause parkinsonism. The individual susceptibility of PD would need to be explained by either chemical or host selectivity. PD is clearly a progressive condition; therefore, the toxin needs to either be present persistently or initiate pathological events that would continue in the absence of the toxin. This putative toxin must, as is the case for MPTP, closely mimic the clinical and pathological changes of PD.

It is likely that more than one toxin will be found that can induce parkinsonism. However, if individual susceptibility plays a major role, it may be very difficult to identify these putative neurotoxins. Classical epidemiologic approaches will probably not identify these chemicals. To date, no specific chemicals or infectious agents have emerged as possible candidates. If epidemiology is to make a contribution to the cause of PD, a long-term prospective study of healthy individuals, some of whom would develop PD, in the future is needed. Possible factors related to PD could therefore be prospectively documented.

References

Aquilonius SM, Hartvig P (1986): A Swedish county with unexpectedly high utilization of anti-parkinsonian drugs. *Acta Neurol Scand* 74:379

Ashok PP, Radhakrishnan K, Sridharan R, Mousa ME (1986): Epidemiology of Parkinson's disease in Benghazi, north-east Libya. *Neurosurgery* 88(2): 109–113

Bademosi O, Al-Rajeh IH, Awada A (1991): Prevalence of Parkinson's disease (PD) in an Arab community: the Thugbah study. In: *Congres de neurologie tropicale, September 26–28, 1991*, p. 27. Recherche en Neurologic Tropicale Press

Barbeau A, Roy M (1985): Uneven prevalence of Parkinson's disease in the province of Quebec. *Can J Neurol Sci* 12:169–170

Barbeau A, Roy M, Bernier G, et al. (1987): Ecogenetics of Parkinson's disease: prevalence and environmental aspects in rural areas. *Can J Neurol Sci* 14:36–41

Baumann RJ, Jamesson HD, McKean HE, Haack DG, Weisburg LM (1980): Cigarette smoking and Parkinson's disease. I. A comparison of cases with matched neighbors. *Neurology* 30:839

Bharucha NE, Bharucha EP, Bharucha AE, Bhise AV, Schoenberg BS (1988): Prevalence of Parkinson's disease in the Parsi community in Bombay, India. *Arch Neurol* 45:1321–1323

Bodmer WF (1973): Population genetics of the HLA system: retrospect and prospect. In: *Histocompatibility Testing 1972*, Dausset J, Colombani J, eds., pp. 611–667. Copenhagen: Munksgaard

Brewis M, Poskanzer DC, Rolland C, Miller H (1966): Neurological disease in an English city. *Acta Neurol Scand* 42(Suppl 24):1–89

Broman T (1963): Parkinson's syndrome, prevalence and incidence in Goteborg. *Acta Neurol Scand* 51(Suppl 4):95–101

Burch PRJ (1981): Cigarette smoking and Parkinson's disease. *Neurology* 31:500.

Burns SP, Chiueh CC, Markey SP, Ebert MH, Jacobowitz DM, Kopin IJ (1983): A primate model of parkinsonism: selective destruction of dopaminergic neurons in the pars compacta of the substantia nigra by *N*-methyl-1,2,3,6-tetrahydropyridine. *Proc Natl Acad Sci USA* 80:4546–4550

Calne DB, Langston JW (1983): Aetiology of Parkinson's disease. *Lancet* 2: 1457–1459

Casetta I, Granieri E, Govoni V, et al. (1990): Epidemiology of Parkinson's disease in Italy. A descriptive survey in the U.S.L. of Cento, province of Ferrara, Emilia-Romagna. *Acta Neurol* (Napoli) 12:284–291

Clifford WB, Heaton TB, Voss PR, Fuguitt GV (1985): The rural elderly in demographic perspective. In: *The Elderly in Rural Society: Every Fourth Elder*, Coward RT, Lee GR, eds., pp. 25–55. New York: Springer

D'Alessandro R, Gamberini G, Granieri E, Benassi G, Naccarato S, Manzaroli D (1987): Prevalence of Parkinson's disease in the Republic of San Marino. *Neurology* 37:1679–1682

Dupont E (1977): Epidemiology of parkinsonism. The Parkinson investigation, Arhus, Denmark (preliminary results). In: *Symposium on Parkinsonism*, Worm-Peterson J, Bottcher J, eds., pp. 65–75. Denmark: Merck, Sharp & Dohme

Golbe LI, Farrell T (1988): Case-control survey of early-adult dietary habits in Parkinson's disease. *Neurology* 38(Suppl 1):204

Granieri E, Carreras M, Casetta I, et al. (1991): Parkinson's disease in Ferrara, Italy, 1967 through 1987. *Arch Neurol* 48:854–857

Gudmundsson KR (1967): A clinical survey of parkinsonism in Iceland. *Acta Neurol Scand* 43(Suppl) 33:1–61

Harado H, Nishikawa S, Takahashi K (1983): Epidemiology of Parkinson's disease in a Japanese city. *Arch Neurol* 40:151–154

Ho SC, Woo J, See CM (1989): Epidemiologic study of Parkinson's disease in Hong Kong. *Neurology* 39:1314–1318

Hughes AJ, Daniel SE, Kilford L, Lees AJ (1992): The accuracy of the clinical diagnosis of Parkinson's disease: a clinicopathological study of 100 cases. *J Neurol Neurosurg Psychiatry* 55:181–184

Jannson B, Jankovic J (1985): Low cancer rates among patients with Parkinson's disease. *Ann Neurol* 17:505

Jenkins AC (1966): Epidemiology of parkinsonism in Victoria. *Med J Aust* 2:496–502

Jenner P, Marsden CD (1988): MPTP-induced parkinsonism in primates and its use in the assessment of novel strategies for the treatment of Parkinson's disease. In: *Current Problems in Neurology (6): Parkinson's Disease: Clinical and Experimental Advances*, Rose FC, ed., pp. 149–162. London: John Libbey

Jimenez-Jimenez FJ, Gonzales DM, Gimenez-Roldan S (1988): Exposure to well water drinking and pesticides in Parkinson's disease. In: *Proceedings of the Ninth International Symposium on Parkinson's Disease*, p. 118, World Congress of Neurology, Jerusalem

Kessler II (1972): Epidemiologic studies of Parkinson's disease. A hospital-based survey. *Am J Epidemiol* 95:308–318

Kessler II (1973): Parkinson's disease: perspectives on epidemiology and pathogenesis. *Prev Med* 2:88–105

Koller WC (1983): Alcoholism in essential tremor. *Neurology* 33:1074

Koller WC (1992): When does Parkinson's disease begin? *Neurology* 43(Suppl 4):27–31

Koller WC, Vetere-Overfield B, Gray C, Alexander C, Chin T, Dolezal, Hassanein R, Tanner C (1990): Environmental risk factors in Parkinson's disease. *Neurology* 40: 1218–1221

Kurland LT (1958): Epidemiology: incidence, geographic distribution and genetic considerations. In: *Pathogenesis and Treatment of Parkinsonism*, Field WS, ed., pp. 5–49. Springfield, IL: Charles C. Thomas

Kurtzke JF, Murphy FM (1990): The changing patterns of death rates in parkinsonism. *Neurology* 40:42–49

Langston JW, Langston EB, Irwin I (1984a): MPTP-induced parkinsonism in human and non-human primates. Clinical and experimental aspects. *Acta Neurol Scand* 70:49–54

Langston JW, Forno LS, Rebert CS, Irwin (1984b): Selective nigral toxicity after systemic administration of 1-methyl-4-phenyl-1,2,3,6-tetrahydropyridine (MPTP) in the squirrel monkey. *Brain Res* 292:390–394

Li SC, Schoenberg BS, Wang CC, et al. (1985): A prevalence survey of Parkinson's disease and other movement disorders in the People's Republic of China. *Arch Neurol* 42:655–657

Marmot M (1981): Mortality and Parkinson's disease. In: *Research Progress in Parkinson's Disease 1980*, Rose F, Capildeo R, eds. pp. 9–16. Kent: Tunbridge Wells

Marttila RJ, Rinne U (1976): Epidemiology of Parkinson's disease in Finland. *Acta Neurol Scand* 53:81–102

Meador KJ, Meador MP, Loring DS, et al. (1987): Neuroepidemiology of Parkinson's disease. *Neurology* 37(Suppl 1):120

Mitchell IJ, Cross AJ, Sambrook MA, Crossman AR (1985): Sites of the neurotoxic action of 1-methyl-4-phenyl-1,2,3,6-tetrahydropyridine in the macaque monkey include the ventral tegmental area and the locus coeruleus. *Neurosci Lett* 61:195–200

Morgante L, Racco WA, Rosa AE (1992): Prevalence of Parkinson's disease and other types of parkinsonism: a door-to-door survey in three Sicilian municipalities. *Neurology* 42: 1901–1906

Nobrega FT, Glattre E, Kurland LT, Okazaki H (1969): Comments on the epidemiology of parkinsonism including prevalence and incidence statistics for Rochester, Minnesota, 1935–1936. In: *Progress in Neuro-Genetics: Proceedings of the International Congress of Neuro-Genetics*, Barbeau A, Brunette JS, eds., pp. 474–485. Amsterdam: Excerpta Medica

Okada K, Kobayashi S, Tsunematsu T (1990): Prevalence of Parkinson's disease in Izumo City, Japan. *Gerontology* 36:340–344

Rajput AH, Stern W, Christ A, Laverty W (1984a): Etiology of Parkinson's disease: environmental factor(s). *Neurology* 34(Suppl 1):207

Rajput AH, Offurd KP, Beard CM, Kurland LT (1984b): Epidemiology of parkinsonism: incidence, classification, and mortality. *Ann Neurol* 16:278–282

Rajput AH, Offurd KP, Beard CM, Kurland LT (1984c): A case-control study of smoking habits, dementia, and other illnesses in idiopathic Parkinson's disease. *Neurology* 37:226

Rajput AH, Uitti RJ, Stern W, et al. (1987b): Geography, drinking water chemistry, pesticides, and herbicides and the etiology of Parkinson's disease. *Can J Neurol Sci* 14:414

Rajput AH, Uitti RJ, Stern W, et al. (1986): Early onset Parkinson's disease in Saskatchewan: environmental considerations for etiology. *Can J Neurol Sci* 13:212–216

Rosati G, Granieri E, Pinna L, et al. (1978): Parkinson's disease. Prevalence and incidence in the province of Sassari, North Sardinia. *Acta Neurol* (Napoli) 33:210–207

Rosati G, Granieri E, Pinna L, Devoto MC (1979): The frequency of Parkinson's disease in the province of Nuoro (Sardinia). *Acta Neurol* 1:303–308

Rosati G, Granieri E, Pinna L, et al. (1980): The risk of Parkinson's disease in Mediterranean people. *Neurology* 30:250–255

Sasco AJ, Paffenberger RS, Jr (1985): Measles infection and Parkinson's disease. *Am J Epidemiol* 122:1017

Schoenberg BS, Anderson DW, Haerer AF (1985): Prevalence of Parkinson's disease in the biracial population of Copiah County, Mississippi. *Neurology* 35:841–845

Schoenberg BS, Osuntokun BO, Adeuja AO, et al. (1988): Comparison of the prevalence of Parkinson's disease in black populations in the rural United States and rural Nigeria: door-to-door community studies. *Neurology* 38:645–646

Semchuck KM, Love EJ, Lee RG (1991): Parkinson's disease and exposure to rural environmental factors: a population based case-control study. *Can J Neurol Sci* 18:279–386

Snow B, Wiens M, Hertzman C, Calne DB (1989): A community survey of Parkinson's disease. *Can Med Assoc* 141:418–422

Spencer PS, Kisby GE, Ludopha AC (1991): Slow toxins, biologic markers, and long-latency neurodegenerative disease in the western Pacific region. *Neurology* 41(Suppl 2):62–66

Steventon GB, Heafield MTE, Waring RH, Williams AC (1989): Xenobiotic metabolism in Parkinson's disease. *Neurology* 39:883–887

Tanner CM, Chen B, Wang WZ, et al. (1987): Environmental factors in the etiology of Parkinson's disease. *Can J Neurol Sci* 14:419

Tanner CM, Cohen JC, Summerville BC, Goetz CG (1988): Vitamin use and Parkinson's disease. *Ann Neurol* 233:182

Teräväinen H, Forgach L, Hietanen M, Schulzer M, Schoenberg BS, Calne DB (1986): The age of onset of Parkinson's disease, etiologic implications. *Can J Neurol Sci* 13:317

Tetrud JW, Langston JW (1987): L-Deprenyl as a possible protective agent in Parkinson's disease. *J Neural transm* 25:69–79

Wang Y, Shi Y, Wu S, He Y, Zhang B (1991): Parkinson's disease in China. *Chin Med J* 33:960–964

Waring RH, Sturman SG, Smith MCG, Steventon GB, Heafield MTE, Williams AC (1989): S-Methylation in motor neuron disease and Parkinson's disease. *Lancet* 2:356–357

Wender M, Pruchnik D, Kowal P, Florczak J, Zalejski M (1989): Epidemiology of Parkinson's disease in the Pozna'n province. *Przegl Epidemiol* 43:150–155

5

Discussion: Session 8 – 9 A.M. – 8 February 1993

RECORDED BY WERNER POEWE

After George-Hyslop's presentation Calne pointed out that genetic heterogeneity in Alzheimer's disease obviously corresponds to clinical heterogeneity. Specifically he wondered how many cases of Alzheimer's disease would fall into the category of genetically determined familial Alzheimer's disease, how many were sporadic cases predominantly caused by environmental factors, and how many cases would fall in between these categories. George-Hyslop thought that "pure" genetic cases of Alzheimer's disease were extremely rare and that the majority are probably caused by an interaction of genetic and environmental factors.

Mizuno invited George-Hyslop to enlarge on possible environmental factors in the pathogenesis of Alzheimer's disease; he then pointed out head injury, premorbid intelligence, schooling, and aluminium exposure as the risk factors most extensively discussed in the literature. George-Hyslop also stated that in his view the critical environmental factors for the development of Alzheimer's disease still remain to be identified.

Beal added to this that the existence of identical twins in any of the known families with chromosome 14 or 19 linkage might help to sort out the role of environmental factors in Alzheimer's disease pathogenesis. While there are no identical twins in the chromosome 14 pedigrees studied by George-Hyslop, his personal series otherwise includes one set of concordant identical twins with late-onset Alzheimer's disease. In the literature there are reports of both concordant and discordant homozygous twins with Alzheimer's disease, but their families have not yet been studied genetically.

Following McGeer's paper, discussion focused on the possible role of bFGF in the diseased and normal substantia nigra. Poewe asked, with respect to the parkinsonian substantia nigra, whether there were differences in the expression of bFGF in early as compared to later disease stages so that changes in bFGF might antedate actual cell loss. Along the same line Hornykiewicz inquired if side-to-side differences had been observed in cases of hemiparkinsonism. McGeer pointed out that so far he had not been able to study these aspects for lack of appropriate post-mortem brain material.

Calne asked whether bFGF reduction in the parkinsonian substantia nigra was a manifestation of diseased neurons no longer producing the factor or rather decreased supply from other cellular sources like glia. McGeer admitted that this was not entirely clear but he favored the idea that neurons expressing reduced amounts of bFGF had actually been starved from the factor as he observed absent bFGF in neurons still expressing TH.

Nagatsu sought clarification on the significance of increases in bFGF in remaining nigral neurons in Parkinson's disease. He pointed out that his group had looked for increases in mRNA expression for TH in dying dopaminergic neurons but rather found the opposite. He wondered whether increased bFGF expression might represent a compensatory mechanism in neurons losing TH. McGeer ruled this out as most dopaminergic neurons in Parkinson's disease lose bFGF and only a small minority showed an increase, which remains poorly understood.

Oertel asked which molecular weight form of bFGF was recognized by the antibody used in McGeer's human studies. McGeer explained that this was a different antibody from the one used in the rat studies and that it recognized the sequence 1–14 of the high molecular weight form but was blind to the C-terminal part of the molecule. Using a different antibody more sensitive to the C-terminal part it had been possible to identify a distinct population of calbindin-positive and bFGF-negative neurons, which corresponded to those projecting to limbic areas and striatal patches but not to the matrix.

Reichmann and Mizuno wanted to know about the regional specificity of nigral bFGF depletion in the parkinsonian brain. McGeer replied that his antibody had not detected any bFGF in the basal ganglia, cortex, cerebellum, or locus coeruleus, which may also be a problem of sensitivity. As for disease specificity he mentioned findings of bFGF depletion in strionigral degeneration but none in ALS.

Mizuno asked about changes in nigral bFGF with normal aging; McGeer mentioned the anecdotal normal findings in the substantia nigra of a 89-year-old but added that systematic studies are lacking.

Following Hefti's presentation, Poewe asked if there are data on the actions of bFGF on cultures of dopaminergic cells. Hefti replied that bFGF was pluripotent and its actions included those of a glial promotor and potent mitogen, but that its action on dopaminergic cells was still poorly defined.

Horowski wanted to know what changes in NGF expression occurred in lesioned cholinergic neurons. Hefti stated that in lesion experiments a transient increase in NGF protein concentration had been observed in the hippocampus. At the same time there was a down-regulation of BDNF expression, and Hefti suggested a cascade of events where cholinergic lesions might first lead to down-regulation of BDNF, which could then have detrimental effects on hippocampal and cortical neurons.

Horowski then turned to therapeutic aspects and mentioned the capacity of certain vitamin D_3 analogs to stimulate the synthesis of growth factors. Hefti agreed that such stimulation could be one approach in the future, as well as direct or indirect activation of growth factor receptors.

Following Reichmann's general comment about the clinical feasibility of growth factor therapy in neurodegenerative disorders, Hefti mentioned blood–brain barrier transport as the most significant problem at present. He thought peripheral applications would therefore have to come first, as already started in clinical trials with CNTF and IGF in ALS. He viewed stroke patients with altered blood–brain barrier permeability as another target of opportunity for growth factor therapy. Further developments might lead to the use of fetal cell transplants together with topical growth factor application, chronic intraventricular infusion pumps, or implantable polymers with sustained growth factor release or even transplantation of genetically engineered cells. He pointed out that there was no simple way forward from findings in cell culture to treatment of patients.

After Koller's paper, Hefti asked if cigarette smoking had a protective effect against Parkinson's disease. Koller stated that an inverse relationship between smoking and Parkinson's disease was firmly established but that the explanation for this was probably psychological and related to the premorbid parkinsonian personality type.

Hefti wondered how firmly the existence of a distinctive premorbid parkinsonian personality had been established, and Koller stated that this concept was difficult to prove retrospectively and that prospective long-term studies were needed.

Poewe added that there might be a correlation between the postulated introverted, rigid, and depressed premorbid personality type of Parkinson's disease patients and certain types of neuropsychological dysfunction – including frontal lobe deficits like set shifting problems – found in early stages of the disease so that premorbid personality features might actually represent early manifestations of the illness. Koller stated that depressive episodes in Parkinson's disease patients may antedate onset of motor symptoms by 10 to 20 years.

Mizuno cited a Japanese case-control study into the childhood life-style of Parkinson's disease patients with their spouses as controls. Patients were found to have been less active in their childhood and had fewer friends but also had consumed fewer milk products. He wondered if similar data existed for a western population. Koller mentioned the study by Golbe and co-workers into dietary risk factors in Parkinson's disease, which had incriminated diets rich in Vitamin E.

Snow also believed that evidence for a premorbid parkinsonian personality was quite persuasive, and raised the issue whether similar personality findings had been obtained in patients with ALS or Alzheimer's disease. The answer was that such studies were lacking.

Eisen took up the issue of the many similarities in the epidemiologies of Parkinson's disease, Alzheimer's disease and ALS. Koller agreed that such similarities were present and speculated about a possible common causative factor for the three neurodegenerative disorders.

With respect to dietary or other life-style risk factors, Gajdusek drew attention to the fact that when the first clusters of ALS and parkinsonism/dementia were described in the Western Pacific, the population involved had never been exposed to any product of western civilization and exhibited essentially Stone Age civilization status. He stated that risk factor discussions for the related neurodegenerative diseases in the western world had to take this into account.

Calne recognized the problem of disease definition in this and raised the question whether Parkinson's disease in the Western Pacific was the same disease as the clinical and pathological entity of idiopathic Parkinson's disease in the western world. He stated that possible overlaps between the neurodegenerative disorders created a major problem for epidemiologic studies.

In the ensuing general discussion, Hornykiewicz raised the issue of the site of the primary insult in neurodegenerative diseases, i.e., the level of the nerve terminals versus cell bodies. This was discussed in relation to idiopathic Parkinson's disease after Hefti and Hornykiewicz had pointed out that the primary site of MPTP toxicity was at the level of striatal nerve terminals.

Hornykiewicz stressed that in MPTP-treated rhesus monkeys there was a mismatch between the magnitude of dopamine depletion in the cell body and nerve terminal regions, i.e., roughly a 95% striatal versus 70% nigral reduction in dopamine concentration.

Poewe added that the human disease is believed to become clinically manifest after about 80% of striatal dopamine had been lost, but the symptomatic threshold of nigral cell loss was only about 50%.

Snow cited further evidence from a study performed in collaboration with the McGeers in which striatal DA loss in 16 cases of idiopathic Parkinson's disease was about 90% versus a 60% neuronal fallout in the substantia nigra.

Olanow took the opposite view and cited evidence from studies of incidental Lewy body cases showing reduced levels of glutathion in the substantia nigra before any significant dopamine loss in the striatum.

Bainbridge cautioned that a mismatch between striatal dopamine and nigral cell loss might eventually resolve if matching striatal projection areas of the different nigral cell groups were considered. Finally, Calne pointed out that even if nerve terminals showed more pronounced changes than the respective cell bodies this was still compatible with a dying back process following primary insults to the cell body.

The second unresolved issue raised in the general discussion related to the progression of neurodegenerative diseases and the ability of experimental models to mimic this aspect. Calne pointed out that in human MPTP parkinsonism progression after discontinuation of exposure was evident in PET studies performed in his laboratory by Snow.

Olanow added evidence from work in his laboratory in which single injections of low-dose iron into the substantia nigra of rodents had led to progressive nigral neuronal loss and striatal dopamine depletion over 6 months.

Youdim found that this fitted well with the brain's ability to sequester iron and other toxins; 90% of iron injected into the brain of 10-year-old rats was still present in the adult animal, so that progression of lesions as observed by Olanow could result from persistence of the toxic agent.

Part II

METALS AND, FREE RADICALS

6

Manganese-Induced Neurotoxicity

C.W. OLANOW, D.B. CALNE, N.S. CHU and D.P. PERL

Manganese is a paramagnetic heavy metal with an atomic number of 25 that was first recognized as an element by the Swedish chemist Schelle in 1771. It is the twelfth most common element in the earth's crust and the fourth most widely used metal in the world. Eight million tons of manganese metal are extracted annually, of which 94% is employed in the manufacture of steel. Electrolytic high-temperature reduction converts manganese oxide to ferromanganese or silicomanganese (alloy) that contains approximately 70% manganese. Manganese dioxide is used in the manufacture of batteries. Potassium permanganate has bactericidal and fungicide properties and is extensively employed in water purification. In addition, the organic compound methylcyclopentadienyl manganese tricarbonyl (MMT) can be used in lieu of lead as an antiknock agent in gasoline.

Manganese neurotoxicity was first described in 1837 by Couper, only 20 years after the original description of Parkinson's disease (PD). Five patients who worked in a manganese ore crushing plant in France developed muscle weakness, a bent posture, whispering speech, limb tremor, and salivation. Other examples of "manganese crusher's disease" were subsequently reported by Embden (1901) and von Jaksh (1907). The first U.S. cases were reported in 1913 by Casamajor. Subsequently, Edsall et al. (1919) described the relationship between manganese exposure, its clinical syndrome, and its pathological effects. During the past 75 years there have been many reports of manganism, particularly in miners, smelters, and workers involved in the manufacture of dry batteries (Abd et al., 1965; Oshizawa, 1927; Canavan et al., 1934; Emara et al., 1971; Ferraz et al., 1988; Flinn et al., 1941; Huang et al., 1989; Mena et al., 1967; Rodier, 1955; Saric et al., 1979; Schuler et al., 1957; Smyth et al., 1973). Manganese toxicity has also been described in patients who received long-term parental nutrition (Ejima et al., 1992) or those ingesting potassium permanganate (Holzgraefe et al., 1986). Much of

ADVANCES IN RESEARCH ON NEURODEGENERATION, II
Y. Mizuno et al.
© 1994 Birkhäuser Boston

the current understanding of the relationship between manganese and neurotoxicity can be attributed to the reports of Cotzias and co-workers who described psychiatric and parkinsonian features in Chilean manganese miners (Cotzias, 1969; Cotzias et al., 1968; Mena et al., 1969).

Clinical features of manganese neurotoxicity resemble PD with dystonia (Barbeau, 1984). The initial stages may include psychiatric features such as behavioral disturbances, hallucinations, and psychoses. This syndrome has been referred to as "manganese madness" or "locura manganica" (Mena et al., 1967; Rodier, 1955). Extrapyramidal features constitute the more typical presentation and, particularly in industrial workers, tend to develop in the absence of "manganese madness" (Cook et al., 1974; Greenhouse, 1971). Clinical features can include bradykinesia, gait dysfunction, postural instability, rigidity, micrographia, masked facies, and speech disturbances. Tremors may be seen but these are typically noted on attempts to maintain a posture or with intentional activity rather than at rest (Casamajor, 1913; Cook et al., 1974; Edsall et al., 1919; Greenhouse, 1991; Mena et al., 1964). There is also a particular propensity for the development of dystonia, usually manifest as a facial grimace or plantar flexion of the foot known as "coq au pied" or "cock walk." This results in a characteristic gait abnormality in which patients strut on their toes with their elbows flexed and their spine erect.

There are conflicting descriptions in the literature regarding the response to levodopa. Individual patients with manganese neurotoxicity are reported to have enjoyed a good response to levodopa (Mena et al., 1970; Rosenstock et al., 1971) while others are reported to have had little if any observable benefit (Cook et al., 1974; Greenhouse, 1971; Huang et al., 1993). Some cases are described in which symptoms persist only as long as exposure continues (Casamajor, 1913; Cook et al., 1974; Edsall et al., 1919; Flinn et al., 1941; Greenhouse, 1971; Huang et al., 1989; Mena et al., 1967; Rodier, 1955; Smyth et al., 1973). Other cases are reported to show progression in neurological dysfunction long after levodopa withdrawal (Canavan et al., 1934; Edsall et al., 1919; Huang et al., 1993; Rosenstock et al., 1971; Tanaka and Lieben, 1969). Levels of manganese in blood, urine, or hair may be elevated in some patients (Cook et al., 1974; Huang et al., 1989; Rodier, 1955; Rosenstock et al., 1971). However, manganese levels may be normal in some affected individuals (Cotzias et al., 1968; Tanaka and Lieben, 1969) and elevated in others who have been exposed but have no clinical dysfunction (Tanaka and Lieben, 1969). This variability in the clinical picture, response to levodopa, and laboratory abnormalities have made it difficult to differentiate basal ganglia damage caused by manganese toxicity from other basal ganglia disorders such as PD, particularly in patients who have been exposed to manganese. This is a problem of considerable practical import as many workers are exposed to low concentrations of manganese and PD is a common disorder that is expected to affect 1%–2% of adults independent of whether they have been exposed to manganese. Recent advances in pathology and brain imaging, coupled with the characterization of a cohort of patients in Taiwan with well-defined manganese neurotoxicity and the development of an animal model of manganese intoxication, have helped to clarify the clinical picture of manganese intoxication and facilitate its distinction from basal ganglia damage caused by PD.

Parkinson's Disease Versus Manganese Neurotoxicity

At the London Brain Bank, pathologic review of 100 brains from patients diagnosed during life as having idiopathic PD detected a misdiagnosis rate of approximately 25% (Hughes et al., 1992). In this study, PD pathology, as evidenced by (SNc) degeneration and Lewy bodies, was most frequently associated with a clinical picture characterized by resting tremor, asymmetric presentation, and a good response to levodopa. Magnetic resonance imaging (MRI) studies suggest that PD with primary involvement of the SNc can be differentiated from atypical parkinsonism with degeneration of the striatum based on the finding of signal hypointensity in the putamen on heavily T_2-weighted high-field-strength images (Drayer et al., 1986). Signal hypointensity is thought to reflect iron accumulation associated with degeneration of the putamen. As observed in the London Brain bank study, parkinsonian patients with normal MRI signal in the putamen indicative of primary degeneration of the SNc have a clinical picture characterized by resting tremor and a good response to levodopa. In contrast, parkinsonian patients with MRI changes in the putamen reflecting striatal degeneration have a syndrome marked by the early appearance of gait and balance disturbance, speech impairment, absence of resting tremor, and little or no response to levodopa (Olanow, 1992).

We have argued that in patients with degeneration confined to the SNc, preservation of striatal neurons (and their dopamine receptors) account for the capacity of these patients to respond to levodopa replacement therapy. In contrast, patients with degeneration involving striatal or pallidal neurons have a lesion that affects either dopamine receptors or downstream neurons, thereby precluding the possibility of a satisfactory response to levodopa therapy. Prospective studies confirmed this interpretation (Olanow et al., 1990). MRI abnormalities in the putamen of patients with early untreated parkinsonism predict a poor response to levodopa and a clinical syndrome characterized by features of atypical parkinsonism rather than PD. These studies suggest that the clinical syndrome and response to levodopa can differentiate disorders such as PD, which primarily affect neurons of the SNc, from disorders such as manganese parkinsonism that primarily involve pallidal or striatal neurons.

Parkinson's disease is characterized by degeneration of the nigrostriatal pathway and a loss of striatal dopamine. Neuronal loss is most prominent in the SNc (Gibb and Lees, 1991; Hassler, 1938; Pakkenburg et al., 1991). Neuronal death may also occur in the locus ceruleus and in the substantia innominata. Lewy bodies are usually found in the SNc; their occurrence is so frequent that most authorities regard them as essential for diagnosis (Duvoisin, 1989). With careful search, Lewy bodies can also be found in the cerebral cortex of virtually all patients with PD, particularly if anti-ubiquitin stains are employed. Occasionally neurofibrillary tangles or activated microglia may be detected (McGeer et al., 1989; Rajput et al., 1989).

In contrast to PD, there is substantial evidence that the globus pallidus (GP) bears the brunt of damage following manganese toxicity. Pathological studies in animal models and in humans demonstrate that following manganese intoxication neuronal loss and gliosis are most prominent in the GP (primarily medial segment) and striatum but not the SNc (Bernheimer et al., 1967; Canavan et al, 1934; Mella, 1924; Pentschew et al., 1963; Yamada et al., 1986). There is also evidence that manganese preferentially accumulates in the GP. In normal individuals, brain manganese levels are highest in the GP (Bonilla et al., 1982; Larsen et al., 1979). Manganese intoxication, but not PD, is associated with an increase in brain manganese concentration that is similarly maximal in the GP (Larson et al., 1981; Suzuki et al., 1975). Administration of radiolabeled manganese results in accumulation of radioactivity in the GP (Dastur et al., 1968). T^1-weighted high-field-strength MRI studies following manganese administration to nonhuman primates demonstrate signal abnormalities in the GP as well as in the striatum and brain stem (Newland et al., 1989). Similar MRI changes have been observed in patients exposed to high concentrations of manganese (Nelson et al., in press).

These findings indicate that, in contrast to PD, manganese preferentially accumulates within and damages the GP and striatum. This difference in the pattern of neuronal degeneration in patients with PD and those with basal ganglia damage from manganese neurotoxicity should permit differentiation of those conditions on the basis of their clinical picture and response to levodopa. Patients with PD who have SNc degeneration would be expected to have a clinical picture characterized by asymmetry, resting tremor, and a good response to levodopa. Patients with manganese-induced damage to the striatum or pallidum would, on the other hand, be more likely to have a clinical picture consisting of gait and balance impairment, speech disturbance, dystonia, absence of resting tremor, and a poor response to levodopa.

Animal models of manganese toxicity provide support for this concept. Mella (1924) described a bradykinetic syndrome coupled with focal dystonia in a series of monkeys who had been chronically treated with manganese chloride ($MnCl_2$) for 18 months. At postmortem examination, degeneration in these animals was primarily localized to the GP and striatum. We treated adult rhesus monkeys with weekly intravenous injections of $MnCl_2$ (Olanow et al., 1993). Cumulative doses of 20 to 40 mg were associated with the development of neurological dysfunction manifested by bradykinesia, rigidity, and facial grimacing but not tremor. None of the animals responded to levodopa. Postmortem degeneration was primarily confined to the GP and was associated with cell loss and gliosis. H & E stains demonstrated focal areas of mineralization distributed predominantly in a perivascular pattern. These deposits stained prominently for iron on Perls stain. Similar changes were noted in the substantia nigra pars recticularis (SNr) and, to a much less pronounced degree, in the SNc. Laser microprobe (LAMMA) studies of mineral deposits within the GP revealed a marked increase in levels of iron and aluminum. It is noteworthy that increased levels of iron and aluminium but not manganese have been found within SNc neurons in PD (Good et al., 1992).

We have examined a cohort of patients with manganese neurotoxicity who worked in a manganese smelting plant in Taiwan (Huang et al., 1989, 1993). Six of 13 individuals who were chronically exposed to an ambient concentration of manganese in excess of $27 \, mg/m^3$ (TLV = $1-5 \, mg/m^3$) developed basal ganglia dysfunction, characterized by gait disturbance with particular difficulty in walking backward, micrographia, and hypophonia. Five had dystonia manifest either as a facial grimace or coq au pied. Postural tremor was observed in 3 but this did not persist; none had resting tremor. Subjective improvement with levodopa was initially reported in 3 patients but did not persist, and by the time of the 3-year follow-up examination, levodopa had been discontinued by all patients because of lack of efficacy (Huang et al., 1993). Further, no patient developed dyskinesia or motor fluctuations. A double-blind study comparing levodopa to placebo showed no benefit in any patient (unpublished observations). MRI studies performed in 2 patients demonstrated signal hyperintensity in the GP, striatum, and SNr on T^1-weighted images consistent with manganese accumulation. Positron emission tomography (PET) scans were also helpful in discriminating these patients. Fluorodopa PET provides an index of the integrity of dopaminergic nigrostriatal neurons (Pate et al., 1992). Fluorodopa PET is abnormal in PD and shows reduced striatal uptake, particularly in the posterior putamen (Calne and Snow, 1993). This finding is in accord with the 60%–80% reduction in dopaminergic cells of the SNc that occurs before the emergence of clinical dysfunction (Bernheimer et al., 1967). In contrast, Taiwanese patients with well-defined basal ganglia dysfunction related to manganese neurotoxicity had normal fluorodopa scans (Wolters et al., 1989) indicative of relative sparing of SNc neurons. In these same patients, PET studies demonstrated decreased F-18 deoxyglucose utilization and decreased raclopride binding in the striatum (Wolters et al., 1989). These observations provide further evidence that manganese neurotoxicity is associated with a clinical syndrome that differs from PD and primarily reflects damage to the GP and striatum.

The mechanism by which manganese induces neurodegeneration is at present unknown. Manganese is a transition metal that theoretically promote the formation of cytotoxic free radicals. Donaldson et al. (1981) have postulated that manganese destroys catecholamines by enhancing their autooxidation. Moreover, the addition of SOD or catalase prevents the death of cultured fibroblasts induced by manganese, and vitamin E administration decreases the loss of striatal dopamine induced by infusion of $MnCl^2$ into the SNc (Parenti et al., 1988). However, manganese does not participate in the Fenton reaction and thus does not directly contribute to the formation of the hydroxyl radical, which is thought to be the prime mediator of tissue damage consequent to oxidant stress. More recent studies suggest that manganese may induce mitochondrial toxicity and a consequent bioenergetic defect with decreased ATP synthesis (Brouillet et al., in press). This could result in the loss of the voltage-dependent magnesium blockade of excitatory amino acid receptors and reduce the capacity of the cell to sequester and extrude calcium. Support for this notion is provided by experiments demonstrating that manganese neurotoxicity can be diminished by pretreatment with an NMDA receptor antagonist or prior decortication (Brouillet et al., 1986). It is noteworthy that other mitochondrial toxins such as cyanide and carbon monoxide cause a pattern of neuronal damage resembling that seen with manganese intoxication. This suggests the possibility that under normal circumstances there may be a relatively high rate of oxidative phosphorylation in the GP and striatum which makes these regions more susceptible to mitochondrial toxins. On the other hand, direct injection of

MnCl^2 into the rat striatum (Lista et al., 1986) or SNc (Daniels and Abarca, 1991) induces a significant but reversible decrease in dopamine concentration. This may reflect the capacity of manganese to cause nonspecific neuronal damage at sites of local accumulation and suggests that the clinical syndrome observed in man following manganese intoxication reflects the propensity of manganese to accumulate in specific regions rather than a particular vulnerability of affected neurons. In this regard it is noteworthy that manganese is thought to gain access to the central nervous system via transferrin receptors and concentrates in areas that are normally rich in iron such as the GP but not the SNc. It is interesting to speculate on the possibility that iron and aluminum contribute to the degeneration associated with manganese toxicity because of their known propensity to promote free radical damage (Gutteridge et al., 1985). The perivascular pattern of accumulation of these metals raises the possibility of a breakdown in the blood–brain barrier.

In summary, current evidence indicates that manganese intoxication can be differentiated from PD because of its predilection to affect the GP and striatum rather than the SNc. The clinical syndrome, response to levodopa, and imaging studies with MRI and PET help to distinguish these two conditions and permit the correct diagnosis to be established. This is of particular relevance in differentiating patients with parkinsonism caused by manganese toxicity from patients with idiopathic PD who have an incidental history of manganese exposure.

References

Abd El, Naby S, Hassanein M (1965): Neuropsychiatric manifestations of chronic manganese poisoning. *J Neurol Neurosurg Psychiatry* 28:128–136

Ashizawa R (1927): Über einen Sektionsfall von chronischer maganvergiftung. *Jpn J Med Sci Trans Intern Med Pediatr Psychiatr* 1:173–191

Barbeau A (1984): Manganese and extrapyramidal disorders. *Neurotoxicology* 5:13–36

Bernheimer H, Birkmayer WA, Hornykiewicz O, Jellinger K, Seitelberger F (1967): Brain dopamine and the syndromes of Parkinson and Huntington. Clinical, morphological, and neurochemical correlations. *J Neurol Sci* 20:415–455

Bonilla E, Salazar E, Villasmil JJ, Villalobos R (1982): The regional distribution of manganese in the normal human brain. *Neurochem Res* 7:221–227

Brouillet BP, Shinobu L, McGarvey U, Hochberg F, Beal MF: Manganese injection into the striatum produces excitotoxic lesions by impairing energy metabolism. *Exp Neurol* (in press)

Calne DB, Snow BJ (1993): PET imaging in parkinsonism. In: *Parkinson's Disease: from Basic Research to Treatment*. Narabayashi H, Nagatsu T, Yanagisawa N, Mizuno Y, eds. *Adv Neurol* 60:484–487

Canavan MM, Cobb S, Drinker CK (1934): Chronic manganese poisoning. *Psychiatry* 32:501–502

Casamajor L (1913): An unusual form of mineral poisoning affecting the nervous system: manganese? *JAMA* 60:646–649

Cook DG, Fahn S, Brait KA (1974): Chronic manganese intoxication. *Arch Neurol* 30:59–64

Cotzias C (1969): Metabolic modification of some neurologic disorders. *JAMA* 210:1255–1262

Cotzias GC, Horiuchi K, Fuenzalida S, Mena I (1968): Chronic manganese poisoning: clearance of tissue manganese concentrations with persistence of the neurological picture. *Neurology* 18:647–651

Couper J (1837): On the effects of black oxide of manganese which inhaled into the lungs. *Br Ann Med Pharm* 1:41–42

Daniels AJ, Abarca J (1991): Effect of intranigral Mn^{2+} on striatal and nigral synthesis and levels of dopamine and cofactor. *Neurotoxicol Teratol* 13:483–487

Dastur DK, Manghani DK, Raghavendran KV, Jeejeebhoy KN (1968): Distribution and fate of the monkey: studies of different parts of the central nervous system and other organs. *J Clin Invest* 50:9–20

Donaldson J, Labella FS, Gesser D (1981): Enhanced autooxidation of dopamine as a possible basis of manganese neurotoxicity. *Neurotoxicology* 2:53–64

Drayer BP, Olanow W, Burger P, Johnson GA, Herfkens R, Riederer S (1986): Parkinson plus syndrome: diagnosis using high field MR imaging of brain iron. *Radiology* 159:493–498

Duvoisin R (1989): Is there a Parkinson's disease? In: *Disorders of Movement*, Quinn NP, Jenner P, eds. Academic Press, London

Edsall DL, Wilbur FP, Drinker CK (1919): The occurrence, course and prevention of chronic manganese poisoning. *J Ind Hyg* 1:183–193

Ejima A, Imamura T, Nakamura S, Saito H, Matsumoto K, Momono S (1992): Manganese intoxication during total parenteral nutrition. *Lancet* 339:426

Emara AM, el-Ghawabi SH, Madkour OI, el-Samra GH (1971): Chronic manganese poisoning in the dry battery industry. *Br J Ind Med* 28: 78–82

Embden H (1901): Zur Kenntnis der metallischen nervengifte. *Dtsch Med Wochenschr* 27:795–796

Ferraz HB, Bertolucci PHG, Pereira JS, Lima JGC, Andrade LAF (1988): Chronic exposure to the fungicide maneb may produce symptoms and signs of CNS manganese intoxication. *Neurology* 38:550–553

Flinn RH, Neal PA, Fulton WB (1941): Industrial manganese poisoning. *J Ind Hyg Toxicol* 23:374–387

Gibb WRG, Lees AJ (1991): Anatomy, pigmentation, ventral and dorsal subpopulations of the substantia nigra, and differential cell death in Parkinson's disease. *J Neurol Neurosurg Psychiatry* 54:388–396

Good PF, Olanow CW, Perl PP (1992): Neuromelanin-containing neurons of the substantia nigra accumulate iron and aluminium in Parkinson's disease: a LAMMA study. *Brain Res* 593:343–346

Greenhouse AH (1971): Manganese intoxication in the United States. *Trans Am Neurol Assoc* 96:248–249

Gutteridge JMC, Quinlan GJ, Clark I, Halliwell B (1985): Aluminum salts accelerate peroxidation of membrane lipids stimulated by iron salts. *Biochem Biophys Acta* 835:441–447

Hassler R (1938): Zur Pathologie der Paralyse agitans und des postenzephalitischen Parkinsonism. *J Psychol Neurol* Leipzig 48:387–476

Holzgraefe R, Poser W, Kijewski H, Beeuche W (1986): Chronic poisoning caused by potassium permanganate: a case report. *Clin Toxicol* 7:235–244

Huang C-C, Chu N-S, Lu C-S, Wang JD, Tsai JL, Tzeng JL, Wolters EC, Calne DB (1989): Chronic manganese intoxication. *Arch Neurol* 46:1104–1106

Huang C-C, Lu C-S, Chu N-S, Hochberg F, Lienfeld D, Olanow CW, Calne DB (1993): Progression after chronic manganese exposure. *Neurology* 43:1479–1483

Hughes AJ, Daniel SE, Kilford L, Lees AJ (1992): Accuracy of clinical diagnosis of idiopathic Parkinson's disease-pathologic study of 100 cases. *J Neurol Neurosurg Psychiatry* 55:181–184

Larsen NA, Pakkenberg H, Damsgaard E, Heydorn K (1979): Topographical distribution of arsenic, manganese, and selenium in the normal human brain. *J Neurol Sci* 42:407–416

Larsen NA, Pakkenberg H, Damsgaard E, Heydorn K, Wold S (1981): Distribution of arsenic, manganese and selenium in the human brain in chronic renal insufficiency, Parkinson's disease, and amyotrophic lateral sclerosis. *J Neurol Sci* 51:437–446

Lista A, Abarca J, Ramos C, Daniels AJ (1986): Rat striatal dopamine and tetrahydrobiopterin content following an intrastriatal injection of manganese chloride. *Life Sci* 38:2121–2127

McGeer PL, Itagaki S, Akiyama H, McGeer EG (1989): Comparison of neuronal loss in Parkinson's disease and aging. *Adv Aging* 36:25–34

Mella H (1924): The experimental production of basal ganglion symptomatology in *Macacus rhesus. Arch Neurol Psychiatry* 11:405–417

Mena I, Marin O, Fuenzalida S, Cotzias GC (1967): Chronic manganese poisoning. Clinical picture and manganese turnover. *Neurology* 17:128–136

Mena I, Court J, Fuenzalida S, Papavasiliou PS, Cotzias GC (1970): Modification of chronic manganese poisoning. Treatment with L-dopa on 5-OH tryptophane. *N Engl J Med* 282:5–10

Nelson K, Golnick J, Kom T, Angle C: Manganese encephalopathy: utility of early magnetic resonance imaging. *Br J Ind Med* (in press)

Newland MC, Ceckler TL, Kordower JH, Weiss B (1989): Visualizing manganese in the primate basal ganglia with magnetic resonance imagining. *Exp Neurol* 106:251–258

Olanow CW (1992): Magnetic resonance imaging in parkinsonism. *Neurol Clin North Am* 10:405–420

Olanow CW, Alberts M, Djang W, Stajich J (1990): MR imaging of putaminal iron predicts response to dopaminergic therapy in parkinsonian patients. In: *Early Markers in Parkinson's and Alzheimer's Diseases*, Dostert P, Riederere P, Strolin B, et al., eds., pp. 99–109. Vienna: Springer-Verlag

Olanow CW, Calne DB, Perl D, Pate B (1993): Does manganese neurotoxicity act by way of iron-induced oxidant stress? *Move Disord* 8:410

Pakkenberg B, Møller A, Gundersen HJG, Dam AM, Pakkenberg H (1991): The absolute number of nerve cells in substantia nigra in normal subjects and in patients with Parkinson's disease estimated with an unbiased stereological method. *J Neurol Neurosurg Psychiatry* 54:30–33

Parenti M, Rusconi L, Cappabianca V, Parati EA, Groppetti A (1988): Role of dopamine in manganese neurotoxicity. *Brain Res* 473:236–240

Pate DB, McGeer EG, Kawamata, T, Yamada T, Snow BJ, Ruth TJ, Calne DB (1992): Neuron density in the SNC, and striatal dopamine, metabolite and synthetic enzyme levels in the unilateral MPTP-monkey SNC, model of parkinsonism. In: 2nd International Congress of Movement Disorders, Munich, Germany. *Move Disord* 7:154

Pentschew A, Ebner FF, Kovatch RM (1963): Experimental manganese encephalopathy in monkeys. A preliminary report. *J Neuropathol Exp Neurol* 22:488–499

Rinne UK, Laihinen A, Rinne JO, Någren K, Bergman J, Ruotsalainen U (1990): Positron emission tomography demonstrates dopamine D2 receptor supersensitivity in the striatum of patients with early Parkinson's disease. *Move Disord* 5:55–59

Rajput AH, Uitti RJ, Sudhakar S, Rozdilsky B (1989): Parkinsonism and neurofibrillary tangle pathology in pigmented nuclei. *Ann Neurol* 25:602–606

Rodier J (1955): Manganese poisoning in Moroccan miners. *Br J Ind Med* 12:21–35

Rosenstock HA, Simons DG, Meyer JS (1971): Chronic manganism. Neurologic and laboratory studies during treatment with levodopa. *JAMA* 217:1354–1358

Saric M, Markicervic A, Hrustic O (1979): Occupational exposure to manganese. *Br J Ind Med* 34:114–118

Schuler P, Oyanguren H, Maturana V, Valenzuela A, Cruz E (1957): Manganese poisoning. Environmental and medical study at Chilean mine. *Int Med Surg* 26:167–173

Smyth LT, Ruhf RC, Whitman NE, Dugan T (1973): Clinical manganism and exposure to manganese in the production and processing of ferromanganese alloy. *J Occup Med* 15:101–109

Suzuki Y, Mouri Y, Suzuki Y, Nishiyama K, Fujii N, Yano H (1975): Study of subacute toxicity of manganese dioxide in monkeys. *Tokwshima J Exp Med* 22:5–10

Tanaka S, Lieben J (1969): Manganese poisoning and exposure in Pennsylvania. *Arch Environ Health* 19:674–684

von Jaksch R (1907): Über Mangantoxikosen und Manganophobie. *Menchen Med Wochenschr* 54:969–972

Woltes ECH, Huang CC, Clark C, Peppard RF, Okada J, Chu NS, Adam MJ, Ruth TJ, Li D, Calne DE (1989): Positron emission tomography in manganese intoxication. *Ann Neurol* 26:647–651

Yamada M, Ohno S, Okayasu I, Okeda R, Hatakeyama S, Watanabe H, Ushio K, Tsukagoshi H (1986): Chronic manganese poisoning: a neuropathological study with determination of manganese distribution in the brain. *Acta Neuropathol* (Berl) 70:273–278

7

Iron and Parkinson's Disease

MOUSSA B.H. YOUDIM, DORIT BEN-SHACHAR, AND PETER RIEDERER

It is difficult to accept the idea that iron, the most prevalent and most utilized transition metal in the body, could be a hazardous factor for brain function related to neurodegenerative diseases, such as Parkinson's disease, Alzheimer's disease, trauma, and brain ischaemia. Nevertheless, abnormalities of iron metabolism (iron deficiency and iron overload) represent the largest metabolic disorders in medicine (see Lauffer, 1992, for review). Indeed, iron plays a crucial role in some of the most important biochemical processes in the body as well as in some of the most deadly and widespread diseases in the world (Lauffer, 1992; Youdim, 1994). Its role in Parkinson's disease has not escaped scrutiny since the first observation by Leheremitte et al. (1924), demonstrating a substantial increase of the iron content in Parkinsonian substantia nigra (SN). This has been confirmed repeatedly, for example, in a series of very recent studies which a variety of techniques including magnetic resonance imaging (MRI) for determination of iron have been used (see Youdim et al., 1993a).

Iron and Transferrin

Little is known or has been studied as regards the mechanism of iron transport and delivery into the central nervous system (CNS), despite the clearly established importance of iron for normal CNS function (Pollit and Metallinos-Katsaras, 1990; Yehuda and Youdim, 1989; Youdim, 1988; Youdim et al., 1989a). Thus, it has been established in rats that the brain, unlike the liver, has a high capacity to maintain its iron stores stable during iron deficiency (ID) (Ben-Shachar et al., 1986). Although the liver iron stores in animals (rats) can be nearly depleted by 1 or 2 weeks of nutritional iron deficiency, the decrease in brain iron can be low, as little as 30% to 35%. Further, while iron repletion of iron-deficient rats can restore the liver iron levels within a few days and even elevate them by a factor of 10 to 20, normalization of brain iron stores takes weeks and its levels cannot be increased beyond the original value (Ben-Shachar et al., 1986; Dwork et al., 1990). Thus the brain maintains its iron homeostasis with very narrow limits. Indeed, it is now apparent that almost all the iron present in adult brain is deposited before the blood–brain barrier is formed, and that brain regulates its iron content conservatively because iron turnover in this tissue is extremely slow as compared to the liver (Banks et al., 1988).

In the young animal (10-day-old rats), iron is rather evenly distributed in the different regions of the brain. However, in the absence of the blood–brain barrier the major uptake of $^{59}Fe^{3+}$ takes place in the cortical regions. This region and the cerebellum have the highest concentration of transferrin (TF), the iron transporter located in oligodendrocytes (Connor, 1992; Connor and Fine, 1986, 1987; Connor et al., 1987, 1990; Mash et al., 1990), but normally these regions have a low iron content in young rats.

In contrast, adult brain (man, monkey, and rat) shows a unique regional pattern of iron distribution that contrasts dramatically with that seen in the young. The pattern consists of extremely high and very localized iron content in the substantia nigra, globus pallidus, red nucleus, interpeduncular nuclei, and dentate gyrus, and of low levels of iron in the TF-rich regions (cerebral cortex, cerebellum, and hippocampus). Indeed, Dwork et al. (1988) have demonstrated a contrasting iron and TF distribution in adult human brains. How this high iron content, comparable to the liver iron level, is accumulated in the extrapyramidal and other regions in the absence of significant amounts of TF is not known. However, the elegant studies of Dwork et al. (1990) have clearly shown that at least in young rat brain iron can be transported from TF-rich cerebral cortex, hippocampus, and cerebellum to the regions which are rich in iron, that is, substantia nigra, globus pallidus, and interpeduncular nuclei, probably by some axonal transport system, until they reach levels observed in the adult. Although in adult brain TF is still present in significant amounts on the capillary endothelial cells (Jefferies et al., 1984), in the different regions iron is barely transported across the blood–brain barrier (Ben-Shachar et al., 1986).

The significance of this phenomenon is not known, but it could be related to some intrinsic cytotoxic property of iron that has caused the brain to protect itself from the action of iron once the normal content of iron has been deposited in those brain regions extremely rich in iron. Mash et al. (1993) have reported an increase of TF in the putamen of patients with Parkinson's disease (PD) as compared to matched controls.

They have suggested that the iron pool is regulated by a receptor-mediated ferrotransferrin uptake and that up-regulation of TF levels may play a role in the pathogenesis of nigral cell damage in PD. Is this the reason why turnover of iron in normal state is so slow and why the brain conserves and reuses its iron and can transport it from one site to another? These are important questions that need to be studied if we are to understand the function of iron in the iron-rich brain regions beyond its well-known roles in the synthesis of DNA, in RNA polymerase, as a cofactor of nonheme and heme proteins, and in a number of other metabolic processes (Youdim, 1988).

Iron in Parkinsonian Brains

Almost all studies so far done on the distribution and brain content of various metals (Fe, Zn, Mn, Mg, and Cu^{2+}) in Parkinsonian brain, as compared to matched controls, agree that iron is selectively increased in Sn and in no other region, and that this increase is associated with a concomitant decrease of Cu^{2+} in this region (Dexter et al., 1989a, 1989b; Riederer et al., 1989) see also Youdim et al., 1993a). Although under normal conditions in control brains there is a significantly higher content of iron in zona reticulata (ZR) than in zona compacta (ZC) of the SN, it is the SNZC that shows the increase of iron content in PD (Jellinger et al., 1990; Sofic et al., 1988, 1992). The rather selective elevation of iron in SNZC would confer a certain specificity to the role of iron in PD because it is the subgroup of melanized dopamine-containing neurons of SNZC that degenerate in PD. Is there a relationship, and is iron a primary cause or a secondary feature of neurodegeneration in PD?

The studies of Jellinger and co-workers (1990) were the first to recognize and demonstrate the cellular localization of increased iron as well as ferritin levels in parkinsonian SN. The histochemical Perl-DAB technique has clearly shown iron to be increased in microglia, macrophages, astrocytes, and oligodendrocytes (which contain TF), as well as outside the degenerated dopamine neurons but not in nonmelanized dopamine neurons. Almost no iron, except as a fine halo, could be shown in Lewy bodies. The absence of Perl stain for iron in highly melanized dopamine neurons of SNZC (Jellinger et al., 1990) has now been attributed to the loss of Perl stain via chelation or binding of iron by neuromelanin (Jellinger et al., 1992). Indeed, in a series of experiments with synthetic dopamine melanin, which can bind with high affinity a significant amount of iron (Ben-Shachar et al., 1991a), Perl stain is lost as a consequence of the complexing of iron. However, x-ray microanalysis of melanized dopamine neurons of SNZC has demonstrated a significant presence of iron bound to neuromelanin in PD that is absent in matched controls (Jellinger et al., 1992). The x-ray microanalysis of the SNZC neuromelanin itself results in a pattern almost identical to synthetic dopamine melanin to which Fe^{3+} is bound (Ben-Shachar et al., 1991a). Iron is not found in the cytoplasm of the neuron, suggesting that it is the neuromelanin-bound iron that could have a functional toxicity.

The studies of Hirsch et al. (1991), Perl et al. (1992) and Good et al. (1992), who employed x-ray microanalysis and the laser microprobe (LAMMA) technique, respectively, have also given support to the concept of a presence of elevated iron levels within the melanized dopamine neurons of SNZC. The fact that iron is shown to be bound to neuromelanin in dopamine neurons of SNZC in PD gives this phenomenon a certain selectivity with regard to the biochemical observation of a degenerating subgroup of dopamine neurons (Jellinger et al., 1992; Youdim et al., 1989b). Whether the accumulation of iron is responsible for the onset of neurodestruction or is the consequence of the disease process cannot be ascertained so far (Youdim et al., 1993b). Nevertheless, interaction of iron with synthetic dopamine melanin results in the potentiation of iron-induced lipid peroxidation of membranes of the cortical synaptosomes of the rat (Ben-Shachar et al., 1991a; Youdim et al., 1993b). This can be inhibited by iron chelators, for example, desferrioxamine (Ben Shachar et al., 1991a).

These sets of findings have been confirmed and extended in the studies of Mochizuki et al. (in press). These authors have demonstrated that the iron–melanin complex has a significantly greater toxicity to dopaminergic neurons of mesencephalon and neostriatum of rats in culture than iron alone. The loss of neurons was correlated with membrane lipid peroxidation as measured by malondialdehyde formation, and this effect could be prevented by the iron chelator desferrioxamine. Thus, melanin can change its normal cytoprotective function and become cytotoxic in the presence of iron (Ben-Shachar et al., 1991a; Youdim et al., 1993b). Further, as is discussed later, in animal models relatively selective dopaminergic neurodegeneration can result in biochemical and behavioral parkinsonism when either SN iron is increased or iron is released from its bound form.

Iron in Cell Toxicity and Death

There have been many studies regarding the toxic effects of ionic iron within the cell and the ability of this transition metal to produce a metabolic disorder that leads to a breakdown of mitochondrial function and eventually cell death, as a consequence of oxygen free radical generation and tissue oxidative stress (see Lauffer, 1992). Diseases in which iron is though to play a direct or indirect role include diabetes, paraquat toxicity to the lung, rheumatoid arthritis, brain and heart ischaemia, trauma, stroke, and radiation-induced skin lesions (Lauffer, 1992).

After the discovery of superoxide dismutase, much investigation was carried out on mechanisms of superoxide (O_2^-) generation within cells and on the nature of the damage that can be induced by this free radical. It is known that O_2^- can accelerate metal ion-dependent formation of the highly reactive hydroxyl radical (OH·) from H_2O_2 according to the Haber–Weiss reaction (Fenton chemistry):

$$O_2^- + Fe^{3+}\text{-chelate} \rightarrow O_2 + Fe^{2+}\text{-chelate}$$

$$Fe^{2+}\text{-chelate} + H_2O_2 \rightarrow Fe^{3+}\text{-chelate} + \cdot OH + OH^-$$

Net reaction:

$$O_2^- + H_2O_2 \xrightarrow[\text{catalyst}]{Fe^{+2}} \cdot OH + OH^- + O_2 + Fe^{3+}$$

The role of OH· and O_2^- has been discussed in numerous diseases. It also has not escaped being implicated in PD. This is quite understandable because the basal ganglia (namely SN) are one of the most metabolically active regions of the brain and contain the highest concentration of iron in the brain. The SN produces a considerable amount of H_2O_2 as a consequence of dopamine metabolism via oxidative deamination by monoamine oxidase and via autoxidation (Youdim et al., 1989). Because of the possible presence of ionic iron in brains of patients with PD, its interaction with H_2O_2 as a consequence of dopamine metabolism has aroused much interest and many studies (Fahn and Cohen, 1992; Olanow, 1990; Youdim et al., 1989). Spina and Cohen (1989) have suggested that the damage to dopamine neurons may result from direct or indirect action of H_2O_2 through the formation of hydroxyl radicals. Transition metals, notably Fe and Cu, can convert a number of less reactive radicals and compounds to more reactive forms including the catecholamines, especially dopamine (Table 1). The formation and deposition of melanin within the dopamine neurons of SNZC is thought to be the consequence of catecholamine autoxidation with formation of semiquinones plus the occurrence of free radical species (O_2^-, H_2O_2, and OH·).

In normal aging, an intact system disposes of radicals and the SN may not be damaged as much as in PD cases. It is well accepted that

Table 1. Conversion of Less Reactive Molecules to More Reactive Molecules by Transition Metal Ions

Superoxide (O_2^-) Hydrogen peroxide	$\xrightarrow{\text{Fe/Cu}}$	Hydroxyl radical (OH·)
Lipid peroxides (ROOH)	$\xrightarrow{\text{Fe/Cu}}$	Aloxy (RO^-) radical Peroxy (RO_2) radical Cytotoxic aldehydes
Catecholamines (autoxidized)[a]	$\xrightarrow[\text{plus } O_2]{\text{Fe/Cu/Mn}}$	O_2^-, H_2O_2, OH· Semiquinones

[a]The autoxidation of catecholamines is potentiated by traces of transition metals, including iron, and proceeds by free radical chain reaction mechanism.

during the course of aging a loss of 8%–13% of the SN sopamine neurons occurs with every decade. This is not sufficient to induce PD, as some 75% of dopaminergic (DA) neurons of the SN need to be lost with aging or for other reasons to produce symptoms of this disease. However, it is more than possible that in the presence of excess iron, as may occur in PD, autoxidation of dopamine is highly activated and the radical scavenging system fails to compensate for the excessive amount of radicals. Such a hypothesis could infer that PD may be an accelerated form of aging induced by iron! Evidence supporting the inability of SN to scavenge free radicals generated by excess H_2O_2 formation has come from reports on a decreased activity of glutathione peroxidase (the most important H_2O_2 scavenger in the CNS) and the loss of its rate-limiting substrate, reduced glutathione (GSH), without a change in oxidized glutathione (GSSG) in this tissue. Indeed it is apparent from the staging of PD that there is a significant increase of iron as well as loss of GSH and that these results correlate with the disappearance of dopamine (degeneration of dopamine neurons in the SN) (Jenner et al., 1992a; Riederer et al., 1989; Youdim et al., 1993a).

At present it is difficult to attribute the loss of GSH in parkinsonian SN to iron "toxicity." There is no clear-cut evidence that reduction of tissue GSH can lead to oxidative stress, because GSH depletion must exceed 90% before lipid peroxidation is initiated. The fall in GSH may result from iron-induced decreased synthesis and increased turnover, rather than from oxidative reactions as suggested by Jenner et al. (1992a). In addition to O_2^-, H_2O_2 and nitric oxide (NO) (Biemond et al., 1988; Mazur et al., 1958; Reif et al., 1988; Reif and Simmons, 1990; Thomas et al., 1985; Youdim and Riederer, 1993) a number of cytotoxins, for example, paraquat, alloxan, and 6-hydroxydopamine, which are known to decompartmentalize ferritin-bound iron, are capable of reducing tissue GSH content. Free radical scavengers can protect tissues against this effect (Gutteridge and Hou, 1986; Montinero and Winterbourne, 1989; Reif et al., 1989; Thomas and Aust, 1986a, 1986b). Thus, iron may participate in the depletion of GSH (Reif et al., 1989). Glutathione peroxidase is found in the cytosolic and mitochondrial fractions of cells and catalyzes the following reaction:

$$2GSH + H_2O_2 \rightarrow GSSG + H_2O$$

The glutathione peroxidase functions with another GSH reductase to generate GSH and remove GSSG, which can be toxic because of the formation of mixed disulfides, or because it dehydrates NADPH:

$$GSSG + 2NADPH \rightarrow 2GSH + 2NADP$$

It has been shown that the concentration of GSSG within the parkinsonian SN is unchanged (Sofic et al., 1992), suggesting an altered GSH reductase activity. Glutathione peroxidase contains selenocysteine at the active site and can also remove lipid and organic hyperoxides in addition to H_2O_2. Conditions of oxidative stress result in depletion of NADPH and GSH. Thus glutathione peroxidase system is important for removal of H_2O_2 produced in the mitochondria, microsomes, and cytosol.

H_2O_2 poses a biological threat not only as a direct oxidant but also because of its potential for releasing free iron through destruction of heme-containing compounds (e.g., hemoglobin) and iron storage proteins (e.g., ferritin). The free ferrous iron would then be available for formation of the hydroxyl radical (OH·) via the Fenton reaction or for production of reactive hypochlorous acid via the myeloperoxidase system. These iron-containing proteins may provide another source of iron, especially when they escape from their usual milieu and from the ultracellular protection afforded by the detoxifying enzymes superoxide dismutase and glutathione peroxidase. The major source of the hydrogen peroxide in SN is probably from spontaneous or enzyme-mediated dismutation of superoxide formed by dopamine oxidation. Thus, in the brain glutathione peroxidase provides the enzymatic protection against hydrogen peroxide. Its inactivation can be the consequence of an iron-induced oxidant stress leading to the consumption of its rate-limiting substrate, reduced glutathione (GSH) (Hallaway and Hedlund, 1992; Liccone and Maines, 1988).

While it is generally accepted that the interaction of iron, hydrogen peroxide, and superoxide generates a potent oxidant stress in tissues, not everyone agrees that the reactive molecule is necessarily hydroxyl radical (OH·) (Halliwell, 1992). Nevertheless, from the physiological and clinical perspective with respect to PD, the important point to appreciate is that iron may seriously exacerbate any oxidative stress in the SN of PD. It is worth noting that higher organisms are especially conservative in the handling of iron. There is little "free" or loosely chelated iron in normal conditions of health. Nowhere in the body is this so well demonstrated as in the brain where the homeostasis of iron is so highly regulated (Youdim, 1993). Iron is transported in the ferric state, bound to transferrin in a complex that is especially difficult to reduce. Likewise, it is stored in the ferric state by ferritin (1 mol of ferritin/4500 atoms of iron), a protein also found in various regions of the brain, including the SN (Hill, 1988).

Source of Increased Iron in PD

In normal cellular homeostasis, uptake of iron via transferrin–transferrin receptors, internalization, and endocytosis occur as described by Crichton and Ward (1992). Under normal conditions, ferritin is the only major iron storage protein so far identified in the brains of controls and Parkinson's disease patients (Connor, 1992; Dexter et al., 1990; Fleming and Joshi, 1987; Hill, 1988; Jellinger et al., 1990; Riederer et al., 1988). There is no evidence for the presence of haemosiderin, the other major iron storage protein, as a consequence of iron overload in the brain (Iancu, Ben-Shachar, and Youdim, unpublished observation). Because iron does not easily cross the blood–brain barrier in the adult brain, during certain pathological conditions (e.g., PD) there may be an up-regulation of transferrin receptors by the diseased cell that could enhance intake of iron taken up by the cells of SN (Mash et al., 1990; see also Connor, 1992). However, initially such excess iron would be successfully sequestered into the iron storage protein ferritin, which in parkinsonian SN was reported to be down-regulated in one study (Dexter et al., 1990) and up-regulated in another (Jellinger et al., 1990; Riederer et al., 1988). This pool may become saturated with a subsequent increase in free iron, the iron pool.

The reported down-regulation of ferritin in parkinsonian SN (Dexter et al., 1990) is difficult to reconcile with already established knowledge for up-regulation of ferritin as a prerequisite for elevated tissue stores of iron. In pioneering studies, Drysdale and Munro (1966) showed that the regulation of ferritin synthesis is operated by iron at the level of translation of the ferritin mRNA and that in the absence of iron within the cell much of this mRNA pool was inactive as regards ferritin protein synthesis (Haile et al., 1989; see Crichton and Ward, 1992, for review). However, it is also possible that under certain other conditions iron may be released from its major store protein, ferritin. Thus, after cellular injury an inflammatory process caused by cytokines may result in perturbation of the normal cellular iron homeostasis. In such a condition there is a decompartmentation of various enzymes that can facilitate the release of iron from ferritin, the major iron storage protein in the brain, including xanthine oxidase (formed by the degradation of xanthine dehydrogenase), which mobilizes iron from ferritin as Fe^{2+} and increases the free ionic Fe^{2+} pool. Importantly, the superoxide radical and H_2O_2 and NO (Hibbs et al., 1984) generated by cytokine or in the disease state are also capable of reducing ferritin-bound iron to the ferrous form so that it can be released.

It is this iron pool when liberated by the pathological condition that is able to catalyze Haber–Weiss (Fenton) chemistry and induce additional cellular havoc (Youdim et al., 1993c). However, consideration should also be given to the possibility of an increased uptake of iron from plasma as a consequence of an alteration in the blood–brain barrier in SN of Parkinson's disease. Indeed, our recent pharmacokinetic studies PET of $^{52}FE^{3+}$ citrate have clearly indicated a significant increase of brain to plasma $^{52}Fe^{3+}$ distribution in parkinsonian subjects as compared to matched controls (Leenders et al., in manuscript). An explanation for this finding is clearly required.

Iron-Induced Oxidative Stress: Parkinson's Disease and Animal Parkinsonism

It is now fashionable to implicate oxidative stress in almost every disease for which no clear etiology can be put forward. PD has not escaped such scrutiny, and the possible involvement of oxidative stress (Fahn and Cohen, 1992; Jenner, 1991; Jenner et al., 1992b; Youdim et al., 1989b) and the roles of iron (Youdim et al., 1993a), melanin (Youdim et al., 1993b), and nitric oxide (NO) (Youdim et al., 1993c) in its initiation have been discussed and reviewed (Fahn and Cohen, 1992; Jenner, 1991; Youdim et al., 1993a, 1993b, 1993c). Although a significant case for oxidative stress in PD has been put forward, this hypothesis has by no means been fully established. Nevertheless, the comparison of data from biochemical changes apparent in the parkinsonian SN with those related to iron-induced tissue oxidative stress show remarkable similarities (see Youdim et al., 1993a). The main biochemical features of PD in the SN are as follow:

A. Increases in
   a. hydrogen peroxide liberated by monoamine oxidase B activity
   b. iron and ferritin
   c. superoxide dismutase activity
   d. lipid peroxidation and lipid hydroperoxides, lipofuscin
   e. ubiquitin

B. Decrease of
   a. glutathione peroxidase activity
   b. reduced glutathione (GSH), the substrate of GSH peroxidase) without a change in oxidized glutathione (GSSG)
   c. mitochondrial electron transport system complex I (NADPH reductase coenzyme Q)
   d. calcium-binding protein (28K) (calbindin)

If a state of oxidative state exists within the SN of the brain in PD then it would be expected that this may result from either an exogenous or endogenous insult (or neurotoxin). To date no such neurotoxin has been identified in the environment or within the basal ganglia of PD patients. However, the synthetic dopaminergic neurotoxins 6-hydroxydopamine (6-OHDA) and 1-methyl-4-phenyl, 1,2,3,6-tetrahydropyridine (MPTP) have provided a wealth of biochemical information on a possible mechanism of neurodegeneration related to the cytotoxic actions of these compounds indicated by generation of superoxide anion, hydrogen peroxide, and hydroxyl radical (OH·) (Cohen et al., 1974). The specificity of 6-OHDA depends on its selective accumulation by dopamine neurons and terminals. Radical scavengers, metal chelators (Ben-Shachar et al., 1991; Cohen et al., 1976) and vitamin E (Cadet et al., 1989) protect mice and rats from peripheral and central neurotoxicity of 6-OHDA. The ability of 6-OHDA to release iron and induce oxidative stress-dependent cell death is not unique (Montinero and Winterbourne, 1989). Thus, paraquat toxicity of lung type II cells (Thomas and Aust, 1986b), adriamycin toxicity in cancer treatment (Thomas and Aust, 1986b), the ability of alloxan to induce diabetes in animals (Reif et al., 1989), and macrophage-induced cell death (Hibbs et al., 1984; Reif and Simmons, 1990) have all been attributed to the release of a reactive (free) form of iron.

Recent detailed study on the mechanism of action of 6-OHDA has indicated that 6-OHDA acts via superoxide- or xanthine oxidase-"like" decompartmentalization of ferritin-bound iron, and alters mitochondrial calcium homeostasis (Ben-Shachar et al., 1991b; Montinero and Winterbourne, 1989). *In vitro* 6-OHDA induces a time- and concentration-dependent release of iron from ferritin–lipid peroxidation (Montinero and Winterbourne, 1989) as well as opening of L-calcium channels in the mitochondria (Frei and Richter, 1989). These findings are compatible with oxidative stress-induced neurodegeneration and particularly with an inherent role of free ionic iron. Support for this hypothesis has come from two sources. First, iron chelator (desferrioxamine desferal) pretreatment of rats completely protects against dopamine neurodegeneration caused by ICV 6-OHDA and significantly decreases the *in vivo* formation of hydroxyl radical (OH·) from 6-OHDA as quantified by the determination of the 2,3-dihydroxybenzoate metabolite of salicylate (Halliwell and Grootveld, 1987) in the striatum (Ben-Shachar et al., 1991b; Eshel, 1993). Second, intranigral iron injection in rats causes a relatively selective degeneration of nigrostriatal dopamine neurons, resulting in biochemical and behavioral "parkinsonism" (Ben-Shachar and Youdim, 1991; Sengstock et al., 1992, in press). There is a threshold effect for dopamine depletion caused by intranigral iron injection. In all probability it is a consequence of first binding of iron to ferritin. Only when ferritin molecules are saturated does free iron become available for oxidative stress. Similarly, the prevention of iron- and oxygen-induced nigrostriatal dopamine neurotoxicity by iron chelators (desferrioxamine and lazaroids) points to the involvement of iron in the neurodegenerative action of 6-OHDA.

It is well known that in both *in vitro* and *in vivo* conditions iron causes a rapid stimulation of lipid peroxidation as measured by oxygen consumption and the formation of thiobarbituric acid-reactive products (malondialdehyde). In rat brain synaptosome preparations, these findings are coupled with a parallel and rapid accumulation of Ca^{2+} (Braughler, 1987; Youdim et al., 1991). It appears that the enhanced permeability of synaptosomal membranes to Ca^{2+} that is induced by iron is directly related to lipid peroxidation caused by hydroxyl radical (OH·) generation. The iron chelator desferrioxamine inhibits lipid peroxidation and prevents the formation of lipid peroxide products. Desferrioxamine and lazaroids block iron-dependent uptake of Ca^{2+} into synaptosomes, but in contrast calcium channel-blocking agents, the dihydropyridines nifediipineand nimodipine do not completely block Ca^{2+} uptake.

The failure of Ca^{2+} channel antagonists to completely inhibit the iron-dependent accumulation of Ca^{2+} within synaptosome suggests that the increase in membrane permeability induced by iron to Ca^{2+} may be nonspecific or caused by holes within the membrane (Braughler, 1987). On the other hand, most of the calcium channel antagonists employed for these experiments were those developed for ischemia of the cardiovascular system. These antagonists may not show the same affinity and specificity for calcium channels of the central nervous system.

In essence, these results have demonstrated a close relationship between the cytotoxic action of free ionic iron and calcium homeostasis. As has been pointed out by Orrenius and his colleagues (see Chapter 9, p. 00, this volume), many toxic drugs that induce cellular membrane damage and finally cell death have a very close connection with altered cellular calcium homeostasis. We may, therefore, have to include iron in this list (Youdim et al., 1991).

Conclusion

The pathophysiology of Parkinson's disease is, at our current level of understanding, a slow complex chain of cellular events that may synergistically lead to the demise of nigrostriatal dopamine neurons. Based on the concept of oxidative stress, an intimate interaction between dopamine oxidation, superoxide, hydrogen peroxide, release of iron, lipid peroxidation, and Ca^{2+} in the pathophysiology of neuronal death fits well into such a scheme. An increased concentration of free ionic iron induced by inflammatory cytokines could theoretically act either too slowly to enhance lipid peroxidation reactions or to stimulate membrane phospholipid degradation. Once the fatty acid begins to be released from membranes, cytokines may bring more Ca^{2+} into the cell to promote further lipid peroxidation. The data summarized in this chapter support the notion that iron must be added to the list of agents which alter cellular calcium homeostasis, and that iron calcium and lipid peroxidation may intimately be involved in dopamine neuron cell death. However, this concept does not necessarily imply a primary role for iron.

Release of iron from ferritin nevertheless may be one important step in a sequence of events that bring about this process. Therefore, preventing its toxic action with iron chelators or inhibitors of lipid peroxidation (lazaroids) could provide neuroprotection not only in Parkinson's disease but also in other neurodegenerative diseases in which oxidative stress has been implicated (Connor, 1992). Certainly further mechanisms including protein oxidation and DNA damage, which are known to be intimately related to ionic iron (Aruoma et al., 1989; Schraufstatter et al., 1987; Trenam et al., 1992), need to be closely examined in the SN of Parkinson's disease if a major role for ionic iron is to be established in this disease.

References

Aruoma OI, Halliwell B, Dizdaroglu M (1989): Iron ion-dependent modification of bases in DNA by the superoxide radical generating system hypoxanthine/xanthine oxidase. *J Biol Chem* 264:13024–13030

Banks WA, Kastin AJ, Fasold MB, Barrera CM (1988): Studies of the slow bidirectional transport of iron and transferrin across the blood brain barrier. *Brain Res Bull* 21:881–885

Ben-Shachar D, Youdim MBH (1991): Intranigral iron injection induces behavioural and biochemical "Parkinsonism" in rats. *J Neurochem* 57:2133–2135

Ben-Shachar D, Ashkenazi R, Youdim MBH (1986): Long-term consequence of early iron deficiency of dopaminergic neurotransmission. *Into J Dev Neurosci* 4:81–88

Ben-Shachar D, Riederer P, Youdim MBH (1991a). Iron-melanin interaction and lipid peroxidation. Implications for Parkinson's disease. *J Neurochem* 57:1609–1614

Ben-Shachar D, Eshel G, Finberg JPM, Youdim MBH (1991b): The iron chelator desferrioxamine (desferal) retards 6-hydroxydopamine-induced degeneration of nigra-striatal dopamine neurons. *J Neurochem* 56:1441–1444

Biemond P, Swaak AJG, Van Eijk HG, Koster JF (1988): Superoxide dependent iron release from ferritin in inflammatory diseases. *Free Radical Biol Med* 4:185–193

Braughler M (1987): Calcium and lipid peroxidation. In: *Oxygen Radicals and Tissue Injury*, Halliwell B, ed. Bethesda: FASEB

Cadet JL, Katz M, Jackson-Lewis V, Fahn S (1989): Vitamin E attenuates the toxic effects of intrastriatal injection of 6-hydroxydopamine in rats: behavioral and biochemical evidence. *Brain Res* 476:10–15

Cohen G, Heikkila RE, McNamee D (1974): The generation of hydrogen peroxide radical and hydroxyl radical by 6-hydroxydopamine dialurgic acid and related cytotoxic agents. *J Biol Chem* 249:2447–2459

Cohen G, Heikkila RE, Allis B (1976): Destruction of sympathetic nerve terminals by 6-hydroxydopamine: protection by 1-phenyl-3-(2-thiazolyl)-2-thiourea, diethyl-dithiocarbamate, methionazole, cysteamine, ethanol and n-butanol. *J Pharmacol Exp Ther* 199:336–352

Connor JR (1992): Proteins of iron regulation in Alzheimer's Disease. In: *Iron and Human Diseases*, Lauffer RB, ed. Boca Raton: CRC Press

Connor JR, Fine RE (1986): The distribution of transferrin immunoreactivity in the rat central nervous system. *Brain Res* 368:319–327

Connor JR, Fine RE (1987): Development of transferrin-positive oligodendrocytes in the rat central nervous system. *J Neurosci Res* 17:51–59

Connor JR, Menzies SL, Martin S, Mufson EJ (1990): The cellular distribution of transferrin, ferritin and iron in the human brain. *J Neurosci Res* 27:595–564

Connor JR, Phillips TM, Laksman MR, Baron KD, Fine RE, Csiza CK (1987): Regional variation in the levels of transferrin in the CNS of normal and myelin-deficient rats. *J Neurochem* 49:1523–1530

Crichton RR, Ward RJ (1992): Structure and molecular biology of iron-binding proteins and the regulation of free iron pools. In: *Iron and Human Disease*, Lauffer RB, ed. Boca Raton: CRC Press

Dexter DT, Wells FR, Lees AJ, Javoy-Agid F, Agid Y, Jenner P, Marsden CD (1989a): Increased nigral iron content and alteration in other metal ions occurring in brain in Parkinson's disease. *J Neurochem* 52:1830–1836

Dexter DT, Carter CJ, Wells FR, Javoy-Agid F, Agid Y, Lees AJ, Jenner P, Marsden CD (1989b): Basal Lipid peroxidation in substantia nigra is increased in Parkinson's disease. *J Neurochem* 52:381–387

Dexter DT, Carayon A, Vidaihet M, Ruberg M, Agid F, Agid Y, Lees AJ, Wells, FR, Jenner P, Marsden CD (1990): Decreased ferritin levels in brain in Parkinson's disease. *J Neurochem* 55:16–20

Drysdale JW, Munro HN (1966): Regulation of synthesis and turnover of ferritin in rat liver. *J Biol Chem* 241:3638–3646

Dwork AJ, Schon EA, Herbert J (1988): Non identical distribution of transferrin and ferric iron in human brain. *Neuroscience* 27:333–345

Dwork AJ, Lawler G, Zybert DA (1990): An autoradiographic study of the uptake and distribution of iron by the brain of the young rat. *Brain Res* 518:31–39

Eshel G (1993): *Mechanism of Action of 6-Hydroxydopamine.* M.Sc. Thesis, Technion, Haifa

Fahn S, Cohen G (1992): The oxidant stress hypothesis in Parkinson's disease: evidence supporting it. *Ann Neurol* 32:804–812

Fleming J, Joshi JG (1987): Ferritin: isolation of aluminum-ferritin complex from brain. *Proc Natl Acad Sci USA* 84:7866–7871

Frei B, Richter C (1989): N-Methyl-4-phenyl pyridine (MPP^+) together with 6-hydroxydopamine or dopamine stimulate Ca^{2+} release from mitochondria. *FEBS Lett* 198:99–102

Good PF, Olanow CW, Perl DP (1992): Neuromelanin-containing neurons of the substantia nigra accumulate iron and aluminium in Parkinson's disease. *Brain Res* 593:343–346

Gutteridge JM, Hou Y (1986): Iron complex and their reactivity in the bleomycin assay for radical promoting loosely-bound iron. *Free Radical Res Commun* 2:143–151

Haile DJ, Hentze MW, Roualt TA, Hartford JB, Klausner RD (1989): Regulation of interaction of iron and responsive element binding protein with iron responsive mRNA elements. *Mol Cell Biol* 9:5055–5064

Hallaway PE, Hedlund BOE (1992): Therapeutic strategies to inhibit iron-catalyzed tissue damage. In: *Iron and Human Disease*, Lauffer RB, ed. Boca Raton: CRC Press

Halliwell B (1992): Iron and damage to biomolecules. In: *Iron and Human Disease*, Lauffer RB, ed. Boca Raton: CRC Press

Halliwell B, Grootveld M (1987): The measurement of free radical reactions in humans. Some thoughts for future experimentation. *FEBS Lett* 213:9–14

Hibbs JB Jr, Traintor RR, Vavrin (1984): Iron depletion: possible cause of tumor cell cytotoxicity induced by activated macrophages. *Biochem Biophys Res Commun* 123:716–723

Hill JM (1988): The distribution of iron in the brain. In: *Brain Iron: Neurochemical and Behavioural Aspects*, Youdim MBH, ed., pp. 1–24. London: Taylor and Francis

Hirsch EC, Brandel JD, Galle P, Javoy-Agid F, Agid Y (1991): Iron and aluminum increase in the substantia nigra of patients with Parkinson's disease. *J Neurochem* 56:446–451

Jefferies WA, Brandon MR, Hunt SV, Williams AF, Getter KC, Mason DY (1984): Transferrin receptor on endothelium of brain capillaries. *Nature* 312:162–165

Jellinger K, Paulus W, Grudke-Iqbal I, Riederer P, Youdim MBH (1990): Brain iron and ferritin in Parkinson's and Alzheimer's diseases. *J Neural Transm* (PD Sect) 2:327–340

Jellinger K, Kienzl E, Rumpelmair G, Riederer P, Stachelberger H, Ben-Shachar D, Youdim MBH (1992): Iron-melanin complex in substantia nigra of Parkinsonian brains: an x-ray microanalysis. *J Neurochem* 59:1168–1171

Jenner P (1991): Oxidative stress as a cause of Parkinson's disease. *Acta Neurol Scand* 84:6–15

Jenner P, Sian D, Dexter D, Schapira DHV, Marsden CD (1992a): Decreased reduced glutathione levels are an early pathological marker of Parkinson's disease. *Mov Dis* 7:288–289

Jenner P, Schapira AHV, Marsden DC (1992b): New insight into the cause of Parkinson's disease. *Neurology* 42:2241–2250

Lauffer RB, ed. (1992): *Iron and Human Diseases*. Boca Raton: CRC Press

Leenders N, Ben-Shachar D, Youdim MBH: $^{52}Fe^{3+}$ citrate brain uptake in Parkinsonian patients (in manuscript)

Lehermitte J, Kraus WM, McAlpine MA (1924): On the occurrence of abnormal deposits of iron in the brain in Parkinson's disease with special reference to its location. *J Neurol Psychopathol* 5:195–208

Liccone JJ, Maines MD (1988): Selectively vulnerability of glutathione metabolism and cellular defence mechanism in rat striatum to manganese. *J Pharmacol Exp Ther* 247:156–163

Mash D, Sanchez-Ramos J, Weiner WJ (1993): Transferrin receptor regulation in Parkinson's disease and MPTP-treated mice. In: *Parkinson's Disease: From Basic Research to Treatment*, Naraboyashi H, Nagatsu T, Yanagisawa N, Mizuno Y, eds., *Advances in Neurology*, Vol. 60. New York: Raven Press

Mash DC, Pablo J, Flynn DD, Efange SMN, Weiner WJ (1990): Characterization and distribution of transferrin receptors in the rat brain. *J Neurochem* 55:1972–1978

Mazur A, Green S, Saha A, Carleton N (1958): Mechanism of release of ferritin iron in vivo by xanthine oxidase. *J Clin Invest* 37:1809–1817

Mochizuki H, Nishi K, Mizuno Y: Iron-melanin complex is toxic to dopaminergic neurons in a nigrostriatal co-culture. *Neurodegeneration* (in press)

Montinero HP, Winterbourne CC (1989): 6-Hydroxydopamine releases iron from ferritin and promotes ferritin-dependent lipid peroxidation. *Biochem Pharmacol* 38:4144–4162

Olanow CW (1990): Oxidation reaction in Parkinson's disease. *Neurology* 40 (suppl 3):32–37

Perl DP, Good PF, Olanow CW (1992): Iron (Fe) and aluminum (Al) accumulate in the neuromelanin granules of the substantia nigra pars compacta (SNC) of idiopathic Parkinson's disease (PD). *Brain Res* 593:343–346

Pollit E, Metallinos-Katsaras E (1990): Iron-deficiency and behavior. In: *Nutrition and the Brain*, Vol. 8, Wurtman JJ, eds. New York: Raven Press

Reif DW, Simmons RD (1990): Nitric oxide mediates iron release from ferritin. *Arch Biochem Biophys* 283:537–541

Reif DW, Schubert J, Aust SD (1988): Iron release from ferritin and lipid peroxidation by radiolytically generated reduced radicals. *Arch Biochem Biophys* 104:238–243

Reif DW, Samokyszyn WM, Miller DM, Aust SD (1989): Alloxan and glutathione-dependent ferritin iron release and lipid peroxidation. *Arch Biochem Biophys* 269:407–515

Riederer P, Rausch WD, Schmidt B (1988): Biochemical fundamentals of Parkinson's disease. *Mount Sinai J Med* 55:21–29

Riederer P, Sofic E, Rausch WD, Youdim MBH (1989): Transitional metals, ferritin, glutathione and ascorbic acid in Parkinsonian brains. *J Neurochem* 52:515–520

Schraufstatter I, Hyslop PA, Jackson J, Cochrane CC (1987): Oxidant-induced DNA damage of target cells. *J Clin Invest* 82:1040–1051

Sengstock GW, Olanow CW, Dunn AJ, Arendash GW (1992): Iron induces degeneration of nigrostriatal neurons. *Brain Res Bull* 28: 645–649

Sengstock GJ, Olanow CW, Menzies RA, Dun AJ, Arendash GW (1993): Infusion of iron into the rat substantia nigra: nigral pathology and dose dependent loss of striatal dopaminergic markers. *J Neurosci Res* 34: 242–254

Sofic E, Lange KW, Jellinger K, Riederer P (1992): Reduced and oxidized glutathione in the substantia nigra of patients with Parkinson's disease. *Neurosci Lett* 142: 128–130

Sofic R, Riederer P, Heinsen H, Youdim MBH (1988): Increased iron (III) and total iron content in post-mortem substantia nigra of parkinsonian brain. *J Neural Transm* 74:199–205

Spina S, Cohen G (1989): Dopamine turnover and glutathione oxidation: implications for Parkinson's disease. *Proc Natl Acad Sci USA* 86:1398–1401

Thomas CE, Aust SD (1986a): Reductive release of iron from ferritin by cation free radicals of paraquat and other bipyridyls. *J Biol Chem* 261:13064–13072

Thomas CE, Aust SD (1986b): Free radicals and environmental toxins. *Ann Emerg Med* 215:1075–1081

Thomas CE, Morehouse LA, Aust SD (1985): Ferritin and superoxide-dependent lipid peroxidation. *J Biol Chem* 260:3275–3281

Trenam CW, Winyard PG, Morris CJ, Blake DR (1992): Iron-promoted oxidative damage in rheumatic disease. In: *Iron and Human Diseases*, Lauffer RB, ed. Boca Raton: CRC Press

Yehuda S, Youdim MBH (1989): Brain iron: a lesson from animal models. *Am J Clin Nutr* (suppl) 50:618–629

Youdim MBH, ed. (1988): *Brain Iron: Neurochemical and Behavioural Aspects.* London: Taylor and Francis

Youdim MBH (1994): Inorganic neurotoxins in neurodegenerative diseases excluding dementia. In: *Neurodegenerative Diseases*, Calne D, ed. New York: Saunders

Youdim MBH, Riederer P (1993): Nitric oxide (NO) and dopaminergic cell death in Parkinson's disease (in manuscript)

Youdim MBH, Ben-Shachar D, Pollard HB (1991): Iron chelators and calcium channel antagonists as inhibitors of iron induced neuronal lipid peroxidation. *Br J Pharmacol* 102:376P

Youdim MBH, Ben-Shachar D, Yehuda S (1989a): Putative biological mechanisms of the effect of iron-deficiency on brain biochemistry and behavior. *Am J Clin Nutr* (suppl) 50:607–617

Youdim MBH, Ben-Shachar D, Riederer P (1989b): Is Parkinson's disease a progressive siderosis of substantia nigra resulting from iron and melanin-induced neurodegeneration? *Acta Neurol Scand* 126:47–54

Youdim MBH, Ben-Shachar D, Riederer P (1993a): The possible role of iron in etiopathology of Parkinson's disease. *Mov Dis* 8:1–14

Youdim MBH, Ben-Shachar D, Riederer P (1993b): Iron-melanin interaction and Parkinson's disease. *News Physiol Sci* 8:45–49

Youdim MBH, Ben-Shachar D, Eshel G, Finberg JPM, Riederer P (1993c): The neurotoxicity of iron and nitric oxide: relevance to the etiology of Parkinson's disease. In: *Parkinson's Disease: From Basic Research to Treatment*, Narabyashi H, Nagatsu T, Yanagisawa N, Mizuno Y, eds., *Advances in Neurology*, Vol. 60. New York: Raven Press

8

Biological Synthesis of Nitric Oxide from L-Arginine

JOHN B. HIBBS, JR.

It has been observed that inorganic nitrogen oxides are enzymatically synthesized from L-arginine (Hibbs et al., 1987a, 1987b; Iyengar et al., 1987; Palmer et al., 1988) (Fig. 1). Nitric oxide (NO·) appears to be the biologically active nitrogen oxide released from the various nitric oxide synthase isoforms. In 1988, two laboratories using different methodology demonstrated that NO· is released from cytokine and lipopolysaccharide-treated murine macrophages (Hibbs et al., 1988; Marletta et al., 1988). These experiments unequivocally established NO· as a low molecular weight biosynthetic product of mammalian cells.

The synthesis of NO· by mammalian cells has been adapted by evolutionary forces for several very different physiological functions (Hibbs et al., 1990; Nathan, 1992). One form of NO· synthesis from L-arginine is immunologically regulated. Cytokines induce high-output NO synthesis in macrophages and in other somatic cells. Induction of the high-output inducible NO synthase (iNOS), a process that requires hours, is controlled at the level of transcription by cytokines. In the presence of necessary cofactors, iNOS continuously synthesizes NO· and is a molecular component of cell-mediated immunity. Second, identity between endothelium-derived relaxation factor (EDRF) and NO· was established (Ignarro et al., 1987; Palmer et al., 1987), and subsequently it was demonstrated that endothelial cell-derived NO· was also synthesized from L-arginine (Palmer et al., 1988). The low-output constitutive NO synthase (cNOS) synthesizes NO from L-arginine within seconds, and for short periods of time, in response to chemical and physical signals in the endothelial cell microenvironment. Two genetically distinct cNOS isoforms (endothelial and neural isoforms) have been identified. Low-output NO· synthesis by cNOS is controlled by a calmodulin cofactor (Bredt and Snyder, 1990; Nathan, 1992). Elevation of intercellular Ca^{2+} induced by appropriate agonists activates cNOS to synthesize NO·. Nitric oxide

ADVANCES IN RESEARCH ON NEURODEGENERATION, II
Y. Mizuno et al.
© 1994 Birkhäuser Boston

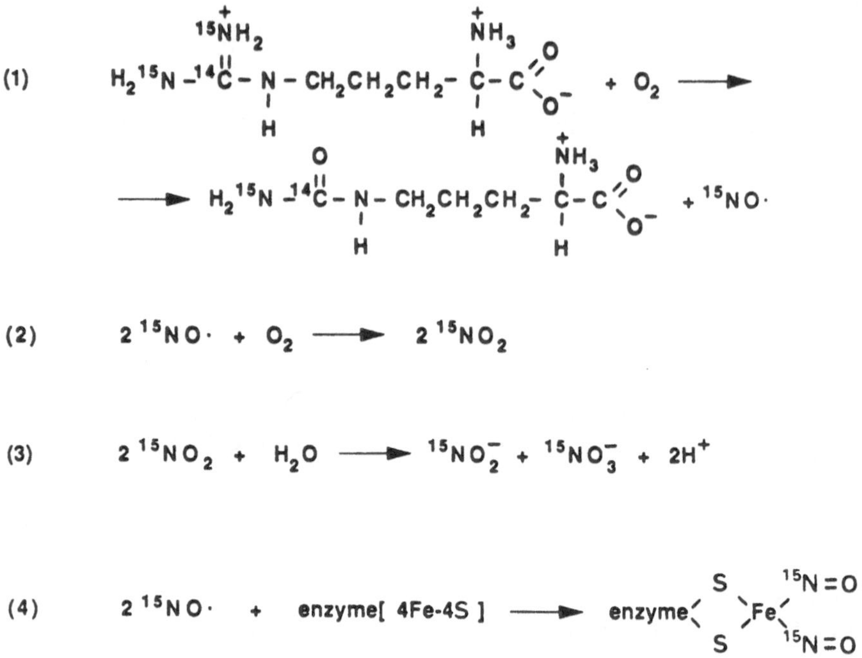

(1)

$$H_2{}^{15}N-{}^{14}\overset{\overset{\displaystyle +}{{}^{15}NH_2}}{\underset{\displaystyle H}{C}}-N-CH_2CH_2CH_2-\underset{\displaystyle H}{\overset{\displaystyle +}{\underset{}{C}}}\overset{\overset{\displaystyle +}{NH_3}}{-}C\overset{\displaystyle O}{\underset{\displaystyle O^-}{\diagup}} + O_2 \longrightarrow$$

$$\longrightarrow H_2{}^{15}N-{}^{14}\overset{\overset{\displaystyle O}{\|}}{C}-\underset{\displaystyle H}{N}-CH_2CH_2CH_2-\underset{\displaystyle H}{\overset{\overset{\displaystyle +}{NH_3}}{C}}-C\overset{\displaystyle O}{\underset{\displaystyle O^-}{\diagup}} + {}^{15}NO\cdot$$

(2) $2\,{}^{15}NO\cdot + O_2 \longrightarrow 2\,{}^{15}NO_2$

(3) $2\,{}^{15}NO_2 + H_2O \longrightarrow {}^{15}NO_2^- + {}^{15}NO_3^- + 2H^+$

(4) $2\,{}^{15}NO\cdot + \text{enzyme[4Fe-4S]} \longrightarrow \text{enzyme}\overset{\displaystyle S}{\underset{\displaystyle S}{\diagup}}Fe\overset{\displaystyle {}^{15}N=O}{\underset{\displaystyle {}^{15}N=O}{\diagup}}$

Figure 1. Precursor and products of the biological synthesis of inorganic nitrogen oxides and L-citrulline from L-arginine. ^{15}N-Containing products derived from L-[guanidino-^{15}N$_2$]-arginine were identified by gas chromatography/mass spectrometry (Hibbs et al., 1988; Iyengar et al., 1987; Marletta et al., 1988; Palmer et al., 1988) or electron paramagnetic resonance spectroscopy (Lancaster and Hibbs, 1990) except for nitrogen dioxide (NO$_2$), which was detected by another method (Hibbs et al., 1988). The direct synthesis of L-citrulline from L-arginine has been identified with several techniques (Amber et al., 1988; Hibbs et al., 1987a, 1988; Iyengar et al., 1987). The experiments utilizing L-[guanidino-^{14}C]-arginine (Amber et al., 1988; Hibbs et al., 1988) are illustrated. NO formed by reaction 1 can undergo oxidative degradation in aqueous solution (reactions 2 and 3 or react with nonheme iron associated with sulfur atoms to form nitrosyl–iron–sulfur complexes (reaction 4)]. Although not shown, certain other forms of intracellular iron, such as heme iron, also complex with NO. NO$_2^-$ that contacts oxyhemoglobin is rapidly oxidized to NO$_3^-$ (Kosaka et al., 1979). Therefore, NO· synthesized from L-arginine by either the cytokine-induced isoform or the constitutive isoforms will be detected in the serum or urine as NO$_3^-$. Abbreviations: nitrite NO$_2^-$; nitrate NO$_3^-$. Modified from Hibbs et al., 1990, with permission of Elsevier Science Publishers.

synthesized by cNOS functions as an intracellular messenger. It is likely that dysregulated activity of both iNOS and cNOS isoforms can cause tissue damage during a number of different pathophysiological situations.

Nitric oxide is a labile, paramagnetic, redox active, and relatively insoluble molecule that has both gas-phase and liquid-phase reactivity. It is membrane permeant, has a half-life measured in seconds, and diffuses isotropically up to several hundred micrometers from its point of synthesis in the tissues. Nitric oxide has the physical and chemical properties needed to create a biological "field effect" coordinating collective cellular function in a volume of tissues, as originally defined by Weiss (Weiss, 1967). Gally et al. (1990) extended the concept of a "field effect" to the function of NO· in the central nervous system. This included NO·-mediated changes of synaptic efficacy (plasticity) (O'dell et al., 1991; Schuman and Madison, 1991) within a volume of neural tissue as well as NO·-mediated signaling that couples blood flow to neural activity. The concept of a NO·-induced field effect is useful in understanding how blood flow and metabolic activity are coordinated spatially in many different tissues in many different physiological situations.

Knowledge of the synthesis of NO· from L-arginine has resulted in a reevaluation of the physiology of virtually every mammalian organ system. We are still in a period when new information implicating NO· in numerous physiological and pathophysiological events is rapidly accumulating. More time and much more work are required before the role of NO· in these many areas of mammalian physiology and pathophysiology is clearly defined. Current evidence suggests that NO· has an important role in both the central nervous system and peripheral nervous system as a messenger molecule (Nathan, 1992; O'dell et al., 1991; Schuman and Madison, 1991; Synder, 1992). However, in this brief review, I focus largely on the role of NO· in vascular functions and as an effector molecule of cell-mediated immunity. It is likely that both vascular cell-derived NO· and cytokine-induced NO· also have important effects on central nervous system function and pathology.

Low-Output Messenger NO· Coordinates Cellular Function Within a Volume of Tissue and Is Synthesized by Constitutive NO Synthase Isoforms

Chemical agonists (acetylchline, bradykinin, ADP, substance P, etc.) and the physical force of shear stress elevate intracellular Ca^{2+} in endothelial cells (Hutcheson and Griffith, 1991; Moncada et al., 1991; Nathan, 1992). In the presence of elevated Ca^{2+}, calmodulin binds to and activates a constitutive nitric oxide synthase. Once activated, the Ca^{2+}/calmodulin-sensitive cNOS synthesizes small quantities of No· from L-arginine. Nitric oxide synthesized by the endothelial cell cNOS diffuses isotropically into both the vessel wall and the vessel lumen (Fig. 2). Nitric oxide diffusing toward the vessel wall penetrates vascular smooth muscle cells and activates cytoplasmic soluble guanylate cyclase, which increases cGMP production. A cascade of biochemical events follow that result in smooth muscle relaxation (Moncada et al., 1991; Nathan, 1992). The molecular target of NO· is a heme prosthetic group of soluble guanylate cyclase

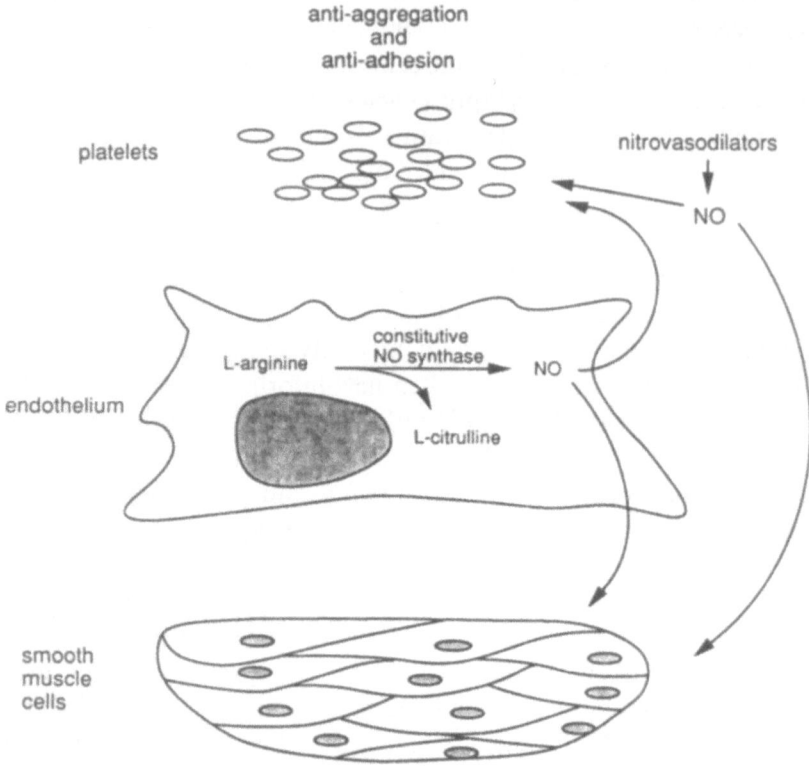

Figure 2. Nitric oxide, endogenously synthesized or pharmacologically derived, regulates vascular flow. (See text for explanation.)

(Ignarro, 1989). The covalent binding of NO· to the heme iron results in a conformational change of the iron-protoporphyrin IX molecule that causes tighter binding to the soluble guanylate cyclase apoenzyme and activation of catalytic activity.

Nitric oxide diffusion directed toward the lumen has an antithrombotic effect by inhibiting platelet aggregation and adhesion to the endothelial surface (Moncada et al., 1991; Nathan, 1992). Therefore, NO· synthesized from L-arginine by the endothelial cell cNOS in response to physiological stimuli acts as a mediator of intercellular communication that functionally links activity of cells in the vessel wall and vessel lumen. The overall effect of NO· synthesis in the vessel is to maintain blood fluidity and adjust flow to meet the metabolic demand of the tissue. It is important to emphasize the central role of NO·-iron interactions in the vessel wall and vessel lumen. Nitric oxide causes vascular smooth muscle relaxation and inhibition of platelet activation by reacting with heme iron of the soluble guanylate cyclase prosthetic group of these key cellular regulators of blood flow (Radomski et al., 1990). In addition, NO· that diffuses into the vessel lumen reacts with erythrocyte oxyhemoglobin to form methemoglobin and nitrate, an inactive degradation product (Doyle and Hoekstra, 1981; Wennmalm et al., 1992). Therefore, in vascular tissue, redox interactions between NO· and iron are important in transduction of the biological message as well as inactivation of the messenger molecule.

Immunologically Regulated High-Output NO· Is an Effector Molecule of Cell-Mediated Immunity and Is Synthesized by the Cytokine-Inducible NO Synthase

In rodent species, NO· is a major molecular component of cell-mediated immune responses (Hibbs et al., 1990; Nathan and Hibbs, 1991), and there is evidence that cytokine-induced NO· synthesis also occurs when cell-mediated immunity is stimulated by interleukin-2 therapy in humans (Hibbs et al., 1992). Currently, not all the biological roles for NO· synthesized from L-arginine by the iNOS are known. However, convincing experimental evidence has been obtained for one immunologically important function for NO· produced during cell-mediated immune reactions. Cytokine-inducible, high-output NO· synthesis appears to have a major role in defense of the intracellular environment against invasion by intracellular pathogens (Hibbs et al., 1990; Nathan and Hibbs, 1991).

Investigation during the 1970s demonstrated that the mechanism of activated macrophage-mediated defense against intracellular pathogens was very similar to activated macrophage-mediated defense to neoplastic cells (Hibbs et al., 1980, 1990). The discovery of the cytokine-induced, high-output L-arginine–NO· pathway identified an effector molecule capable of targeting both intracellular microbes and neoplastic cells (Hibbs et al., 1987a, 1987b, 1988, 1990; Iyengar et al., 1987; Marletta et al., 1988). Further, immunologically induced synthesis of NO· from L-arginine provided a biochemical explanation for an unusual pattern of metabolic perturbation that had been described previously in tumor target cells of activated macrophages (Drapier and Hibbs, 1986, 1988; Granger and Lehninger, 1982; Granger et al., 1980; Hibbs et al., 1990) (Fig. 3). Prominent among the metabolic changes induced in target cells of activated macrophages were inhibition of DNA replication and inhibition of mitochondrial respiration. This observation was based on demonstrations that cytotoxic activated macrophages caused inhibition of complex I and complex II of the mitochondrial electron transport

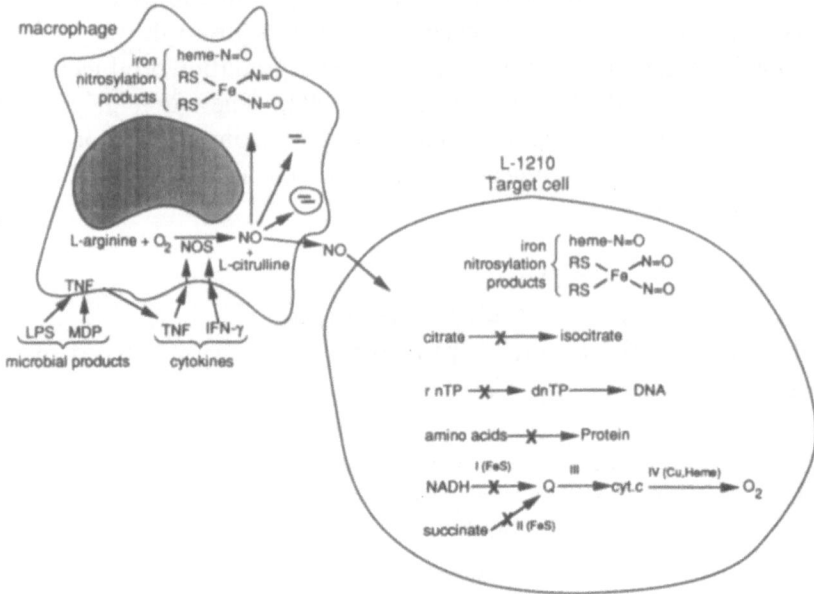

Figure 3. Cytokine-induced NO· synthesis by macrophages as an effector molecule of cell-medicated immunity. Expression of L-arginine-dependent cytotoxicity by activated macrophages is the result of phenotypic changes induced by at least two differentiation signals. Macrophages from normal mice are not activated and are not cytotoxic for intracellular pathogens or mammalian cells. Acquisition of cytotoxic activity, now known to be L-arginine dependent, by macrophages requires several signals (Hibbs et al., 1980, 1990). The first signal produces primed macrophages (noncytotoxic activated macrophages). Primed macrophages are produced *in vitro* by treatment of peritoneal macrophages from normal mice with interferon-γ (IFN-γ). However, full induction of the high-output L-arginine–NO pathway and expression of L-arginine-dependent cytotoxicity requires a cosignal, for example, exposure to a microbial product such as lipopolysaccharide (LPS) (Drapier and Hibbs, 1988; Hibbs et al., 1987a, 1987b, 1988, 1990; Stuehr and Nathan, 1989). Recent studies show that TNF is a potent cosignal (Drapier et al., 1991). Microbial products such as muramyl dipeptide or LPS act, at least in part, by inducing TNF synthesis, which is a physiologic final inducer of the high-output L-arginine–NO pathway in activated macrophages (Drapier et al., 1991). Therefore, classical cell-mediated immune mechanisms (in the presence of absence of certain microbial components) induce the high-output L-arginine–NO pathway in macrophages. Cytokine-induced synthesis of NO· by macrophages causes the pattern of metabolic inhibition described in the text in both activated macrophages (autocrine effects) and target cells (paracrine effects). Protein synthesis also is inhibited by NO· by an unknown mechanism (Curran et al., 1989; Hibbs et al., 1984). Cytokines induce the high-output NO synthase in most tumor and normal murine cells (see text and Fig. 4) but not in L1210 murine leukemia cells. Abbreviations: muramyl dipeptide, MDP; interferon-gamma, IFN-γ; tumor necrosis factor, TNF.

systems as well as the citric acid cycle enzyme aconitase (Drapier and Hibbs, 1986, 1988). These three enzymes all have [4Fe–4S] prosthetic groups that are essential for their catalytic function. These studies also showed that enzymatic inhibition involved the [4Fe–4S] prosthetic group rather than the apoenzyme. In addition, it was observed that tumor cells cocultivated with cytotoxic activated macrophages released a significant fraction of their intracellular iron in parallel with development of inhibition of DNA synthesis, inhibition of protein synthesis, and inhibition of mitochondrial respiration (Hibbs et al., 1984). It is important to point out that cytotoxic activated macrophages develop the same pattern of metabolic inhibition as their target cells (Drapier and Hills, 1988). Discovery of the cytokine-induced L-arginine–NO pathway provided an effector mechanism capable of causing the biochemical changes that had been observed (Drapier and Hibbs, 1986, 1988; Granger and Lehninger, 1982; Granger et al., 1980; Hibbs et al., 1984, 1987a, 1987b; Stuehr and Nathan, 1989) (see Fig. 3). The identification of nitrosyl–iron–sulfur complex formation (in both cytotoxic activated macrophages and in their target cells) links inhibition of enzymes with [4Fe–4S] prosthetic groups and NO synthesis by cytotoxic activated macrophages (Drapier et al., 1991; Lancaster and Hibbs, 1990).

The observation that N^{ω}-monomethyl-L-arginine (MLA) is a potent competitive inhibitor of the NO· synthase (Hibbs et al., 1987a, 1987b) provided a useful experimental tool for demonstrating which effector functions of the cell-mediated immune response were mediated by iNOS. In addition to mediating L-arginine-dependent cytotoxicity for mammalian cells, this pathway has antimicrobial activity (Granger et al., 1988, 1990; James and Glaven, 1989). We think it likely that the cytokine-induced L-arginine–NO· pathway is a primary defense against intracellular microorganisms as well as pathogens that are too large to be phagocytized (e.g., large fungal elements and certain helminthic parasites). We speculate that cytokine-induced NO· synthesis from L-arginine could represent a major biochemical defense of the intracellular environment. Results obtained to date are consistent with this hypothesis. This pathway has potent cytotoxic effects for the facultative intracellular fungal pathogen *Cryptococcus neoformans* (Granger et al., 1988, 1990), schistosomula of *Schistosoma mansoni* (James and Glaven, 1989), intracellular amastigotes of *Leishmania major* (Green et al., 1990; Liew et al., 1990), intracellular trophozoites of *Toxoplasma gondii* (Adams et al., 1990), plasmodia (Nussler et al., 1991), the obligate intracellular bacteria *Chlamydia trachomatis* (Mayer et al., 1993), as well as the facultative intracellular bacteria *Mycobacterium leprae* (Adams et al., 1991), *Mycobacterium tuberculosis* (Chan et al., 1992; Denis, 1991); *Francisella tularensis* (Fortier et al., 1992), and *Listeria monocytogenes* (Beckerman et al., 1993).

It is important to emphasize that cytokines also induce the high-output NOS in nonmacrophage cells (Amber et al., 1988; Hibbs et al., 1990) (Fig. 4). This causes the same reproducible pattern of metabolic

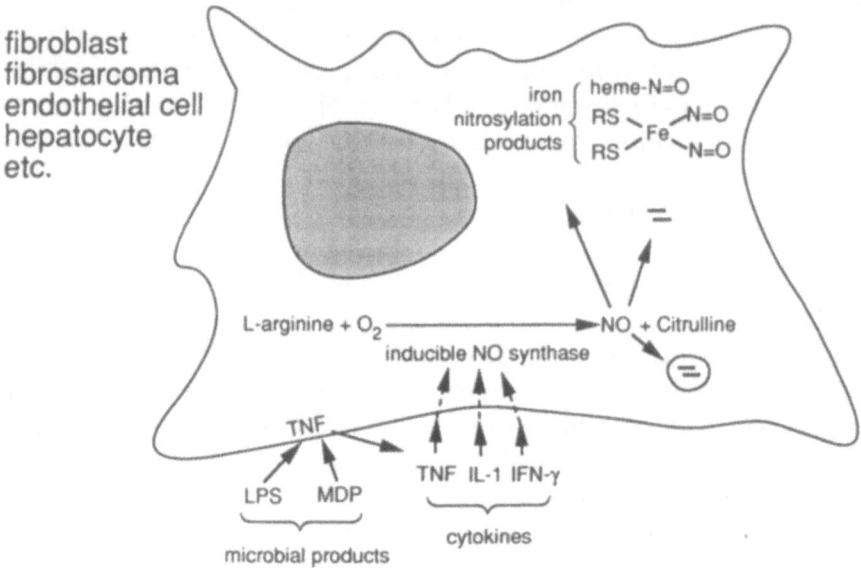

Figure 4. Cytokine-induced NO· synthesis by nonmacrophage cells as an effector molecule of cell-medicated immunity. Cytokines can induce synthesis of the high-output NO· synthase in many nonmacrophage cell lines. The cytokine signals inducing iNOS are the same for macrophages and nonmacrophages, with the exception that IL-1 is a potent cosignal for nonmacrophage cells but is inactive as a cosignal for macrophages (Amber et al., 1988; Drapier et al., 1991; Hibbs et al., 1990). Although not illustrated, induction of high-output NO· synthesis by cytokines in nonmacrophage cells and subsequent iron nitrosylation causes the same pattern of metabolic inhibition in the cytokine-stimulated nonmacrophage cells as occurs in macrophages and their targets (Amber et al., 1988; Hibbs et al., 1990). The figure shows that cytokines can induce a potent NO·-mediated defense against intracellular microbes in nonmacrophage cells. Abbreviations: interleukin 1, Il-1.

inhibition as described (see Fig. 3) in the nonmacrophage cell phenotype in which the iNOS has been induced. The ability of cytokines to induce iNOS in most or all somatic cells could markedly enhance the efficiency of cell-mediated immunity. Signals generated by a cell-mediated immune response could cause NO-induced biochemical changes locally in non-macrophage cells of tissues invaded by certain microbes or within nonmacrophage cells comprising a tumor mass. Treatment of murine EMT-6 mammary adenocarcinoma cells with cytokines caused release of [55]Fe label, inhibition of DNA replication, and inhibition of aconitase activity (Amber et al., 1988). In addition, the same combination of cytokines induced EMT-6 cells to synthesize nitrite, nitrate, and L-citrulline from L-arginine (Amber et al., 1988, 1991; Lepoivre et al., 1989). These findings are identical to those obtained when macrophages are treated with cytokines. The high-output iNOS has been induced in a number of other nonmacrophage somatic cell phenotypes, including hepatocytes (Nussler et al., 1991; Curran et al., 1989) and endothelial cells (Kilbourn and Belloni, 1990). Therefore, the awareness that cytokines can induce iNOS activity in many, if not most, somatic cells changes our view of cell-mediated immune responses. Cytokine-inducible, high-output NO· synthesis is not just an activity of cells recruited from the bone marrow and specialized for host defense such as macrophages, but potentially an activity of most somatic cells of a tissue involved in a cell-mediated immune reaction.

Synthesis of NO· from L-arginine in the Central Nervous System

It was recognized very soon after the biological synthase of NO· was discovered that NO· or a closely related molecule has a role in neuro-physiology (Bredt and Snyder, 1989; Garthwaite et al., 1988; Knowles et al., 1989). In the cerebellum, cGMP rapidly increases when the N-methyl-D aspartate (NMDA) subtype of glutamate receptor is activated (Bredt and Synder, 1989; Knowles et al., 1989). Glutamate-induced elevation of cerebellar cGMP was inhibited by MLA, a potent inhibitor of all NOS isoforms (Bredt and synder, 1990; Hibbs et al., 1987a, 1987b). Using rat cerebellar tissue, Bredt and Synder were the first to biochemically isolate and purify a NOS isoform. In these experiments, they demonstrated for the first time that cNOS isoforms are Ca^{2+} calmodulin-dependent enzymes. These experiments identified the Ca^{2+} calmodulin requirement of the cerebellar cNOS and explained how glutamate, via interaction with NMDA receptors, caused rapid (within seconds) synthesis of NO· from L-arginine. Interaction of glutamate with NMDA receptors opens Ca^{2+} channels. This elevates intracellular Ca^{2+}, which binds to calmodulin and activates the cNOS (Bredt and Synder, 1990). The distribution of cNOS in the CNS appears to be localized to a few cell types, although isoforms may exist that cannot be identified with currently used immunochemical or histochemical techniques (Bredt et al., 1990; Dawson et al., 1991; Hope et al., 1991; Synder, 1992). In the cerebellum, the cNOS was identified in basket and granule cells. In the hippocampus, corpus striation, and cerebral cortex, cNOS localizes in aspiny neurons that represent only 1% to 2% of neurons. However, their cell extensions arborize extensively and make contact with most other neurons in the brain.

During normal physiological activity, NO· is synthesized in very small quantities by a cNOS isoform in the brain and, similar to its role in vascular tissue, functions as an intercellular messenger that may produce a "field effect" within a three-dimensional matrix of tissue. Again, similar

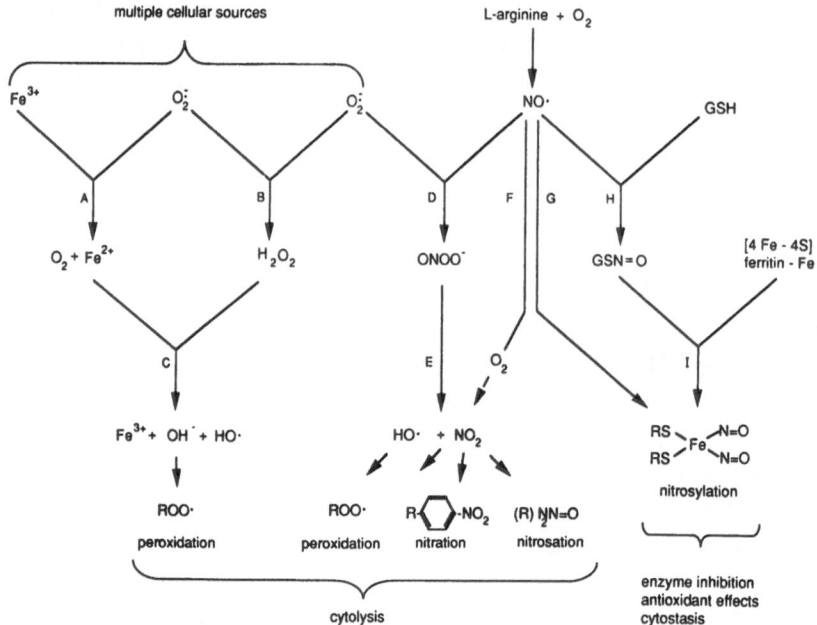

Figure 5. Schematic representation of pathways synthesizing low molecular weight reactive molecules active in host defense. We have arbitrarily termed addition of the nitroso group to iron and thiols as *nitrosylation* and to other atoms as *nitrosation*. Additional products of pathway F include N_2O_3, N_2O_4, NO_2^-, and NO_3^- (Hibbs et al., 1990; Leaf et al., 1990). GSH may not react directly with NO flowing through pathway H, but with NO metabolites such as N_2O_3 and N_2O_4. (Unpaired electrons are symbolized by ·) Abbreviations: nitrogen dioxide, NO_2·; reduced glutathione, GSH; *S*-nitrosoglutathione, GSN=O; paramagnetic mononuclear iron sulfur dinitrosyl complexes, $(RS)_2Fe(No·)_2^-$. Heme nitrosyl complexes, also formed by pathways G, H, and I (Hibbs et al., 1992), are not shown. From Hibbs, 1992, with permission of Portland Press.

to vascular tissue, and at least in certain instances in the brain, the information encoded in NO· is transduced by a redox reaction with the iron atom of the heme prosthetic group of soluble guanylate cyclase (Bredt and Synder, 1989; Knowles et al., 1989). Other targets may exist for NO synthesized in the brain. Information also could be transduced by NO·-mediated activation of ADP ribosylation or by other as yet undefined mechanisms (Brune and Lapetina, 1989; Zhang and Synder, 1992). It is likely that inappropriate activation in the CNS of cNOS isoforms in both vascular tissue and neurons during certain pathophysiological situations, or of iNOS by cytokines, can result in neurotoxicity. For example, redox reactions of NO· with O_2 and superoxide anion (O_2^-) could readily occur if NO· is inappropriately synthesized from L-arginine in the CNS (Fig. 5). The interaction of NO· with O_2 and O_2^- can produce very toxic products capable of causing indiscriminant damage in the tissues (Beckman et al., 1990; Hibbs, 1992; Wink et al., 1992). Further, inappropriate high-output synthesis of NO· flowing into the iron nitrosylation pathway could cause enzymatic inhibition (see Fig. 3) that results in neurotoxicity. I am certain that studies performed during the next several years will better define both the physiological and pathophysiological role of NO· in the CNS.

References

Adams LB, Hibbs JB Jr, Taintor RR, Krahenbuhl JL (1990): Microbiostatic effect of murine macrophages for *Toxoplasma gondii*: role of synthesis of inorganic nitrogen oxides from L-arginine. *J Immunol* 144:2725–2729

Adams LB, Franzblau AG, Vavrin Z, Hibbs JB Jr, Krahenbuhl JL (1991): L-Arginine-dependent macrophage effector functions inhibit metabolic activity of *Mycobacterium leprae*. *J Immunol* 147:1642–1646

Amber IJ, Hibbs JB Jr, Taintor RR, Vavrin Z (1988): Cytokines induce an L-arginine-dependent effector system in non-macrophage cells. *J Leukocyte Biol* 44:58–65

Amber IJ, Hibbs JB Jr, Parker CJ, Johnson BB, Taintor RR, Vavrin Z (1991): Activated macrophage conditioned medium: Identification of the soluble factors inducing cytotoxicity and the L-arginine dependent effector mechanism. *J Leukocyte Biol* 49:610–620

Beckerman KP, Rogers HW, Corbett JA, Schreiber RD, McDaniel ML, Unanue ER (1993): Release of nitric oxide during the T cell-independent pathway of macrophage activation: Its role in resistance to *Listeria monocytogenes*. *J Immunol* 150:888–895

Beckman JS, Beckman TW, Chen J, Marshall PA, Freeman BA (1990): Apparent hydroxyl radical production by peroxynitrite: implications for endothelial injury from nitric oxide and superoxide. *Proc Natl Acad Sci USA* 87: 1620–1624

Bredt DS, Snyder SH (1989): Nitric oxide mediates glutamate-linked enhancement of cGMP levels in the cerebellum. *Proc Natl Acad Sci USA* 86:9030–9033

Bredt DS, Synder SH (1990): Isolation of nitric oxide synthetase, a calmodulin-requiring enzyme. *Proc Natl Acad Sci USA* 87:682–685

Bredt DS, Hwang PM, Synder SH (1990): Localization of nitric oxide synthase indicating a neural role for nitric oxide. *Nature* 347:768–770

Brune G, Lapetina EG (1989): *J Biol Chem* 264:8455–8458

Chan J, Xing Y, Magliozzo RS, Bloom BR (1992): Killing of virulent *Mycobacterium tuberculosis* by reactive nitrogen intermediates produced by activated murine macrophages. *J Exp Med* 175:1111–1122

Curran RD, Billiar TR, Stuehr DJ, Simmons RL (1989): Hepatocytes produce nitrogen oxides from L-arginine in response to inflammatory products of kupffer cells. *J Exp Med* 170: 1796–1774

Dawson TM, Bredt DS, Fotuhi M, Hwang PM, Snyder RH (1991): Nitric oxide synthase and neuronal NADPH diaphorase are identical in brain and peripheral tissues. *Proc Natl Acad Sci USA* 88:7797–7801

Denis M (1991): Interferon-gamma-treated murine macrophages inhibit growth of tubercle bacilli via the generation of reactive nitrogen intermediates. *Cell Immunol* 132:150–157

Doyle MP, Hoekstra JW (1981): Oxidation of nitrogen oxides by bound dioxygen in hemoproteins. *J Inorg Biochem* 14:351–358

Drapier J-C, Hibbs JB Jr (1986): Murine cytotoxic activated macrophages inhibit aconitase in tumor cells. Inhibition involves the iron-sulfur prosthetic group and is reversible. *J Clin Invest* 78:790–797

Drapier J-C, Hibbs JB Jr (1988): Differentiation of murine macrophages to express nonspecific cytotoxicity for tumor cells results in L-arginine-dependent inhibition of mitochondrial iron-sulfur enzymes in the macrophage effect cells. *J Immunol* 140:2829–2838

Drapier J-C, Pellat C, Yann H (1991): Generation of EPR-detectable nitrosyl-iron complexes in tumor target cells cocultured with activated macrophages. *J Biol Chem* 266:10162–10167

Fortier AH, Polsinelli T, Green SJ, Nacy CA (1992): Activation of macrophages for destruction of *Francisella tularensis*: identification of cytokines, effector cells, and effector molecules. *Infect Immunol* 60:817–825

Gally JA, Montague PR, Reeke GN, Edelman GM (1990): The NO hypothesis: possible effects of a short-lived, rapidly diffusible signal in the development and function of the nervous system. *Proc Natl Acad Sci USA* 87: 3547–3551

Garthwaite J, Charles SL, Chess-Williams R (1988): Endothelium-derived relaxing factor on activation of NMDA receptors suggests role as intercellular messenger in the brain. *Nature* 336:385–388

Granger DL, Lehninger AI (1982): Sites of inhibition of mitochondrial electron transport in macrophage-injured neoplastic cells. *J Cell Biol* 95:527–535

Granger DL, Hibbs JB Jr, Perfect JR, Durack DT (1988): Specific amino acid (L-arginine) requirement for the microbiostatic activity of murine macrophages. *J Clin Invest* 81:1129–1136

Granger DL, Hibbs JB Jr, Perfect JR, Durack DT (1990): Metabolic fate of L-arginine in relation to microbiostatic capability of macrophages. *J Clin Invest* 85:264–273

Granger DL, Taintor RR, Cook JL, Hibbs JB Jr (1980): Injury of neoplastic cells by murine macrophages leads to inhibition of mitochondrial respiration. *J Clin Invest* 65:357–370

Green SJ, Meltzer MS, Hibbs JB Jr, Nacy CA (1990): Activated macrophages destroy intracellular. *Leishmania major* amastigotes by an L-arginine dependent killing mechanism. *J Immunol* 144:278–283

Hibbs JB Jr (1992): Overview of cytotoxic mechanisms and defense of the intracellular environment against microbes. In: *The Biology of Nitric Oxide, 2: Enzymology, Biochemistry and Immunology*, Moncada S, Marletta MA, Hibbs JB Jr, Higgs EA, eds. London and Chapel Hill: Portland Press

Hibbs JB Jr, Remington JS, Stewart CC (1980): Modulation of immunity and host resistance by micro-organisms. *Pharmacol Ther* 8:37–69

Hibbs JB Jr, Taintor RR, Vavrin Z (1984): Iron depletion: possible cause of tumor cell cytotoxicity induced by activated macrophages. *Biochem Biophys Res Commun* 123:716–723

Hibbs JB Jr, Taintor RR, Vavrin Z (1987a): Macrophage cytotoxicity: role for L-arginine deiminase activity and imino nitrogen oxidation to nitrite. *Science* 235:473–476

Hibbs JB Jr, Vavrin Z, Taintor RR (1987b): L-Arginine is required for expression of the activated macrophage effector mechanism causing selective metabolic inhibition in target cells. *J Immunol* 138:550–565

Hibbs JB Jr, Taintor RR, Vavrin Z, Rachlin EM (1988): Nitric oxide: a cytotoxic activated macrophage effector molecule. *Biochem Biophys Res Commun* 157:87–94. [Erratum *Biochem Biophys Res Commun* 1989) 158:624]

Hibbs JB Jr, Taintor RR, Vavrin Z, Granger DL, Drapier J-C, Amber IJ, Lancaster JR Jr (1990): Synthesis of nitric oxide from a terminal guanidino nitrogen atom of L-arginine: a molecular mechanism regulating cellular proliferation that targets intracellular iron. In: *Nitric Oxide from L-Arginine: A Bioregulatory System*. New York: Elsevier

Hibbs JB Jr, Westenfelder C, Taintor RR, Vavrin Z, Kablitz G, Baranowski RL, Ward JH, Menlove RL, McMurray MP, Kushner JP, Samlowski W (1992): Evidence for cytokine-inducible nitric oxide synthesis from L-arginine in patients receiving interleukin-2 therapy. *J Clin Invest* 89:867–877

Hope BR, Michael GJ, Knigge KM, Vincent SR (1991): Neuronal NADPH diaphorase is a nitric oxide synthase. *Proc Natl Acad Sci USA* 88:2811–2814

Hutcheson IR, Griffith TM (1991): Release of endothelium-derived relaxing factor is modulated by both frequency and amplitude of pulsatile flow. *Am J Physiol* 261:H257–H262

Ignarro LJ (1989): Heme-dependent activation of soluble guanylate cyclase by nitric oxide: regulation of enzyme activity by porphyrins and metalloporphyrins. *Semin Hematol* 26:63–76

Ignarro LJ, Buga GM, Wood KS, Byrns RE, Chaudhuri G (1987): Endothelium-derived relaxing factor produced and released from artery and vein in nitric oxide. *Proc Natl Acad Sci USA* 84:9265–9269

Iyengar R, Stuehr DR, Marletta MA (1987): Macrophage synthesis of nitrite, nitrate, and *N*-nitrosamines: precursors and role of the respiratory burst. *Proc Natl Acad Sci USA* 84:6369–6373

James SI, Glaven J (1989): Macrophage cytotoxicity against schistosomula of *Schistosoma mansoni* involves arginine-dependent production of reactive nitrogen intermediates. *J Immunol* 143:4208–4212

Kilbourn RG, Belloni P (1990): Endothelial cell production of nitrogen oxides in response to interferon-γ in combination with tumor necrosis factor, interleukin-1, or endotoxin. *J Natl Cancer Inst* 82:772–776

Knowles RG, Palacios GM, Palmer RMJ, Moncada S (1989): Formation of nitric oxide from L-arginine in the central nervous system: a transduction mechanism for stimulation of the soluble guanylate cyclase. *Proc Natl Acad Sci USA* 86:5159–5162

Kosaka H, Kazuhiko I, Kiyohiro I, Itiro T (1979): Stoichiometry of the reaction of exyhemoglobin with nitrite. *Biochim Biophys Acta* 581:184–188

Lancaster JR Jr, Hibbs JB Jr (1990): EPR demonstration of iron-nitrosyl complex formation by cytotoxic activated macrophages. *Proc Natl Acad Sci USA* 87:1223–1227

Leaf CD, Wishnok JS, Tannenbaum SR (1990): In: Nitric Oxide from L-Arginine: A Bioregulatory System, Moncada S, Higgs EA, eds., pp. 291–299. Amsterdam: Elsevier Science Publishers B.V. (Biomedical Division)

Lepoivre M, Boudbid H, Petit JF (1989): Antiproliferative activity of γ-interferon combined with lipopolysaccharide on murine adenocarcinoma: dependence on an L-arginine metabolism with production of nitrite and citrulline. *Can Res* 49:1970–1976

Liew FY, Millott S, Parkinson C, Palmer RMJ, Moncada S (1990): Macrophage killing of *Leishmania* parasite *in vivo* is mediated by nitric oxide from L-arginine. *J Immunol* 144:4794–4797

Marletta MA, Yoon PS, Iyengar R, Leaf CD, Wishnock JS (1988): Macrophage oxidation of L-arginine to nitrite and nitrate: nitric oxide is an intermediate. *Biochemistry* 27:8706–8711

Mayer J, Woods M, Vavrin Z, Hibbs JB Jr (1993): Gamma interferon-induced nitric oxide production reduces *Chlamydia trachomatis* infectivity in McCoy cells. *Infect Immun* 61: 491–497

Moncada S, Palmer RMJ, Higgs EA (1991): Nitric oxide: physiology, pathology, and pharmacology. *Pharmacol Rev* 43:109–142

Nathan CF (1992): Nitric oxide as a secretory product of mammalian cells: *FASEB J* 6:3051–3064

Nathan CF, Hibbs JB Jr (1991): Role of nitric oxide synthesis in macrophage antimicrobial activity. *Curr Opin Immunol* 3:65–70

Nussler A, Drapier J-C, Renia L, Pied S, Miltgen F, Gentilini M, Maxier D (1991): L-Arginine-dependent destruction of intrahepatic malaria parasites in response to tumor necrosis factor and/or interleukin 6 stimulation. *Eur J Immunol* 21:227–230

O'dell TJ, Hawkins RD, Kandel ER, Arancio O (1991): Tests of the roles of two diffusible substances in long-term potentiation: evidence for nitric oxide as a possible early retrograde messenger. *Proc Natl Acad Sci USA* 88:11285–11289

Palmer RMJ, Ashton DS, Moncada S (1988): Vascular endothelial cells synthesize nitric oxide from L-arginine. *Nature* 333:664–666

Palmer RMJ, Ferrige AG, Moncada S (1987): Nitric oxide release accounts for the biological activity of endothelium-derived relaxing factor. *Nature* 327:524–526

Radomski MW, Palmer RMJ, Moncada S (1990): L-Arginine/nitric oxide pathway present in human platelets regulates aggregation. *Proc Natl Acad Sci USA* 87:5193–5197

Schuman EM, Madison DV (1991): A requirement for the intercellular messenger nitric oxide in long-term potentiation. *Science* 254:1503–1506

Stuehr DJ, Nathan CF (1989): A macrophage product responsible for cytostasis and respiratory inhibition in tumor target cells. *J Exp Med* 169:1543–1555

Synder SH (1992): Nitric oxide: first of a new class of neurotransmitters. *Science* 257:494–496

Weiss PA (1967): $1 + 1 \neq 2$ (When one plus one does not equal two). In: *The Neurosciences: A Study Program*, Quarton GE, Melnechuck T, eds. New York: Rockefeller University Press

Wennmalm A, Benthin G, Petersson AS (1992): Dependence of the metabolism of nitric oxide (NO·) in healthy human whole blood on the oxygenation of its red cell haemoglobin. *Br J Pharmacol* 106:507–508

Wink DA, Kasprzak KS, Maragos CM, Elespuru RK, Misra J, Dunams TM, Cebula TA, Koch WH, Andrews AW, Allen JS, Keefer LK (1992): DNA deaminating ability and genotoxicity of nitric oxide and its progenitors. *Science* 254:1001–1003

Zhang J, Synder SH (1992): Nitric oxide stimulates auto-ADP-ribosylation of glyceraldehyde-3-phosphate dehydrogenase. *Proc Natl Acad Sci USA* 89:9382–9385

9

Multiple Roles of the Calcium Ion in Cell Killing

Sten Orrenius and Pierluigi Nicotera

The realization that the calcium ion is involved in the regulation of a large number of physiological processes has included the understanding that Ca^{2+} can play a determinant role in a variety of pathological and toxicological conditions. It has long been recognized that Ca^{2+} accumulates in necrotic tissue, and subsequent work has revealed that a disruption of intracellular Ca^{2+} homeostasis is frequently associated with the early development of cell injury (Fleckenstein et al., 1983; Jewell et al., 1982; Schanne et al., 1979). This led to the formulation of the calcium hypothesis of cell injury, which proposes that perturbation of the intracellular Ca^{2+} homeostasis may be a common step in the development of cytotoxicity.

During recent years it has become progressively clear that multiple mechanisms may be involved in Ca^{2+}-mediated cell killing, including Ca^{2+} overload and Ca^{2+} signaling for cell deletion (Fig. 1). Thus, Ca^{2+} appears to mediate the neurotoxicity of cyanide, chlordecone, and heavy metals, including lead, mercury, and organotin compounds (Komulainen

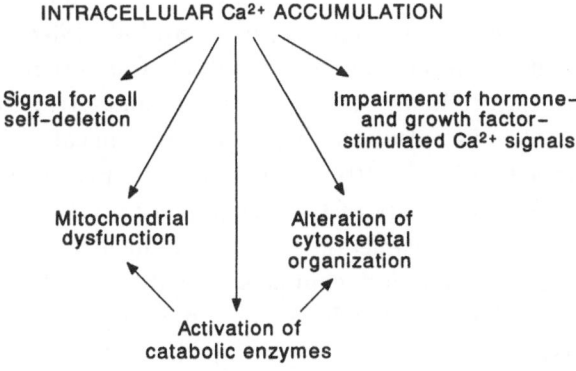

Figure 1. Multiple roles of Ca^{2+} in cell killing.

ADVANCES IN RESEARCH ON NEURODEGENERATION, II
Y. Mizuno et al.
© 1994 Birkhäuser Boston

and Bondy, 1988). In addition, intracellular Ca^{2+} overload caused by excessive stimulation of excitatory amino acid receptors and enhanced Ca^{2+} influx through membrane channels seems to play an important role in ischemic brain damage (Manev et al., 1990). An elevation of intracellular Ca^{2+} also seems to contribute to cell killing by several hepatotoxic agents and to trigger thymocyte killing by the environmental contaminants 2,3,7,8-tetrachlorodibenzo-p-dioxin (TCDD) and tributyltin (see Nicotera et al., 1990a, for review). There is also increasing evidence that Ca^{2+} plays an important role in both physiological and pathological cell killing in the immune system. Thus, the killing of immature thymocytes by glucocorticoids (McConkey et al., 1989), and the killing of target cells by cytotoxic T lymphocytes (Berke, 1989) and by natural killer cells (McConkey et al., 1990) all appear to be Ca^{2+} dependent. Finally, recent studies have suggested that both bacterial toxins (Caspar et al., 1987) and viral components such as the human immunodeficiency virus (HIV) envelope glycoprotein, gp 120 (Dreyer et al., 1990), can promote killing of infected cells by increasing intracellular Ca^{2+} levels.

Intracellular Ca^{2+} homeostasis is normally maintained by the concerted operation of cellular transport and compartmentalization systems. Impairment of these processes during cell injury, however, can result in enhanced Ca^{2+} influx, release of Ca^{2+} from intracellular stores, or inhibition of Ca^{2+} extrusion at the plasma membrane. This can lead to an uncontrolled, sustained rise in intracellular Ca^{2+} concentration and subsequent loss of cell viability.

Regulation of Intracellular Ca^{2+} Homeostasis

The Ca^{2+} concentration in the cytosol ($[Ca^{2+}]_i$) of unstimulated cells is maintained between 0.05 and 0.2 μM (Carafoli, 1989). Consequently there is a concentration difference of about four orders of magnitude between the extracellular Ca^{2+} level (approximately 1.3 mM) and the cytosolic Ca^{2+} concentration. This electrochemical driving force is balanced by active Ca^{2+} extrusion through the plasma membrane and by the coordinated activity of Ca^{2+}-sequestering systems located in the mitochondrial, endoplasmic reticular, and nuclear membranes. Ca^{2+} uptake occurs through ion channels and different types of voltage-operated Ca^{2+} channels that have been identified and characterized in excitable tissues. In addition, receptor-operated channels are involved in Ca^{2+} entry during hormone stimulation.

Although isolated mitochondria can accumulate large amounts of Ca^{2+}, the affinity of their uniport carrier for Ca^{2+} uptake is low, and they appear to play a minor role in buffering cytosolic Ca^{2+} under normal conditions. In addition, electron probe x-ray microanalysis of rapidly frozen liver sections has shown that mitochondria contain little Ca^{2+} *in situ* (about 1 nmol Ca^{2+}/mg protein), whereas the endoplasmic reticulum represents the major intracellular Ca^{2+} store. We have shown that liver nuclei possess an ATP-stimulated Ca^{2+}-uptake system responsible for intranuclear Ca^{2+} accumulation and that Ca^{2+} can be released from a nuclear compartment in response to intracellular messengers (Nicotera et al., 1989a, 1990b).

The mechanisms by which Ca^{2+}-mobilizing hormones produce $[Ca^{2+}]_i$ transients have been extensively studied in recent years (Berridge, 1987). The signal transduction pathway leading to the elevation of $[Ca^{2+}]_i$ can be summarized as follows. On binding of the agonist to its plasma membrane receptor, a specific phospholipase C becomes activated via stimulation of a G protein, resulting in the hydrolysis of phosphatidylinositol 4,5-bisphosphate to generate two second messengers, inositol 1,4,5-trisphosphate and diacylglycerol. Diacylglycerol is a potent activator of protein kinase C and inositol 1,4,5-trisphosphate is the mediator for Ca^{2+} release from a nonmitochondrial intracellular store; this release of Ca^{2+} is responsible for the initial rapid elevation of $[Ca^{2+}]_i$. The exact intracellular localization of the inositol 1,4,5-trisphosphate-sensitive Ca^{2+} pool is not known, but it appears that at least part of this pool is located within the endoplasmic reticulum.

In addition to mobilizing Ca^{2+} from intracellular stores, hormones can stimulate Ca^{2+} influx from the extracellular compartment through specific receptor-operated Ca^{2+} channels (Barritt et al., 1981). With the recent development of digital imaging techniques, it has become possible to study $[Ca^{2+}]_i$ transients in individual cells. This has led to the observation that at low, close-to-threshold concentrations of Ca^{2+}-mobilizing hormones, many cells respond to these agents with oscillating $[Ca^{2+}]_i$ spikes (Woods et al., 1986). It has been suggested that such oscillatory patterns may carry a frequency-encoded message (Berridge, 1990); however, the possible pathophysiological implications of this phenomenon have yet to be identified.

Disruption of Intracellular Ca^{2+} Homeostasis by Toxic Agents

Cellular Ca^{2+} overload can result from either an enhanced influx of extracellular Ca^{2+} or an impairment of Ca^{2+} extrusion from the cell. In addition, interference with individual Ca^{2+} translocases can compromise the ability of the cell to buffer cytosolic Ca^{2+} changes and can contribute to an increase in cytosolic Ca^{2+} level. A number of hepatotoxins have been found to impair Ca^{2+} sequestration by the isolated microsomal fraction or by the endoplasmic reticulum in intact cells. However, recent work in our laboratory has shown that the antioxidant, 2,5-di-(*tert*-butyl)-1,4-benzohydroquinone (*t*-BuBHQ), which selectively inhibits both the microsomal Ca^{2+}-ATPase and Ca^{2+} uptake by the endoplasmic reticulum (Kass et al., 1989), rapidly releases endoplasmic reticular Ca^{2+} without producing hepatotoxicity in the isolated perfused rat liver (Farrell et al., 1990). Hence, the sole interference with Ca^{2+} sequestration by the endoplasmic reticulum does not appear to play a major role in the development of acute hepatotoxicity.

The role of mitochondria in toxin-induced perturbation of Ca^{2+} homeostasis is still unclear. As discussed previously, mitochondria contain only little Ca^{2+} under physiological conditions. However, they have the capacity to sequester large quantities of Ca^{2+} and could therefore act as efficient buffers of $[Ca^{2+}]_i$ under toxic conditions. Unfortunately, this potentially important line of defense does not appear to be operational in many instances because toxins frequently stimulate Ca^{2+} release from the mitochondria. In addition, the release and reuptake of Ca^{2+} through separate routes results in Ca^{2+} cycling that can lead to membrane damage, mitochondrial swelling, uncoupling of respiration, and loss of intracellular ATP. This, in turn, will further compromise cell survival.

There is compelling evidence that many hepatotoxins interfere with Ca^{2+} uptake and extrusion mechanisms (Orrenius et al., 1989). Inhibition of Ca^{2+} efflux will result in the net accumulation of Ca^{2+} and in a pathological elevation of $[Ca^{2+}]_i$ (Nicotera et al., 1989b). In addition, it has become clear that chemical toxins can stimulate Ca^{2+} entry by interacting with existing Ca^{2+} channels or by increasing the plasma membrane permeability to Ca^{2+}. The resulting Ca^{2+} overload can activate several cytotoxic mechanisms that can cause cell death.

The importance of Ca^{2+} overload in cell killing is illustrated by experiments in which removal of extracellular Ca^{2+}, or loading of cells with intracellular Ca^{2+} chelators, has caused cytoprotection. Intracellular Ca^{2+} chelators such as quin-2 or BAPTA have been employed to buffer increases in cytosolic Ca^{2+} in a variety of experimental systems, and such treatment has prevented, or delayed, cell killing induced by various agents (Nicotera et al., 1990a). In addition to Ca^{2+} chelators, Ca^{2+} channel blockers have also been used to prevent Ca^{2+} overload and cell death in several studies.

Mechanisms of Ca^{2+}-Mediated Cell Killing

Both the duration and the extent of the increase in $[Ca^{2+}]_i$ appear to be critical for the development of cytotoxicity. Even moderate increases in cytosolic Ca^{2+} can impair the ability of the cell to respond adequately to agonist stimulation and thereby interfere with cell control by hormones and growth factors. Another early effect of a sustained elevation of the cytosolic free Ca^{2+} concentration is the impairment of mitochondrial functions. In addition, more intense increases in cytosolic Ca^{2+} will result in the disruption of cytoskeletal organization and in the activation of a number of Ca^{2+}-stimulated catabolic processes such as proteolysis, membrane degradation, and chromatin fragmentation.

Mitochondrial Damage

Work from several laboratories has indicated that mitochondrial damage may represent a common event in cell injury caused by a variety of toxic agents. Mitochondrial damage is initially manifested by a decrease in the mitochondrial membrane potential followed by a decline in adenosine diphosphate (ADP) phosphorylation, eventually resulting in adenosine triphosphate (ATP) depletion. As described earlier, Ca^{2+} can be actively transported into mitochondria via an electrophoretic uniporter. The driving force for continuous Ca^{2+} pumping is provided by the transmembrane potential. However, studies performed in isolated mitochondria have demonstrated that during Ca^{2+} uptake the membrane potential decreases and that the extent of this decrease is proportional to the amount of Ca^{2+} taken up by the mitochondria (Gunther and Pfeiffer, 1990). It thus appears that under conditions which cause massive amount of Ca^{2+} to accumulate in the mitochondria that the mitochondrial membrane potential would collapse.

The existence of different Ca^{2+} uptake and release pathways in mitochondria provides a basis for Ca^{2+} cycling. This process continuously utilizes energy that is supplied by the membrane potential. Oxidation of intramitochondrial NAD(P)H can activate the release route and acelerate Ca^{2+} cycling across the mitochondrial membrane (Lehninger et al., 1978). This condition is associated with a decrease in the mitochondrial membrane potential that parallels the rate of Ca^{2+} cycling. Moreover, chelation of extramitochondrial Ca^{2+} with EGTA (ethylene glycol-bis(β-aminoethyl ether)-N,N,N',N'-tetraacetic acid) or inclusion of ruthenium red in the incubation medium, to abolish the reuptake of the released Ca^{2+}, completely prevents the collapse of the membrane potential (Moore et al.,

1983). Evidence that this mechanism is also operational in intact cells has been obtained using cultured hepatocytes loaded with rhodamine 123 and video imaging analysis (Nicotera et al., 1990a).

Cytoskeletal Alterations

One of the early signs of cell injury caused by a variety of toxic agents is the appearance of multiple surface protrusions (blebs) (Jewell et al., 1982). The events leading to bleb formation have not yet been fully elucidated, and several mechanisms may independently contribute to their formation. However, it is generally accepted that a perturbation of cytoskeletal organization and of the interaction between the cytoskeleton and the plasma membrane plays an important role. Evidence for this assumption is provided by the observation that agents which modify the cytoskeleton, such as cytochalasins and phalloidin, stimulate bleb formation and by the demonstration that the bundles of actin microfilaments present at the base of the bleb appear to be totally dissociated from the bleb-forming portion of the plasma membrane (Phelps et al., 1989). The finding that treatment of cells with a Ca^{2+} ionophore was able to induce similar blebbing, and that this was prevented by the omission of Ca^{2+} from the incubation medium, led to the proposal that Ca^{2+} is involved in the cytoskeletal alterations associated with the formation of surface blebs during cell injury (Jewell et al., 1982).

The cytoskeleton is organized into a complex array of fibers, including microfilaments, microtubules, and intermediate filaments. Microfilaments are mainly composed of actin and several actin-binding proteins. Many of the actin-binding proteins require Ca^{2+} to be able to interact with other cytoskeletal constituents. Moreover, Ca^{2+} regulates the function of three actin-binding proteins that are directly involved in the association of microfilaments with the plasma membrane. Among these proteins, α-actinin is involved in the normal organization of actin filaments into regular, parallel arrays. The other two actin-binding proteins, vinculin and actin-binding protein (ABP; in platelets), are substrates for Ca^{2+}-dependent proteases, and an increase in the cytosolic free Ca^{2+} concentration to micromolar levels results in the proteolysis of these two polypeptides.

Evidence for the involvement of Ca^{2+} in the toxic alterations of actin microfilaments and actin-binding proteins has been provided; for example, the incubation of human platelets with menadione resulted in the dissociation of α-actinin from the whole cytoskeleton and the proteolysis of the ABP (Mirabelli et al., 1989). These changes were largely prevented in cells preloaded with intracellular Ca^{2+} chelators. Further, immunocytochemical investigations using anti-α-actinin antibodies and NBD-phallacidin to stain actin, revealed that dissociation of the α-actinin from the actin filaments may be responsible for bleb formation (Bellomo et al., 1990).

Ca^{2+}-Dependent Degradative Enzymes

The catabolism of phospholipids, proteins, and nuclei acids involves enzymes, most of which require Ca^{2+} for activity. Ca^{2+} overload can result in sustained activation of these enzymes and in the degradation of cell constituents, which may ultimately lead to cell death.

Phospholipases are widely distributed in biological membranes and generally required Ca^{2+} for activation. A specific subset of phospholipases, collectively designated phospholipase A_2, have been proposed to function in the detoxication of phospholipid hydroperoxides by releasing fatty acids from peroxidized membranes (Van Kuijk et al., 1991). However, phospholipase activation can also mediate pathophysiological reactions by stimulating membrane breakdown or by generating toxic metabolites. Therefore, phospholipase activation has been proposed as an important mechanism of cell killing under conditions of cellular Ca^{2+} overload. Although a number of studies have indicated that accelerated phospholipid turnover occurs during anoxia or toxic cell injury, the importance of phospholipase activation in the development of cell damage remains to be established.

During the past 10 years, the involvement of nonlysosomal proteolysis in several cell processes has become progressively clear. Proteases with a neutral pH optimum include the ATP- and ubiquitin-dependent proteases and the calcium-dependent proteases, or calpains. Calpains are present in virtually all mammalian cells and appear to be largely associated with membranes in conjunction with a specific inhibitory protein (calpastatin). The extralysosomal localization of this proteolytic system allows the proteases to participate in several specialized cell functions, including cytoskeletal and cell membrane remodeling, receptor cleavage and turnover, enzyme activation, and modulation of cell mitosis. Cellular targets for those enzymes include cytoskeletal elements and membrane integral proteins. Thus, the activation of Ca^{2+} proteases causes modification of microfilaments in platelets and is apparently involved in cell degeneration during muscle dystrophy (see Imahori, 1982, for review). Extensive proteolysis has also been implicated in the development of ischemic injury in nervous tissue (Manev et al., 1990).

Studies from our and other laboratories have suggested the involvement of Ca^{2+}-activated proteases in the toxicity of certain agents in hepatocytes, myocardial cells, and platelets (Nicotera et al., 1990a). Although the substrates for protease activity during cell injury remain largely unidentified, it appears that cytoskeletal proteins may be a major target.

Alterations of Ca^{2+} Signaling

One of the primary consequences of a pathological modification of signal transduction systems can be the loss of the normal Ca^{2+} responses to hormones and growth factors. Several reports have indicated that toxic agent, including metals, can interfere with Ca^{2+} signaling. Thus, it has been found that micromolar $HgCl_2$ concentrations can block specific binding to high-affinity receptor sites in rat brain. Muscarinic (Von Burg et al., 1980) and α-adrenergic (Bondy and Agrawaal, 1980) receptors, whose stimulation couples with phosphatidyl inositol breakdown and Ca^{2+} increase, appear to be particularly sensitive. Recent results in our laboratory have shown that 50 to 300nM $HgCl_2$ can affect the active state of L-type channels in PC12 cells. This reflects in the potentiation of the Ca^{2+} signals caused by certain agonists or during depolarization. Interestingly, this is associated with a potentiation of the differentiation induced by nerve growth factor (NGF) in the PC12 cell line. Increasing the $HgCl_2$ concentration cause instead a modification of the L-type channel at the resting state, which results in Ca^{2+} overload and cell death (Rossi et al., 1993).

Activation of Apoptosis as Consequence of Alterations in Ca^{2+} Signaling

During physiological cell killing, a suicide process is activated in affected cells which is known as "apoptosis" or programmed cell death. Several early morphological changes occur within apoptotic cells, including widespread plasma and nuclear membrane blebbing, compacting of organelles, and chromatin condensation (Arends et al., 1990). The most characteristic marker for this process is the activation of a Ca^{2+}-dependent endonuclease that results in the cleavage of cell chromatin into oligonucleosome-length fragments (Wyllie, 1980). Endonuclease activation has been implicated in the killing of target cells by cytotoxic T lymphocytes and natural killer cells, and in thymocytes exposed to glucocorticoid hormones or to any antibody to the CD3/T cell receptor complex (Nicotera et al., 1990a).

The results of several studies have shown that Ca^{2+} overload can trigger endonuclease activation. The Ca^{2+} ionophore A23187 stimulates apoptosis in thymocytes, and characteristic endonuclease activity in isolated nuclei is dependent on Ca^{2+} (Jones et al., 1989). In addition, Ca^{2+}-mediated endonuclease activation appears to be involved in the cytotoxicity of TCDD and tributyltin in thymocytes (Aw et al., 1990; McConkey et al., 1988). Although Ca^{2+}-dependent endonuclease activation has been most extensively studied in thymocytes, it appears that this process may also be important in a variety of other tissues. Endonuclease activation has been implicated in damage to macrophages by oxidative stress (Waring et al., 1988) and in glutamate neurotoxicity (Kure et al., 1991). More recently, we found that exposure of human adenocarcinoma cells to tumor necrosis factor causes intracellular Ca^{2+} accumulation and endonuclease activation (Bellomo et al., 1992). Interestingly, in many cells the initial Ca^{2+} increase was found in the nucleus. This suggests that selective elevation of the nuclear Ca^{2+} concentration may be sufficient to stimulate DNA fragmentation. However, although the responsible endonuclease requires Ca^{2+} for activity, its regulation appears to be more complex and to involve additional signals.

Summary

It appears safe to conclude that calcium ions play an important role in both toxic cell killing and programmed cell death. Recent research has revealed some of the biochemical mechanisms by which intracellular Ca^{2+} overload can cause cytoxicity. However, the relative importance of the various Ca^{2+}-dependent processes in toxic cell killing needs to be further clarified. Finally, it should be emphasized that cell death can occur without any apparent early change in intracellular Ca^{2+} homeostasis, and that mechanism other than overload are also important in cell killing.

References

Arends MJ, Morros RG, Wyllie AH (1990): Apoptosis – the role of the endonuclease. *Am J Pathol* 136:593–608

Aw TY, Nicotera P, Manzo L, Orrenius S (1990): Tributyltin stimulates apoptosis in rat thymocytes. *Arch Biochem Biophys* 283:46–50

Barritt GJ, Parker JC, Wadsworth JC (1981): A kinetic analysis of the effect of adrenalin on calcium distribution in isolated rat liver parenchymal cells. *J Physiol* 312:29–55

Bellomo G, Mirabelli F, Richelmi P, Malorni W, Iosi F, Orrenius S (1990): The cytoskeleton as a target in quinone toxicity. *Free Radical Res Commun* 8:391–399

Bellomo G, Perotti M, Taddei F, Mirabelli F, Finardi G, Nicotera P, Orrenius S

(1992): Tumor necrosis factor α induces apoptosis in mammary adenocarcinoma cells by an increase in intranuclear free Ca^{2+} concentration and DNA fragmentation. *Cancer Res* 52:1342–1346

Berke G (1989): The cytolytic T lymphocyte and its mode of action. *Immunol Lett* 20:169–178

Berridge MJ (1987): Inositol trisphosphate and diacylgycerol: two interacting second messengers. *J Biol Chem* 56:159–193

Berridge MJ (1990): Calcium oscillations. *J Biol Chem* 265:9583–9586

Bondy SC, Agrawal AK (1980): The inhibition of cerebral high affinity receptor sites by lead and mercury compounds. *Arch Toxicol* 46:249–256

Carafoli E (1989): Intracellular Ca^{2+} homeostasis. *Annu Rev Biochem* 56:395–433

Caspar M, Florin I, Thelestam M (1987): Calcium and calmodulin in cellular intoxication with clostridium difficile toxin B. *J Cell Physiol* 132:168–172

Dreyer EB, Kaiser PK, Offerman JT, Lipton SA (1990): HIV-1 coat protein neurotoxicity prevented by calcium channel antagonists. *Science* 248:364–367

Farrell GC, Duddy SK, Kass GE, Llopis, J, Gahm A, Orrenius S (1990): Release of Ca^{2+} from the endoplasmic reticulum is not the mechanism for bile acid-induced cholestasis and hepatotoxicity in the intact rat liver. *J Clin Invest* 85:1255–1259

Fleckenstein A, Frey M, Fleckenstein-Grün G (1983): Cellular injury by cytosolic calcium overload and its prevention by calcium antagonists – a new principle of tissue protection. In: *Mechanisms of Hepatocyte Injury and Death*, Keppler D, Popper H, Bianchi L, et al., eds., pp. 321–335. Lancaster: MTP Press Limited

Gunther TE, Pfeiffer DR (1990): Mechanisms by which mitochondria transport calcium. *Am J Physiol* 258:c755–786

Imahori K (1982): Calcium-dependent neutral protease: its characterization and regulation. In: *Calcium and Cell Function*, Cheung WY, ed., Vol. III. Orlando: Academic Press

Jewell SA, Bellomo G, Thor H, Orrenius S, Smith MT (1982): Bleb formation in hepatocytes during drug metabolism is caused by disturbances in thiol and calcium ion homeostasis. *Science* 217:1257–1259

Jones DP, McConkey DJ, Nicotera P, Orrenius S (1989): Calcium-activated DNA fragmentation in rat liver nuclei. *J Biol Chem* 264:6398–6403

Kass GEN, Duddy SK, Moore GA, Orrenius S (1989): Di-(*tert*-butyl)-1,4-benzohydroquinone rapidly elevates cytosolic Ca^{2+} concentration by mobilizing the inositol 1,4,5-trisphosphate-sensitive Ca^{2+} pool. *J Biol Chem* 264:15192

Komulainen H, Bondy SC (1988): Increased free intracellular Ca^{2+} by toxic agents: an index of potential neurotoxicity? *Trends Pharmacol Sci* 9:154–156

Kure S, Tominaga T, Yoshimoto T, Tada K, Narisawa K (1991): Glutumate triggers internucleosomal DNA cleavage in neuronal cells. *Biochem Biophys Res Commun* 179:39–45

Lehninger AL, Vercesi A, Bababunmi EA (1978): Regulation of Ca^{2+} release from mitochondria by the oxidation-reduction state of pyridine nucleotides. *Proc Natl Acad Sci USA* 75:1690–1694

Manev H, Costa E, Wroblewski JT, Guidotti A (1990): Abusive stimulation of excitatory amino acid receptors: a strategy to limit neurotoxicity. *FASEB J* 4:2789–2797

McConkey DJ, Chow SC, Orrenius S, Jondal M (1990): NK cell-induced cytotoxicity is dependent on a Ca^{2+} increase in the target. *FASEB J* 4:2661–2664

McConkey DJ, Hartzell P, Duddy SK, Håkansson H, Orrenius S (1988): 2,3,7,8-

Tetrachlorodibenzo-*p*-dioxin kills immature thymocytes by Ca^{2+}-mediated endonuclease activation. *Science* 242:256–258

McConkey DJ, Nicotera P, Hartzell P, Bellomo G, Wyllie AH, Orrenius S (1989): Glucocorticoids activate a suicide process in thymocytes through an elevation of cytosolic Ca^{2+} concentration. *Arch Biochem Biophys* 269:365–370

Mirabelli F, Salis A, Vairetti M, Bellomo G, Thor H, Orrenius S (1989): Cytoskeletal alterations in human platelets exposed to oxidative stress are mediated by oxidative and Ca^{2+}-dependent mechanisms. *Arch Biochem Biophys* 270:478–488

Moore GA, Jewell SA, Bellomo G, Orrenius S (1983): On the relationship between Ca^{2+} efflux and membrane damage during *tert*-butyl hydroperoxide metabolism by liver motochondira. *FEBS Lett* 153:289–292

Nicotera P, McConkey DJ, Jones DP, Orrenius S (1989a): ATP stimulates Ca^{2+} uptake and increases the free Ca^{2+} concentration in isolated liver nuclei. *Proc Natl Acad Sci USA* 86:453–57

Nicotera P, Rundgren M, Porubek DJ, Cotgreave I, Moldeus P, Orrenius S, Nelson SD (1989b): On the role of Ca^{2+} in the toxicity of alkylating and oxidizing quinone imines in isolated hepatocytes. *Chem Res Toxicol* 2:46–50

Nicotera P, Bellomo G, Orrenius S (1990a): The role of Ca^{2+} in cell killing. *Chem Res Toxicol* 3:484–494

Nicotera P, Orrenius S, Nilsson T, Berggren P-O (1990b): An inositol 1,4,5-trisphosphate-sensitive Ca^{2+} pool in liver nuclei. *Proc Natl Acad Sci USA* 87:6858–6862

Orrenius S, McConkey DJ, Bellomo G, Nicotera P (1989): Role of Ca^{2+} in toxic cell killing. *Trends Pharmacol Sci* 10:281–285

Phelps PC, Smith MW, Trump BF (1989): Cytosolic ionized calcium and bleb formation after acute cell injury of cultured rabbit renal tubule cells. *Lab Invest* 60:630–642

Rossi AD, Larsson O, Manzo L, Orrenius S, Vahter M, Berggren P-O, Nicotera P (1993): Modifications of Ca^{2+} signalling by inorganic mercury in PC12 cells. *FASEB J* 7:1507:1514

Schanne FAX, Kane AB, Young EE, Farber JL (1979): Calcium dependence of toxic cell death: a final common pathway. *Science* 206:700–702

Somylo AP, Bond M, Somylo AV (1985): Calcium content of mitochondria and endoplasmic reticulum in liver frozen rapidly in vivo. *Nature* 314:622–625

Van Kuijk FJGM, Sevanian A, Handleman GJ, Dratz EA (1991): A new role for phospholipase A2: protection of membrane from lipid peroxidation damage. *Trends Biochem Sci* 12:31–34

Von Burg R, Northington FK, Shamoo A (1980): Methylmercury inhibition of rat brain muscarinic receptors. *Toxicol Appl Pharmacol* 53:285–292

Waring P, Eichner RD, Mullbacher A, Sjaarda A (1988): Gliotoxin induced apoptosis in macrophages unrelated to its antiphagocytic properties. *Science* 263:18493–18499

Woods NM, Cuthbertson KSR, Cobbold PE (1986): Repetitive transient rises in cytoplasmic free calcium in hormone-stimulated hepatozytes. *Nature* 319:600–602

Wyllie AG (1980): Glucocorticoid-induced thymocyte apoptosis is associated with endogenous endonuclease activation. *Nature* 284:555–556

10

Discussion: Session 5 – 8 P.M. – 8 February 1993

RECORDED BY PETER RIEDERER AND MOUSSA B.H. YOUDIM

After Olanow's paper, Baimbridge (Vancouver) asked why manganese intoxication as a pallidal disease is not a hyperkinetic movement disorder. Olanow said that if the dorsal pallidum is involved, hypokinesia appears.

Calne raised the issue of early manganese patients and the problem of a dose relationship in the nigrostriatal system with regard to dopamine depletion. Olanow answered that dopamine depletion as result of manganese intoxication has been described. He pointed out that manganese intoxicates the pallidum first while substantia nigra is involved later and to a lesser extent.

Koller (Kansas) wondered that while he had substantial experience with atypical parkinsonian patients, he was not aware of any "manganese parkinsonism." Olanow said that there are only occupational case reports. Studies on low-level toxins, especially manganese, are rare while in high-level manganese patients the syndrome looks like atypical parkinsonism. MRI studies can discriminate both. While atypical parkinsonism shows signal hypointensity in putamen on T_2-weighted scans, in manganese intoxication the signal is hyperintense in the putamen on T_1-weighted scans.

The chairman mentioned two patients with gait disturbances and asked whether this might result from damage of the motor cortex. If this occurs the (motor) cortex cannot be stimulated by using transcranial stimulation technique. These early gait disturbances in conjunction with extrapyramidal gait disturbances make it difficult to detect pyramidal disturbances. Therefore, there should be a more diffuse lesion than you see at the moment. Olanow and Perl mentioned no changes in the motor cortex and that the pathology is confined to the regions described.

The question whether manganese opens the blood–brain barrier has been addressed in Olanow's lecture. Whether these observations are

similar to those described by Youdim and colleagues for phenothiazine-
and butyrophonone-induced iron uptake across the blood–brain barrier
and its deposition in the pallidum remains to be elucidated in further
studies (Olanow).

Youdim said that manganese depletes glutathione (GSH) thus
leading to oxidative stress and depletion of iron. Olanow answered that
any mitochondrial damage depletes GSH.

Mizuno mentioned a paper by Martin from 1950 indicating dystonic
flexion posture (DFP) in patients with pallidal lesion. He wondered if
DFP occurs in Olanow's patients described here. In a second question
Mizuno asked what may be the mechanism for high signal intensity of T_1-
weighted images in manganese patients. Olanow speculated that iron
might be a candidate to be discussed here.

Riederer asked whether respiratory chain enzymes are changed in
manganese patients and whether iron is exchanged by manganese in such
enzymes. Olanow said that such experiments are missing so far.

Reichmann asked whether the patients feel better after removal of
manganese. Olanow said that the patients removed from the source of
intoxication stay the same or do better. While animals worsen after each
injection, many patients show a slow deterioration after years when they
were exposed to high concentrations of low-particle manganese.

The question whether manganese intoxication is the result of a special
and regional blood-brain barrier disturbance (Perl) or not (Olanow)
could not be solved.

After Youdim's paper Orrenius asked about the origin of nitrogen
oxide (NO) and whether it is generated from neurons or from extraneuronal cells. Youdim said that it seems to come from either of these and that
there is the suggestion that it is connected to the glutamatergic system,
which in the striatum makes contact to the dopaminergic nerve endings.
By this NO has to penetrate only a small distance to be toxic at
dopaminergic nerve terminals. Orrenius mentioned that NO release
might then be the result of an increase of calcium. Youdim agreed with
that.

Olanow then raised the question whether any toxin to the cell has a
capacity to potentially degrade ferritin and release iron. Youdim stated
that there are not too many toxins having the capacity to release iron as 6-
hydroxy-dopamine. Further studies are required to get a better insight
into this problem (Youdim), and especially studies are needed to show
that the iron released is reactive iron (Olanow). Youdim mentioned the
toxicity of 6-hydroxydopamine and NO and that both intoxications could
be blocked by iron-chelators, indicating that reactive iron causes both
intoxications. In Parkinson's disease this is not as clear, but as Perl stain

does not stain ferritin iron it seems that again reactive iron is seen with this method (Youdim).

Calne mentioned that by using Perl stain or MRI a lot of iron is seen in the red nucleus (RN). He regarded this as being important because no cells are dying in the RN (as is the case in the globus pallidus and dentate nucleus (Youdim). But if the concept is true that iron really is driving cell death, this should occur in a number of brain regions and not only in the substantia nigra (SN). Youdim said that decompartmentalisation of iron in the SN seems to be connected to the special "biochemistry" of this brain region (neuromelanin, catecholamines etc.) and that other complementary reactions such as NO release should not be underestimated in this regard. Also a selective iron transport to the SN seems possible according to Youdim's studies with neuroleptics, which (except clozapine) transport iron selectively to the globus pallidus.

Perl raised the question about the cells that contain iron. Youdim said that macrophages and glial cells especially contain iron but that it is also seen in neurons. Perl mentioned his own study indicating that both iron and aluminium have been detected in the neuromelanin of PD-SN. Aluminium potentiates the toxicity of iron significantly.

After Hibbs' paper, Youdim raised the point that "killers" seem to survive and he wanted to know how macrophages defend themselves against NO. Further, he said that NO has so many functions and that it is not clear why it is beneficial in one cell type and deleterious in another. Hibbs answered that NO is important for all organisms and that it is unique as a messenger molecule. NO differs from other messengers because it is a gas, has a short half-life, permeates membranes easily, and is very reactive, for example, with iron.

Riederer raised the question whether in pathological conditions like Parkinson's disease, in which a disturbed iron and calcium metabolism and homeostasis, respectively, can be detected, NO synthesis is expected to be enhanced or reduced. Hibbs pointed out that this is hard to predict for this disease. But in the ischemica reperfusion oxygen increases. This causes an increase of intracellular calcium and NO. NO is extremely reactive and damages cells leading finally to cell death. In general, if calcium homeostasis is disturbed, NO is disregulated.

Reichmann wanted to know whether NO plays a role in brain tumors, which show increased glycolytic activity, while the mitochondrial activity including all complexes of the respiratory chain decreases. (As an answer could not be found this issue seems to be worth to be followed in upcoming studies.)

Nagatsu raised the question about the role of tetrahydrobiopterin (BH_4) as a cofactor of NO synthase. On the other hand calmoduline housekeeping enzyme does not require BH_4. Hibbs said that BH_4 is necessary for both enzymes and that NO synthase requires a number of cofactors/cosubstrates.

Olanow said that SOD which is enhanced in Parkinson's disease might be protective for cells because it could form peroxynitrate. After Orrenius paper Youdim asked whether heat-inactivated serum has the same effect, namely killing cells. Orrenius said that this is not the case, indicating that there must be something bioactive (Youdim).

There was a question about evidences for apoptosis in age-related and neurodegenerative processes and whether under such circumstances DNA fragmentation occurs or fine structural information exists. Orrenius said that there is little evidence for this at this time. Evidence for killing of neuronal cells by apoptotic mechanisms comes from experiments with mercury. Here low concentrations disturb calcium homeostasis of neuronal cells, leading to apoptotic cell killing. Also glutamatergic toxicity in diaphorase positive neurons may occur by apoptotic cell killing, and DNA fragmentation is probable.

Nagatsu said that MPTP kills nigrostriatal dopamine neurons by apoptosis and DNA fragmentation has been demonstrated. Orrenius mentioned that DNA fragmentation is probable if MPTP leads to a perturbation of calcium.

Baimbridge raised the issue of early neurodegeneration, starting at birth, and Calne hypothesized that people might be born with a low nigral neuron number because of excessive apoptosis during neurodevelopment. If this is the case, PET studies should be able to show this in the normal population. Baimbridge said that there are no double peaks in normals.

Calne said that the tools are extremely limited in cell cultures as cell death is very slow in neurological diseases. Orrenius agreed in this. There is a time lag between the initial signal and cell killing from about 0.5 hours to days or longer depending on the cell system. Oxidative stress undergoes a dose–response relationship. Oxidative stress causes first proliferation (stimulation of cell growth), then apoptotic cell killing, and finally necrotic cell killing.

Nagatsu said that intracellular increase of calcium causes increase in calpain and cell death follows. Inhibition of calpain inhibits cell death.

Part III

ENERGY METABOLISM AND NEUROTOXINS

11

Mitochondrial Dysfunction, Aging, and Huntington's Disease

M. Flint Beal

An essential feature of neurodegenerative diseases is their delayed onset and relentless inexorable progression. The most important risk factor for Alzheimer's disease is advancing age. Huntington's disease typically has a onset in the thirties and forties. A number of studies show age-dependent increases in mitochondrial DNA deletions, oxidative damage to mitochondrial DNA, and reductions in activities of mitochondrial enzymes.

Structure and Function of Mitochondria

Mitochondria vary widely in size, shape, and number in differing cell types (Hatefi, 1985; Wallace, 1986). Each mitochondrion has an outer membrane, which is freely permeable to large molecules and surrounds the mitochondrion, and an inner membrane that is relatively impermeable and contains the electron transport chain enzyme complexes. The inner compartment of the mitochondrion, enclosed by the inner membrane, is the matrix in which the Kreb's cycle takes place. Reduced nicotinamide adenine dinucleotide (NADH) and reduced flavin adenine dinucleotide ($FADH_2$) generated from the Kreb's cycle donate electrons that are carried through the series of transport enzymes (complexes I–IV) of the inner mitochondrial membrane (Fig. 1). Concomitantly, ejection of protons across the inner mitochondrial membrane results in an electrochemical proton gradient, which stores potential energy that is then converted to adenosine triphosphate (ATP) by ATP synthase (complex V), the last enzyme complex involved in oxidative phosphorylation. Oxidative phosphorylation is the coupling of the transfer of reducing equivalents (electrons) to oxygen with the synthesis of ATP.

The oxidative phosphorylation system consists of a complex array of enzymes (Hatefi, 1985; Wallace, 1986). Complex I (NADH-ubiquinone

ADVANCES IN RESEARCH ON NEURODEGENERATION, II
Y. Mizuno et al.
© 1994 Birkhäuser Boston

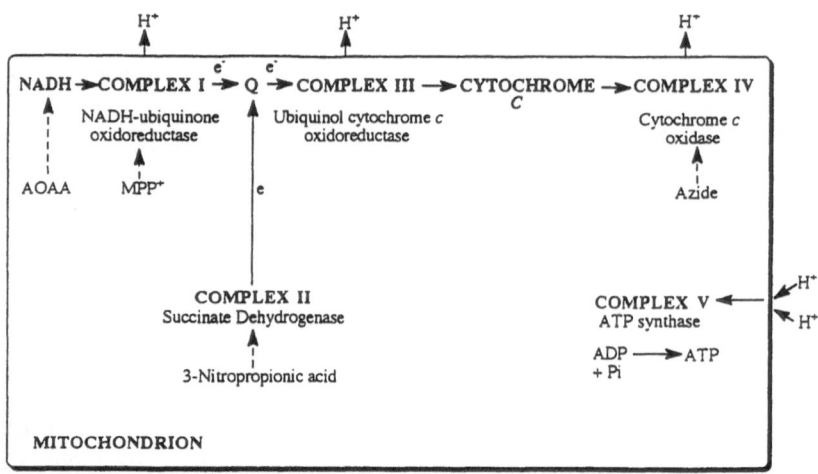

Figure 1. Schematic diagram of oxidative phosphorylation shows sites at which mitochondrial inhibitors act.

reductase), the main entrance to the electron transport chain, is composed of 26 subunits, 7 of which are encoded by mitochondrial DNA. Complex II (succinate ubiquinol oxidoreductase), another entrance to the electron transport unit, consists of 5 subunits of which all are nuclear encoded. Complex III (ubiquinol cytochrome c oxidoreductase) has 11 subunits with 1 (cytochrome b) that is encoded by mitochondrial DNA. Complex IV (cytochrome c oxidase) is composed of 13 subunits, with 3 encoded by mitochondrial DNA; complex V (ATP synthase) is composed of 12 subunits with 2 mitochondrially encoded subunits.

Effects of Aging on Mitochondrial Energy Metabolism

One theory to account for age-dependent onset of degenerative diseases such as Alzheimer's disease (AD) and Huntington's disease is that mitochondrial dysfunction may hasten neuronal death (Linnane et al., 1989; Miquel, 1991; Wallace, 1992). It has been proposed that the accumulation of mitochondrial genome mutations during life results in a progressive impairment of oxidative phosphorylation. The rate of mutations in mitochondrial DNA is about 10 fold greater than that in chromosomal DNA (Linnane et al., 1989). A high rate of mutation has been suggested by extensive restriction fragment polymorphism among individual human beings (Brown et al., 1979). Further, mutations in mitochondrial DNA are more likely to have functional consequences because mitochondrial DNA has no noncoding sequences, except for a small segment involved in the replication of mitochondrial DNA. There also appear to be limited repair mechanisms for mitochondrial DNA (Clayton et al., 1974). Mitochondrial DNA may be particularly susceptible to damage because of its lack of protective histones and its close proximity to the inner mitochondrial membrane where reactive oxygen species are generated (Linnane et al., 1989; Micquel, 1991; Wallace, 1992).

Recent studies have demonstrated the presence of an age-dependent deletion between nucleotide positions 8470 and 13459 of the mitochondrial genome (Cortopassi and Arnheim, Linnane et al., 1990; Simonetta et al., 1992). In the heart, the deletion, which has been detected in individuals starting at age 30, increases exponentially with advancing age (Corral-Debrinski et al., 1991; Hattori et al., 1991). A recent quantitative study showed that the deletion was estimated at 3% and 9% in patients of ages 80 and 90 years, respectively (Sugiyama et al., 1991). Further, deletions are much more frequent in patients with ischemic heart disease (Corral-Debrinski et al., 1991). We and others have recently shown that there are marked increases in the deletion in human postmortem brain tissue with normal aging (Corral-Debrinski et al., 1992; Soong et al., 1992). This finding is consistent with the suggestion that patients with defects in oxidative phosphorylation generate increased amounts of oxygen free radicals that result in mitochondrial DNA damage (Linnane et al., 1989). Mitochondrial oxidative phosphorylation generates most of the free radicals in the cell, and mitochondrial DNA is particularly susceptible to oxidative damage (Richter et al., 1988). The respiratory chain components that make the greatest contribution to production of free radicals are ubiquinone and cytochrome b_{566} of complex III (Nohl et al., 1978). An increase in production of superoxide radicals by cytochrome b_{566} occurs with normal aging (Nohl, 1986).

Recent studies show that 8-hydroxy-2-deoxyguanosine is a biomarker of oxidative DNA damage (Shigenaga et al., 1990). Of 13 base adducts formed after exposing purified mammalian chromatin to ionizing radiation-generated free radicals, 8-hydroxy-2-deoxyguanosine is the most frequent (Dizdaroglu, 1991). Several studies indicate that 8-hydroxy-2-deoxyguanosine most frequently codes correctly for cytosine, but also has the monospecific mutagenic ability to pair with adenine about 1% of the time (Cheng et al., 1992; Kuchino et al., 1987; Shibutani et al., 1991; Wood et al., 1990). It also results in misreading at adjacent residues (Kuchino et al., 1987). Inhibitors of the electron transport chain increase the amount of 8-hydroxy-2-deoxyguanosine in mitochondrial DNA (Hayakawa et al., 1991a). Concentrations of 8-hydroxy-2-deoxyguanosine increase with normal aging in several rat tissues and in mitochondrial DNA isolated from human diaphragm and heart muscle

(Fraga et al., 1990; Hayakawa et al., 1991b; 1992). In heart muscle, the amount of mitochondrial deletions correlates with 8-hydroxy-2-deoxy-guanosine concentrations in mitochondrial DNA (Hayakawa et al., 1992). It is possible that these changes may be exacerbated in AD because there are reports of impaired DNA repair in lymphoblasts of AD patients (Robinson et al., 1987).

Several studies have shown a reduction in capacity for oxidative phosphorylation with normal aging in both animal and human tissues. In aged rat brain, variable results have been obtained, but the activity of complex IV appears to reduced (Curti et al., 1990). In rat brain, there are age-dependent decreases in mitochondrial respiration with complex I substrates but not with complex II substrates (Harmon et al., 1987). A study of aged rat muscle showed the activities of complex I and complex IV were reduced, but the activity of complex II–III was unchanged (Torri et al., 1992). The numbers of cytochrome c oxidase-deficient cardiomyo-cytes in the human heart increases with aging (Muller-Hocker, 1989). A study of muscle biopsies in 29 subjects between ages 16 and 92 showed a significant negative correlation between activated mitochondrial respira-tion rates and age with all substrates tested (Trounce et al., 1989). Similar observations were made in human liver biopsy samples (Yen et al., 1989).

In a recent study of human muscle biopsies, the activities of complex I and complex IV were decreased while complex II–III activity was unaffected (Cooper et al., 1992). The decrease in activity in skeletal muscle is not associated with decreases in respiratory chain protein content, suggesting that it is not caused by impaired mitochondrial DNA transcription or translation (Byrne et al., 1991). Metabolic studies of oxygen utilization in human skeletal muscle and brain have also confirmed a decline with normal aging (Astrand et al., 1973; Pantano et al., 1984). The results of prior studies indicate that complex I and complex IV in brain and muscle may be particularly vulnerable to age-dependent decreases in activity, while complex II–III activity is relatively preserved. The finding of an age-related decline in complex I and complex IV activities is consistent with damage to mitochondrial DNA because it encodes 7 subunits of complex 1 and 3 subunits of complex IV, whereas complex II is encoded exclusively by nuclear DNA (Wallace, 1992).

We have carried out studies of electron transport chain enzymes in cerebral cortex obtained from rhesus monkeys (*Macaca mulatta*) ranging in age over the life span of this species (Bowling et al., 1993). Frontopar-ietal cortex was obtained from 20 rhesus monkeys who were divided into three groups: group 1 (mean $\pm$ SEM $= 6.9 \pm 0.9$ years; $n = 7$, 4 male, 3 female); group II (22.5 ± 0.9 years; $n = 6$, 4 male, 2 female); group III (30.7 ± 0.9 years; $n = 7$, 2 male, 5 female). Crude mitochondrial preparations were obtained from approximately 1 g of frontoparietal cortex by applying the P_2 pellet to a discontinuous Ficoll gradient. Enzymes were assayed spectrophotometrically by minor modifications of established procedures for complex I (Hatefi and Stiggal, 1978), complex II–III (Zheng et al., 1989), complex IV (Darley-Usmar et al., 1987), complex V (Darley-Usmar et al., 1987), and citrate synthase (Shepherd and Garland, 1969). The data were analyzed by two statistical methods. First, linear regression analysis was employed to determine correlation of age with enzyme activity. Second, differences in activity between the groups were determined by analysis of variance followed by Fisher's PLSD post hoc test.

Although analysis of enzyme activities (expressed as nmol/min/mg protein) showed neither correlations with age by linear regression analysis nor any differences between the three age by linear regression analysis nor any differences between the three age groups, citrate synthase activity and some of the oxidative phosphorylation enzyme activities showed significant negative correlations with protein concentration (r values of -0.87, -0.67, -0.70, -0.23, and -0.70 for complex I, complex II–III, complex IV, complex V, and citrate synthase, respectively). This effect did not appear to be caused by an endogenous inhibitor or lack of linearity of activity with protein concentration because several enzymes were affected and enzyme activities were linear with protein concentration for individual samples. There was no significant correlation of age with protein concentration ($r = 0.06$). It was assumed that this correlation of enzyme activities with protein concentration resulted from a lower mitochondrial enrichment in samples that initially contained more tissue. Larger amounts of tissue may reduce the effectiveness of the differential centrifugation or the Ficoll gradient.

Because it appeared that the samples exhibited variable degrees of mitochondrial enrichment, the activities of the oxidative phosphorylation enzymes present in each sample were "corrected" by dividing the enzyme activity of citrate synthase, a well-accepted mitochondrial matrix marker. When these citrate synthase-corrected activities were analyzed, linear regression analysis demonstrated a significant negative correlation of complex I ($p < .002$) and complex IV ($p < .03$) with age, but no significant correlation was obtained with complex II–III or complex V. Complex I activity was reduced by 13% in group II ($p < .05$) and by 22% in group III relative to group 1 ($p < .01$). In addition, relative to group I, complex IV activity exhibited nonsignificant reductions of 21% in group II ($p = .11$) and 22% in group III ($p = .08$). These findings show an age-associated progressive impairment of mitochondrial complex I and complex IV activities in cerebral cortices of primates.

Evidence for Impaired Energy Metabolism in Huntington's Disease

The largest body of evidence suggesting an impairment of energy metabolism has come from studies of glucose metabolism using positron emission tomography. The major difficulty with these studies is that it is difficult to determine whether changes play a role in the disease process or are merely secondary. In Huntington's disease (HD) there is a decrease in glucose utilization in the caudate and putamen, and the hypometabolism appears early and precedes bulk tissue loss (Kuhl et al., 1990). In a study of asymptomatic patients at risk for HD, 31% showed bilaterally reduced glucose metabolism (Mazziotta et al., 1987). Of 8 asymptomatic persons at risk who had positive DNA polymorphisms, 3 of the 8 showed glucose metabolism 2 SD below controls, while the remaining persons showed reduced glucose metabolism 1–2 SD below controls (Hayden et al., 1987). In a similar study, 15 to 20 patients (75%) with a positive test had reduced caudate metabolism (Grafton et al., 1990). Recent studies documented reduced glucose metabolism in cerebral cortex as compared with normal controls (Kuwert et al., 1990; Martin et al., 1992). The degree of dementia was significantly correlated with the reductions in cortical glucose utilization.

Biochemical studies have shown reduced pyruvate dehydrogenase and succinate dehydrogenase activity in the basal ganglia in HD, but not in other brain regions (Butterworth et al., 1985; Sorbi et al., 1983). Decreased complex II/III activity has been reported in the caudate but not in the putamen or cortex (Mann et al., 1990). A decrease in complex I activity in platelets was reported in patients with HD, but not in family members at risk for HD (Parker et al., 1990). In the caudate nucleus, a significant reduction in cytochrome oxidase activity and cytochrome aa_3 were found, whereas cytochromes b and cc_1 were normal (Brennan et al., 1985). Ultrastructural studies of cortical biopsies from patients with both juvenile and adult-onset HD have shown abnormal mitochondria (Goebel et al., 1978; Tellez-Nagel et al., 1974). One patient was reported with clinical manifestations resembling HD (but no family history of the illness) who had abnormal "tweed ball mitochondria" on skin biopsy (Lewitt et al., 1989).

We have recently obtained direct evidence for a defect in oxidative phosphorylation in HD (Koroshetz et al., 1992). We performed magnetic resonance spectroscopy in 16 HD and 12 control patients. We observed elevated lactate concentrations in the occipital cortex of 16 of 16 HD patients. More recent studies showed consistent lactate increases in the basal ganglia in 8 patients. Concentrations were increased about three-fold as compared with controls, and were significantly correlated with duration of disease. In addition, preliminary studies of lactate:pyruvate ratios in the cerebrospinal fluid (CSF) of HD patients show an increase as compared with normal controls (Beal and Koroshetz, unpublished findings). We therefore have obtained the first direct *in vivo* evidence for a defect in oxidative phosphorylation in HD.

Effects of Inhibitors of Mitochondrial Energy Metabolism in Experimental Animals and Man

There have been scattered reports of striatal lesions with metabolic inhibitors for many years. About 50 years ago, Hurst (1942) examined the effects of several different metabolic toxins on the central nervous system in monkeys. He noted that repeated doses of potassium cyanide would produce severe bilateral lesions in the basal ganglia as well as areas of necrosis in the white matter. Sodium azide was also found to produce bilateral necrotic lesions in the basal ganglia, with the caudate affected more than the globus pallidus. Bilateral striatal lesions in rats were produced with sodium azide by Hicks (1950) and by Miyoshi (1967).

Hurst noted that azide administration to monkeys resulted in "attacks" of abnormal movements (Hurst, 1942). This was subsequently investigated further by Mettler (1972), who found that intramuscular injections of sodium azide for 8 to 10 weeks to monkeys produced episodic variable dyskinesia. This dyskinesia was characterized as choreoathetosis. Histologically there were symmetrical lesions in the putamen and retrograde changes in the substantia nigra.

Additional evidence that some toxins cause lesions largely confined to the basal ganglia comes from studies of the plant-derived toxin 3-nitropropionic acid. This compound causes a variety of motor disturbances in livestock. It also caused putaminal necrosis and delayed dystonia in Chinese children, where it has been found as a fungal contaminant of sugar cane (Ludolph et al., 1991b). It is an irreversible inhibitor of succinate dehydrogenase, and therefore will interfere with the tricarboxylic acid cycle, as well as with complex II of mitochondrial respiration. In mice and rats large doses have been shown to produce a symmetrical striatal degeneration (Gould and Gustine, 1982; Hamilton and Gould, 1987). The neuronal degeneration was characterized by swollen cell processes and neurons, similar to changes observed with excitotoxins. *In vitro* studies have shown that 3-nitropropionic acid toxicity can be partially blocked with kynurenic acid (Ludolph et al., 1991a). These studies therefore show that inhibitors of mitochondrial energy metabolism can produce selective striatal lesions in both experimental animals and in man.

Role of Mitochondrial Dysfunction in Producing Excitotoxin Lesions In Vivo

Mitochondria are essential to the cell for maintaining the normal voltage gradient across the cell membrane as well as a number of processes controlling intracellular calcium. An impairment of energy metabolism with reduced adenosine triphosphate (ATP) levels leads to several consequences (Blaustein, 1988; Choi, 1988). Impairment of normal sodium–potassium adenosine triphosphatase function depolarizes cell membranes, which permits intracellular sodium accumulation. This can relieve the voltage-dependent Mg^{2+} block of N-methyl-D-aspartate (NMDA) channels, cause the opening of voltage-dependent calcium channels and reverse the sodium–calcium antiport system, such that calcium enters the cell as sodium is extruded. This would prevent ATP-dependent extrusion of calcium and the storage of excess intracellular calcium in the endoplasmic reticulum by ATP-dependent mechanisms. The mitochondria also contain a high-capacity uniport mechanism for calcium uptake, which relies on the potential across the inner mitochondrial membrane to transport calcium internally. The intramitochondrial calcium levels can be regulated by an antiport system exchanging 2 sodium ions for 1 calcium ion. ATP is also necessary for high-affinity reuptake of glutamate by glial cells.

In cultured neurons, inhibitors of oxidative phosphorylation or of the sodium–potassium pump allow subtoxic amounts of NMDA or glutamate to become neurotoxic (Novelli et al., 1988). Depolarization and ischemia also result in enhancement of NMDA receptor-mediated neurotoxicity in the hippocampal slice (Vornov and Coyle, 1991). This presumably results from a reduction in resting membrane potential (above -60 to -30 mV), which is then insufficient to maintain the voltage-dependent Mg^{2+} block of the NMDA receptor leading to persistent receptor activation. Consistent with this notion, Olney and colleagues found that depolarization of chick retina with potassium produced a lesion that histologically resembled an excitotoxic lesion (Olney et al., 1986), and potassium channel activators can prevent excitotoxicity *in vitro* (Abele and Miller, 1990). Recent work in chicken retina showed that both chemically induced hypoglycemia and blockers of electron transport (potassium cyanide) resulted in excitotoxic lesions blockable with NMDA antagonists that were not accompanied by increases in glutamate release (Zeevalk and Nicklas, 1990). Graded titration of membrane potential with potassium mimicked the toxicity produced with graded metabolic inhibition (Zeevalk and Nicklas, 1991). These results indicate that ambient glutamate can cause excitotoxic damage if intracellular energy metabolism is compromised. Electrophysiological studies in both hippocampus and neocortex show that there is sufficient ambient glutamate to tonically activate NMDA receptors (Sah et al., 1989).

Aminooxyacetic Acid Lesions

We have recently obtained the first *in vivo* findings that inhibitors of oxidative phosphorylation produce secondary excitotoxic lesions. We initially studied aminooxyacetic acid (AOAA), which is an inhibitor of enzymes utilizing pyridoxal phosphate as a cofactor. Aminooxyacetic acid is a potent inhibitor of aspartate transaminase, which is an essential component of the malate–aspartate shunt across mitochondrial membranes (Cheeseman and Clark, 1988). In 1951, Lehninger demonstrated that intact rat liver mitochondria are unable to oxidize externally added NADH. It is now generally accepted that oxidation of NADH from the cytoplasm is accomplished by transport of reducing equivalents from the cytoplasm to the mitochondria. The malate–aspartate shunt is the predominant shuttle in the brain. A block of aspartate aminotransferase with AOAA in both brain slices and synaptosomes results in decreased oxygen consumption, decreased glucose and pyruvate oxidation, and an increase in NADH/NAD in the cytosol (Cheeseman and Clark, 1988; Kauppinen et al., 1987).

We found that AOAA produces excitotoxin lesions *in vivo* that can be blocked by NMDA antagonists or prior decortication, removing the striatal glutamate input (Beal et al., 1991). Electrophysiological studies showed that AOAA does not directly activate ligand-gated ion channels in cultured cortical or striatal neurons (Beal et al., 1991). Lesions with AOAA produced marked sparing of NADPH-diaphorase and large neurons, which was more striking than that we have seen with NMDA agonists. The lesions therefore closely resemble HD. We used the freeze-clamp procedure to directly measure the effects of AOAA on lactate and ATP following intrastriatal injections (Beal et al., 1991). The injections resulted in fourfold increases in lactate and 50% depletions of ATP levels. AOAA therefore appears to cause excitotoxic lesions *in vivo* by impairing mitochondrial energy metabolism. Consistent with this possibility, pentobarbital anesthesia, which reduces brain energy requirement, attenuated the size of the lesions as well as the reductions in ATP and the increases in lactate.

MPP⁺ Lesions

We have also examined the effects of MPP$^+$ in rat striatum (Storey et al., 1992). Using freeze-clamp and microwave sacrifice there were marked increases in lactate and depletions of ATP in the striatum to 48 hours after the injections. This finding was also confirmed using water-suppressed proton chemical shift magnetic resonance imaging at 3 hours after injections. MPP$^+$ produced dose-dependent depletions of dopamine, serotonin, γ-amino butyric acid (GABA), and substance P that were partially blocked at 1 week by prior decortication or completely blocked by MK-801 at 24 hours. Both neurochemical measurements and somatostatin immunocytochemistry showed relative sparing of somatostatin-neuropeptide Y neurons, consistent with an NMDA receptor excitotoxic process. These findings show that specific blockers of mitochondrial complex I can produce lesions that are neurochemically and histologically similar to HD. Furthermore the MPP$^+$ lesions were blocked by prior decortication and MK-801. This finding is consistent with the observation of L. Turski that NMDA antagonists can block the MPP$^+$-induced damage in the substantia nigra (Turski et al., 1991).

3-Nitropropionic Acid Lesions

We have also examined the effects of aging on 3-nitropropionic acid-induced lesions (Brouillet et al., 1993). Mitochondrial dysfunction, which occurs with normal aging, may play a role in the delayed onset and age-dependent incidence of HD and PD. Following local administration of 500 nmol of 3-nitropropionic acid into the left striatum there was a marked increase in lactate using *in vivo* chemical shift magnetic resonance imaging in 4- and 12-month-old animals as compared with 1-month-old animals. Direct measurements of ATP and lactate using the freeze-clamp technique confirmed a greater impairment of oxidative phosphorylation in the older animals. The entire striatum was processed, and the volume of the lesions was measured using the Cavalieri estimator. The volume of the lesions measured on Nissl-stained sections was significantly less ($p < .01$) in 1-month-old animals than in 4- and 12-month-old animals. The lesion volumes in the three groups were 1 month, $0.61 \pm 0.24 \, \text{mm}^3$; 4 months, $14.28 \pm 2/22 \, \text{mm}^3$; and 12 months, $40.27 \pm 4.10 \, \text{mm}^3$ (X $\pm$ SE, $n = 3, 4, 4$). 3-Nitropropionic acid is the first neurotoxin to show an age-dependent neurotoxicity in young adult rodents, which is similar to the typical age of onset in HD.

Our most exciting findings are that chronic administration of low doses of 3-nitropropionic acid for 1 month can produce selective striatal lesions which replicate many of the characteristic histological and neurochemical features of HD (Brouillet et al., 1993). This mode of administration produces lesions confined to the striatum in which there are growth-related proliferative changes in dendrites of spiny neurons similar to changes that occur in HD. In addition, these lesions are axon sparing as assessed with tyrosine-hydroxylase immunocytochemistry. Our preliminary findings indicate that this mode of administration of 3-nitropropionic acid results in relative sparing of NADPH-diaphorase neurons as compared with Nissl-stained neurons. Following subacute administration of 3-nitropropionic acid, animals showed a movement disorder, with dystonic posturing of the hind limbs. These lesions therefore reproduce the following characteristic features of HD: striatal vulnerability, age dependence, movement disorders, sparing of striatal afferents, loss of spiny projection neurons, spiny neuron dendritic abnormalities, and relative sparing of NADPH-diaphorase neurons. As such they appear to be an improved animal model for many of the characteristic features of HD.

Conclusion

This chapter reviews evidence that mitochondrial dysfunction may play a role in the physiological changes associated with normal aging and in neurodegenerative diseases. An impairment of energy metabolism could potentially explain both the delayed onset, the age dependence, and the slow progression of neurodegenerative illnesses. It is possible that a mild defect in energy metabolism may exert no deleterious effects until it interacts with the effects of normal aging to pass a critical threshold in energy production. At this point impaired mitochondrial function may lead to the generation of free radicals, which may further impair mitochondrial function. If this is the case, one should be able to model neurodegenerative diseases with mitochondrial toxins. Our recent studies with 3-nitropropionic acid suggest that chronic administration produces an excellent model for Huntington's disease. Continuous administration of low doses of this compound to rats produced selective striatal lesions showing age-dependence, sparing of striatal interneurons, and spiny neuron dendritic changes characteristic of Huntington's disease. We therefore believe that this type of model may lead to new insights into the pathogenesis ofneurodegenerative diseases, and may prove useful in testing new therapeutic approaches.

References

Abele AE, Miller RJ (1990): Potassium channel activators abolish excitotoxicity in cultured hippocampal pyramidal neurons. *Neurosci Lett* 115:195–200

Astrand I, Astrand P-O, Hallback I, Kilbom A (1973): Reduction in maximal oxygen uptake with age. *J Appl Physiol* 35:649–654

Beal MF, Swartz KJ, Hyman BT, Storey E, Finn SF, Koroshetz W (1991): Aminooxyacetic acid results in excitotoxin lesions by a novel indirect mechanism. *J Neurochem* 57:1068–1073

Blaustein MP (1988): Calcium transport and buffering in neurons. *Trends Neurosci* 11:438–443

Bowling AC, Mutisya E, Walker LC, Price DL, Cork LC, Beal MF (1993): Age-dependent impairment of mitochondrial function in primate brain. *J Neurochem* 60:1964–1967

Brennan WA, Bird ED, Aprille JR (1985): Regional mitochondrial respiratory activity in Huntington's disease brain. *J Neurochem* 44:1948–1950

Brouillet E, Jenkins BG, Hyman BT, Ferrante RJ, Kowall NW, Srivastava R, Samanta Roy D, Rosen BR, Beal MF (1993): Age-dependent vulnerability of the striatum to the mitochondrial toxin 3-nitropropionic acid. *J Neurochem* 60:356–359

Brown AW, Aldridge WN, Street BW, Veschoyle RD (1979): The behavioral and neuropathologic sequelae of intoxication by trimethyltin compounds in the rat. *Am J Pathol* 97:59–81

Butterworth J, Yates CM, Reynolds GP (1985): Distribution of phosphate-activated glutaminase, succinic dehydrogenase, pyruvate dehydrogenase, and α-glutamyl transpeptidase in postmortem brain from Huntington's disease and agonal cases. *J Neurol Sci* 67:161–171

Byrne E, Trounce I, Dennett X (1991): Mitochondrial theory of senescence: respiratory chain protein studies in human skeletal muscle. *Mech Aging Dev* 60:295–302

Cheeseman AJ, Clar JB (1988): Influence of the malate-aspartate shuttle on oxidative metabolism in synaptosomes. *J Neurochem* 50:1559–1565

Cheng KC, Cahill DS, Kasai H, Nishimura S, Loeb LA (1992): 8-hydroxy-2-deoxyguanosine, an abundant form of oxidative DNA damage causes G $\rightarrow$ T and A $\rightarrow$ C substitutions. *J Biol Chem* 267:166–172

Choi DW (1988): Calcium-mediated neurotoxicity: relationship to specific channel types and role in isochemic damage. *Trends Neurosci* 11:465–469

Clayton DA, Doda JN, Freiberg EC (1974): The absence of a pyrimidine dimer repair mechanism in mammalian mitochondria. *Proc Natl Acad Sci USA* 71:2777–2781

Cooper JM, Mann VM, Schapira AHV (1992): Analyses of mitochondrial respiratory chain function and mitochondrial DNA deletion in human skeletal muscle: effect of aging. *J Neurol Sci* 13:91–98

Corral-Debrinski M, Horton T, Lott MT, Shoffner JM, Beal MF, Wallace DW (1992): Mitochondrial deletions in human brain: regional variability and increase with advanced age. *Nature Genet* 2:324–329

Corral-Debrinski M, Stepien G, Shoffner JM, Lott MT, Kanter K, Wallace DC (1991): Hypoxemia is associated with mitochondrial DNA damage and gene induction: implications for cardiac disease. *JAMA* 266: 1812–1816

Cortopassi GA, Arnheim N (1987): Detection of a specific mitochondrial DNA deletion in tissues of older humans. *Nucleic Acids Res* 18:6927–6933

Curti D, Giangare MC, Redolfi ME, Fugaccia I, Benzi G (1990): Age-related modifications of cytochrome c oxidase activity in discrete brain regions. *Mech Aging Dev* 55:171–180

Darley-Usmar VM, Rickwood D, Wilson MT (1987): *Mitochondria: a Practical Approach.* Oxford, England: IRL Press

Dizdaroglu M (1991): Chemical determination of free radical-induced damage to DNA. *Free Radical Biol Med* 10:225–242

Fraga CG, Shigenaga MK, Park J-W, Degan P, Ames BN (1990): Oxidative damage to DNA during aging: 8-hydroxy-2-deoxyguanosine in rat organ DNA and urine. *Proc Natl Acad Sci USA* 87:4533–4537

Goebel HH, Heipertz R, Scholz W, Iqbal K, Tellez-Nagel I (1978): Juvenile Huntington chorea: clinical, ultrastructural, and biochemical studies. *Neurology* 28:23–31

Gould DH, Gustine DL (1982): Basal ganglia degeneration, myelin alterations, and enzyme inhibition induced in mice by the plant toxin 3-nitropropanoic acid. *Neuropathol Appl Neurobiol* 8:377–393

Grafton ST, Mazziotta JC, Pahl JJ, St. George-Hyslop P, Haines JL, Gusella J, Hoffman JM, Baxter LR, Phelphs ME (1990): A comparison of neurological, metabolic, structural and genetic evaluations in persons at risk for Huntington's disease. *Ann Neurol* 28:614–621

Hamilton BF, Gould DH (1987): Nature and distribution of brain lesions in rats intoxicated with 3-nitropropionic acid: a type of hypoxic (energy deficient) brain damage. *Acta Neuropathol* 72:286–297

Harmon HJ, Nank S, Floyd RA (1987): Age-dependent changes in rat brain mitochondria of synaptic and non-synaptic origins. *Mech Aging Dev* 38:167–177

Hatefi Y (1985): Mitochondrial electron transport and oxidative phosphorylation system. *Annu Rev Biochem* 54:1015–1069

Hatefi Y, Stiggal DL (1978): Preparations and properties of NADH: ubiquinone oxidoreductase (complex I). In: *Methods in Enzymology*, Fleischer S, Packer C, eds. New York: Academic Press

Hattori K, Tanaka M, Sugiyama S, Obayash T, Ito T, Satake T, Hanaki Y, Asai J, Nagaon M, Ozawa T (1991): Age-dependent increase in deleted mitochondrial DNA in the human heart: possible contributory factor to presbycardia. *Am Heart J* 121:1735–1742

Hayakawa M, Hattori K, Sugiyama S, Ozawa T (1992): Age-associated oxygen damage and mutations in mitochondrial DNA in human hearts. *Biochem Biophys Res Commun* 189:979–985

Hayakawa M, Ogawa T, Sugiyama S, Tanaka M, Ozawa T (1991a): Massive conversion of guanosine to 8-hydroxy-2-deoxyguanosine in mouse liver mitochondrial DNA by administration of azidothymidine. *Biochem Biophys Res Commun* 176:87–93

Hayakawa M, Torii K, Sugiyama S, Tanaka M, Ozawa T (1991b): Age-associated accumulation of 8-hydroxy-2-deoxyguanosine in mitochondrial DNA of human diaphragm. *Biochem Biophys Res Commun* 179:1023–1029

Hayden MR, Hewitt J, Stoessel AJ, Clark C, Amman W, Martin WRW (1987): The combined use of positron emission tomography and DNA polymorphisms for preclinical detection of Huntington's disease. *Neurology* 37:1441–1447

Hicks SP (1950): Brain metabolism in vivo. II. *Arch Pathol* 50:545–561

Hurst EW (1942): Experimental demyelination of the central nervous system. 3. Poisoning with potassium cyanide, sodium azide, hydroxylamine, narcotics, carbon monoxide, etc., with some consideration of bilateral necrosis occurring in the basal nuclei. *Aust J Exp Biol Med Sci* 20:297–312

Kauppinen RA, Sihra TS, Nichols DG (1987): Aminooxyacetic acid inhibits the malate-aspartate shuttle in isolated nerve terminals and prevents the mitochondria from utilizing glycolytic substrates. *Biochem Biophys Acta* 930:173–178

Koroshetz WJ, Jenkins BG, Beal MF, Rosen BR (1992): Localizing proton-NMR spectroscopy in patients with Huntington's disease (HD) demonstrates abnormal lactate levels in occipital cortex: evidence for compromised metabolism in HD. *Neurology* 42 (suppl. 3):319

Kuchino Y, Mori F, Kasai H, Inoue H, Iwai S, Miura K, Ohtsuka E, Nishimura S (1987): Misreading of DNA templates containing 8-hydroxy-2-deoxyguanosine at the modified base and at the adjacent residues. *Nature* 327:77–79

Kuhl DE, Phelps ME, Markham CH, Metter EJ, Riege WH, Winter J (1990): Cerebral metabolism and atrophy in Huntington's disease determined by [18]FDG and computed tomographic scan. *Ann Neurol* 12:425–434

Kuwert T, Lange HW, Langer K-J, Herzog H, Aulich A, Feinendegen LE (1990): Cortical and subcortical glucose consumption measured by PET in patients with Huntington's disease. *Brain* 113:1405–1423

Lehninger AL (1951): Phosphorylation coupled to oxidation of dihydrodiphosphopyridine nucleotide. *J Biol Chem* 190:345–359

Lewitt PA, Truong DD, Hashimoto K, Kareti D, Young AB (1989). "Tweed ball" mitochondropathy with a unique neurodegenerative disorder. *Ann Neurol* 26:122

Linnane AW, Marzuki S, Ozawa T, Tanaka M (1989): Mitochondrial DNA mutations as an important contribution to aging and degenerative diseases. *Lancet* i:642–645

Linnane AW, Baumer A, Maxwell RJ, Preston H, Zhang C, Marzuki S (1990): Mitochondrial gene mutation: the aging process and degenerative diseases. *Biochem Int* 22:1067–1076

Ludolph AC, Ludolph AG, Sabri MI (1991a): 3-Ntropropionic acid-abundant xenobiotic excitotoxin linked to putaminal necrosis and tardive dystonia. *Ann Neurol* 30:253

Ludolph AC, He F, Spencer PS, Hammerstad J, Sabri M (1991b): 3-Nitropropionic acid-exogenous animal neurotoxin and possible human striatal toxin. *Can J Neurol Sci* 18:492–498

Mann VM, Cooper JM, Javoy-Agid F, Agid F, Jenner P, Schapira AHV (1990): Mitochondrial function and parental sex effect in Huntington's disease. *Lancet* 336:749

Martin WRW, Clark C, Ammann W, Stoessl AJ, Shtybel W, Hayden MR (1992): Cortical glucose metabolism in Huntington's disease. *Neurology* 42:223–229

Mazziotta JC, Phelps ME, Pahl JI, Huang S-C, Baxter LR, Riege WH, Hoffman JM, Kuhl DE, Lanto AB, Wapenski JA, Markham CH (1987): Reduced cerebral glucose metabolism in asymptomatic subjects at risk for Huntington's disease. *N Engl J Med* 316:356–362

Mettler FA (1972): Choreoathetosis and striopalllidal necrosis due to sodium azide. *Exp Neurol* 34:291–308

Miquel J (1991): An integrated theory of aging as the result of mitochondrial-DNA mutation in differentiated cells. *Arch Gerontol Geriatr* 12:99–117

Miyoshi K (1967): Experimental striatal necrosis induced by sodium azide. *Acta Neuropathol (Berl)* 9:199–216

Muller-Hocker J (1989): Cytochrome-c-oxidase deficient cardiomyocytes in the human heart, an age-related phenomenon. *Am J Pathol* 134:1167–1173

Nohl H (1986): Oxygen radical release in mitochondria: influence of age. In: *Free Radicals, Aging, and Degenerative Diseases*, Johnson JE Jr, Walford R, Harman D, Miquel J, eds. New York: Alan R. Liss

Nohl H, Breuninger V, Hegner D (1978): Influence of mitochondrial radical formation of energy-linked respiration. *Eur J Biochem* 90:385–390

Novelli A, Reilly JA, Lysko PG, Henneberry RC (1988): Glutamate becomes neurotoxic via the *N*-methyl-D-aspartate receptor when intracellular energy levels are reduced. *Brain Res* 451:205–212

Olney JW, Price MT, Samson L, LeBruyere J (1986): The role of specific ions in glutamate neurotoxicity. *Neurosci Lett* 65:65–71

Pantano P, Baron J-C, Lebrun-Grandié P, Duquesnoy N, Bousser M-G, Comar D (1984): Regional cerebral blood flow and oxygen consumption in human aging. *Stroke* 15:635–641

Parker WD, Filley CM, Parks JM (1990): Cytochrome oxidase deficiency in Alzheimer's disease. *Neurology* 40:1302–1303

Richter C, Park J-W, Ames BN (1988): Normal oxidative damage to mitochondrial and nuclear DNA is extensive. *Proc Natl Acad Sci USA* 85:6465–6467

Robinson SH, Munzer TS, Tandan R, Bradley WG (1987): Alzheimer's disease cells exhibit defective repair of alkylating agent-induced DNA damage. *Ann Neurol* 21:205–258

Sah P, Hestrin S, Nicoll RA (1989): Tonic activation of NMDA receptors by ambient glutamate enhances excitability of neurons. *Science* 246:815–818

Shepherd D, Garland PB (1969): Citrate synthase from rat liver. *Methods Enzymol* 13:11–16

Shibutani S, Takeshita M, Grollman AP (1991): Insertion of specific bases during DNA synthesis past the oxidation damage base 8-OXOdG. *Nature* 349:431–434

Shigenaga MR, Park J-W, Cundy KC, Gimeno CJ, Ames BN (1990): In vivo oxidative DNA damage: measurement of 8-hydroxy-2-deoxyguanosine in DNA and urine by high-performance liquid chromatography with electrochemical detection. *Methods Enzymol* 186:521–530

Simonetta S, Chen X, DiMauro S, Schon EA (1992): Accumulation of deletions in human mitochondrial DNA during normal aging: analysis by quantitative PCR. *Biochem Biophys Acta* 1180:113–122

Soong NW, Hinton DR, Cortopassi G, Arnheim N (1992): Mosaicism for a specific somatic mitochondrial NDA mutation in adult human brain. *Nature Genet* 2:318–323

Sorbi S, Bird ED, Blass JP (1983): Decreased pyruvate dehydrogenase complex activity in Huntington and Alzheimer brain. *Ann Neurol* 13: 72–78

Storey E, Hyman BT, Jenkins BT, Rosen BR, Beal MF (1992): MPP$^+$ produces excitotoxic lesions in rat striatum due to impairment of oxidative metabolism. *J Neurochem* 58:1975–1978

Sugiyama S, Hattori K, Hayakawa M, Ozawa T (1991): Quantitative analysis of age-associated accumulation of mitochondrial DNA with deletion in human hearts. *Biochem Biophys Res Commun* 180:894–899

Tellez-Nagel I, Johnson AB, Terry RD (1974): Studies on brain biopsies of patients with Huntington's chorea. *J Neuropathol Exp Neurol* 33:178–184

Torri K, Sugiyama S, Takagi K, Satake T, Ozawa T (1992): Age-related decreases in respiratory muscle mitochondrial function in rats. *Am J Respir Cell Mol Biol* 6:88–92

Trounce I, Byrne E, Marzuki S (1989): Decline in skeletal muscle mitochondrial respiratory chain function: possible factor in aging. *Lancet* 1:637–639

Turski L, Bressler K, Rettig K-J, Löschmann P-A, Wachtel H (1991): Protection of substantia nigra from MPP$^+$ neurotoxicity by N-methyl-D-aspartate antagonists. *Nature* 349:414–418

Vornov JJ, Coyle JT (1991): Enhancement of NMDA receptor-mediated neurotoxicity in the hippochampal slice by depolarization and ischemia. *Brain Res* 555:99–106

Wallace DC (1986): Mitochondrial genes and disease. *Hosp Pract* 21:77–92

Wallace DW (1992): Mitochondrial genetics: a paradigm for aging and degenerative diseases? *Science* 256:628–632

Wood ML, Dizdaroglu M, Gajewski E, Essigmann JM (1990): Mechanistic studies of ionizing radiation and oxidative mutagenesis: genetic effects of a single 8-hydroxyguanine residue inserted at a unique site in a viral genome. *Biochemistry* 29:7024–7032

Yen T-C, Chen Y-S, King K-L, Yeh S-H, Wei Y-H (1989): Liver mitochondrial respiratory functions decline with age. *Biochem Biophys Res Commun* 165:994–1003

Zeevalk GD, Nicklas WJ (1990): Chemically induced hypoglycemia and anoxia: relationship to glutamate receptor-mediated toxicity in retina. *J Pharmacol Exp Ther* 253:1285–1292

Zeevalk GD, Nicklas WJ (1991): Mechanisms underlying initiation of excitotoxicity associated with metabolic inhibition. *J Pharmacol Exp Ther* 257:870–878

Zheng X, Shoffner JM, Lott MT, Voljavec AS, Krawiecki NS, Winn K, Wallace DC (1989): Evidence in a lethal infantile mitochondrial disease for a nuclear mutation affecting respiratory complexes I and IV. *Neurology* 39:1203–1209

12

Energy Failure, Glutamate and Neuropathology: Relevance to Neurodegenerative Disorders

LECHOSLAW TURSKI AND CHRYSANTHY IKONOMIDOU

Impairment of energy metabolism resulting in deterioration of the function of membranes, leading to loss of the Mg^{2+} block on N-methyl-D-aspartate (NMDA) receptors, allowing persistent activation of these receptors by endogenous glutamate is postulated as a mechanism to explain slow neuronal death in neurodegenerative disorders. Studies in rodents with mitochondrial respiratory chain toxins, aminooxyacetic acid, 1-methyl-4-phenylpyridinium ion, and 3-nitropropionic acid, suggest that such mechanisms may indeed be involved in neurotoxicity produced by these agents. Nigral and striatal neurotoxicity induced by mitochondrial toxins in rodents reproduces neuropathology similar to that seen in humans suffering from Parkinson's or Huntington's disease, and can be prevented by NMDA receptor antagonists. Such observations indicate that glutamate may be involved in slow neuronal death leading to abiotrophic disorders and suggest the use of glutamate antagonists as potential neuroprotective agents to prevent or retard neuronal damage and death in relevant regions of the brain. Such an approach would consequently slow the rate of progression of these disabling disorders.

Mitochondrial Energy Metabolism and the Concept of Delayed and Slow-Onset Neurotoxicity: Where Does It Come From?

In Vitro

In 1988, Henneberry and his associates (Novelli et al., 1988) reported that impairment of energy metabolism in cell cultures increases vulnerability of neurons to the toxic action of excitatory amino acids and demonstrated that NMDA gated ion channels are primarily involved. Subsequently, Zeevalk and Nicklas (1990), experimenting with cultured chick embryo retina, showed that compromising the energy supply of neurons with cyanide triggers excitotoxic lesions sensitive to NMDA antagonists. Consistent with these observations was the demonstration that toxicity induced by metabolic inhibition can be mimicked by membrane depolarization with potassium or relief of the Mg^{2+} block of the NMDA receptor (Zeevalk and Nicklas, 1991).

In Vivo

In 1989, we communicated that aminooxyacetic acid (AOAA), a non-selective inhibitor of transaminases, induces axon-sparing lesions in the rat striatum that can be blocked by NMDA antagonists and prior decortication (Turski et al., 1992; Urbańska et al., 1989, 1991). The behavioral consequences of such lesions were similar to those reported following striatal lesions with kainic or quinolinic acids in rodents (Schwarcz et al., 1990; Urbańska et al., 1991), well established and widely accepted animal models of Huntington's disease.

Two different facts led to the investigation of the neurotoxic potential of AOAA (Turski et al., 1992). The first one was the evidence that AOAA blocks *in vitro* kynurenate transaminase activity and decreases the endogenous concentrations of the glutamate antagonist kynurenic acid (Schwarcz et al., 1990). The second one was the fact that AOAA blocks the malate–aspartate shunt across mitochondrial membranes, which leads to an insufficient supply of mitochondrial NADH in reducing equivalents necessary for oxygenation (Beal et al., 1991; Wallace, 1992). The breakthrough in understanding the mechanisms involved in AOAA toxicity was achieved when the data on nigral neurotoxicity of 1-methyl-4-phenylpyridinium ion (MPP^+; active metabolite of the parkinsonism-inducing compound MPTP) and the protective action of NMDA antagonists against it were published (Turski et al., 1991).

At first, there was no reason to believe that there is a relationship between the action of AOAA and MPP^+. However, it has been recognized that MPP^+ is a specific mitochondrial complex I toxin (Di Monte et al., 1986; Mizuno et al., 1988; Nicklas et al., 1985). AOAA, which inhibits the malate–aspartate shunt in the mitochondria, may indirectly produce results very similar to those of MPP^+ on the mitochondrial respiratory chain.

The inference has been experimentally confirmed by Beal and associates (Beal et al., 1991), who initially extended observations on

AOAA toxicity in the rat striatum showing similarity of its anatomical profile to that of quinolinate-induced lesions (sparing NADPH-diaphorase-containing neurons). They also demonstrated the lack of effect of AOAA in activating NMDA receptors in electrophysiological tests (Beal et al., 1991). Further, these authors provided evidence that AOAA concentrations necessary to trigger striatal lesions do not significantly affect kynurenate transaminase activity in the rat brain (Beal et al., 1991). It was subsequently demonstrated that MPP^+ can induce striatal lesions with morphological and pharmacological profiles similar to those induced by AOAA (Storey et al., 1992). Striatal lesions induced by MPP^+ in rats, as well as those triggered by AOAA, were found to be sensitive to NMDA antagonists and to depend on intact corticostriatal innervation (Beal et al., 1991; Srivastava et al., 1993; Urbańska et al., 1991). Finally, it was demonstrated that AOAA may induce nigral lesions that are sensitive to NMDA antagonists (Turski, 1991).

The mitochondrial complex II toxin, 3-nitropropionic acid (3-NP), has recently been reported to be a selective striatal neurotoxin in rodents provided it is given to rats in sufficiently low doses and over a period of weeks (Brouillet et al., 1993). Chronic systemic administration of 3-NP to rats for as long as 1 month leads to low-grade metabolic disturbances in the striatum and subsequently to selective damage of striatal neurons (sparing NADPH-diaphorase-containing neurons). This effect is blocked by prior decortication (Beal et al., 1993; Brouillet et al., 1993).

These observations (Figs. 1 and 2) founded and experimentally confirmed the hypothesis that disturbances in mitochondrial energy metabolism can lead to axon-sparing, glutamate-like toxicity in the brain and that such processes may eventually be involved in the pathogenesis of chronic neurodegenerative disorders in man.

Mitochondrial Respiratory Chain: How Does It Work?

The mitochondria supply cells, including neurons, with energy (Wallace, 1992). In the mitochondrial matrix, energy carriers such as reduced nicotinamide adenine dinucleotide ($NADH_2$) and flavin adenine dinucleotide ($FADH_2$) are formed in the Krebs cycle. $NADH_2$ and $FADH_2$ donate electrons necessary for the generation of an electrochemical gradient across the inner membrane of the mitochondrion and for the synthesis of ATP. The enzymes responsible for the transport of electrons are located in the inner mitochondrial membrane (Figs. 3A and B). Two very important members of this highly organized and hierarchical enzyme system are NADH–ubiquinone oxidoreductase (complex I)

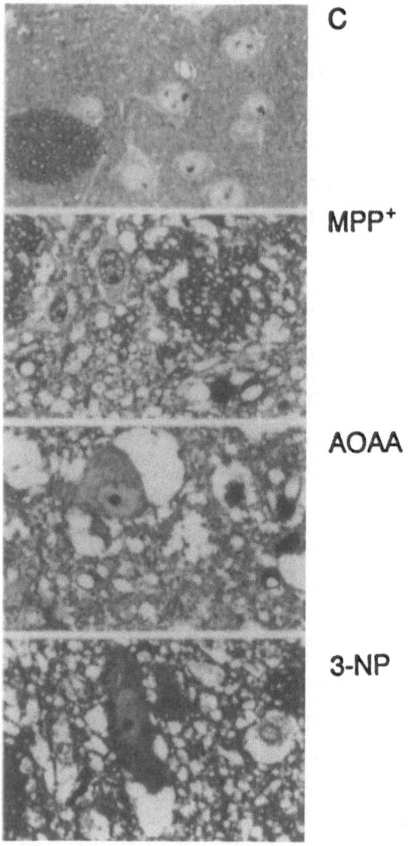

Figure 1. Neuropathological sequelae of 1-methyl-4-phenylpyridinium ion (MPP^+), aminooxyacetic acid (AOAA), and 3-nitropropionic acid (3-NP) in the rodent striatum after microinjection of MPP^+ or AOAA, or systemic administration of 3-NP. C: Normal cytoarchitecture of the mouse striatum 72 h after intrastriatal microinjection of saline. MPP^+: Mouse striatum with breakdown of the morphological structure in the transition zone of neuronal loss 72 h after microinjection of 45 nmol of MPP^+. There appears to be a relative sparing of large neurons. AOAA: Destruction of the striatum in a rat microinjected with 500 nmol of AOAA observed 72 h after treatment. Relative sparing of large neurons in the transition zone of neuronal loss is apparent. 3-NP: Pathological reaction to 3-NP seen in the rat striatum after 7 daily IP injections of 15 mg/kg. The type and pattern of morphological changes seen in the transition zone are very similar to those observed with MPP^+ and AOAA. Methylene blue/azure II stain, ×400.

and succinate–ubiquinone oxidoreductase (complex II) (Fig. 3C). The electrons entering the system are transported via flavin mononucleotides (FMN) and multiple iron–sulphur centers of complex I or II and passed to ubiquinone (coenzyme Q; CoQ). The electrons then are transported to the ubiquinol:cytochrome C oxidoreductase (complex III) and encompass cytochromes B, Rieske-iron–sulphur protein and cytochrome C_1. From complex III, electrons are transferred via cytochrome C to cytochrome C oxidase (complex IV), containing cytochromes A and A_3 equipped with copper atoms, and finally passed on to oxygen (Fig. 3C). Concomitantly to the traveling of electrons through complexes I/II, III, and IV, protons cross the inner mitochondrial membrane creating an electrochemical gradient. This energy is used by adenosine triphosphate (ATP) synthase (complex V) for the synthesis of ATP (Fig. 3C). The adenine nucleotide translocator exchanges then ATP for cytosolic ADP (Fig. 3C).

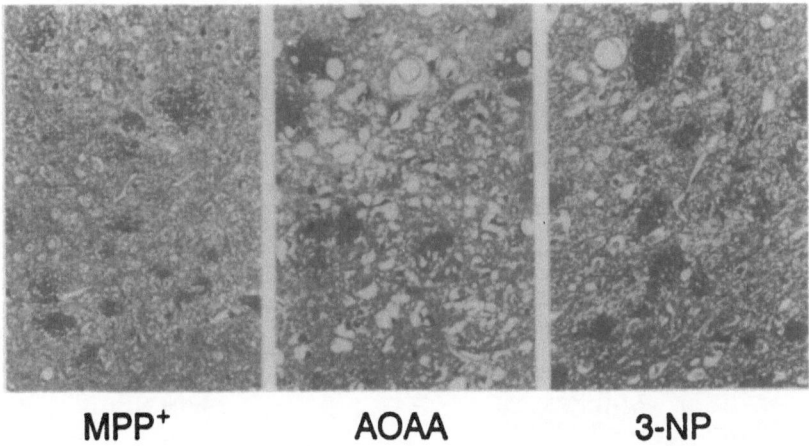

MPP⁺   **AOAA**   **3-NP**

Figure 2. Neuropathological sequelae of 1-methyl-4-phenylpyridinium ion (MPP⁺), aminooxyacetic acid (AOAA), and 3-nitropropionic acid (3-NP) in the rodent striatum (central core of the lesion) after microinjection of MPP⁺ or AOAA, or systemic administration of 3-NP. MPP⁺: Breakdown of the cell structure, massive edematous changes, and extensive disintegration of neuropil 72 h after intrastriatal microinjection of 45 nmol of MPP⁺ in a mouse. AOAA: Severe neuronal loss in the rat striatum seen 72 h after microinjection of 500 nmol of AOAA. 3-NP: Destruction of the striatal tissue seen in the rat striatum after 7 daily IP injections of 15 mg/kg of 3-NP. The type and pattern of morphological changes seen in the central core of the lesion are similar to those observed with MPP⁺ and AOAA. Methylene blue/azure II stain, ×100.

Sites of Action of Mitochondrial Toxins

AOAA prevents electron supply to mitochondrial NADH, which indirectly leads to relative insufficiency of the function of complex I because reducing equivalents necessary for oxygenation do not enter the respiratory chain (Beal et al., 1991). MPP⁺ is a specific complex I toxin blocking one of the two major pathways for electrons entering the mitochondrial respiratory chain (Jenner et al., 1992; Srivastava et al., 1993). 3-NP is an inhibitor of the activity of complex II and therefore blocks another entrance for electrons into the mitochondrial respiratory chain (Alston et al., 1977; Gould and Gustine, 1982; Ludolph et al., 1991). The obvious consequence of the action of all these three toxins is deficient electron supply for CoQ and prevention of its reduction to ubiquinol, which immediately leads to major dysfunction of complexes III and IV and loss of the electrochemical gradient across the inner mitochondrial membrane. Consequently, the energy-dependent synthesis of ATP is reduced, and if deleterious processes remain, it may cease completely. Such major changes in mitochondrial energy metabolism lead to disturbances of the functions of the entire cell and may result in cell death if the toxic impact persists.

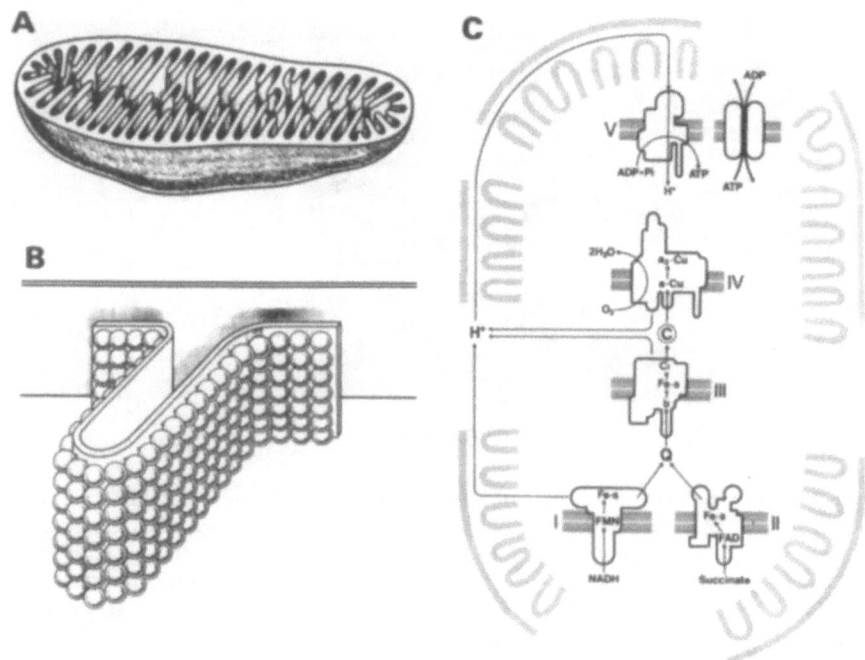

Figure 3. A: Schematic diagram of the mitochondrion. B: Morphology of the internal mitochondrial wall containing respiratory chain enzymes. C: Schematic diagram of mitochondrial electron transport complexes. Abbreviations: NADH, nicotinamide adenine dinucleotide reduced; FAD, flavin adenine dinucleotide; FMN, flavin mononucleotide; Fe-S, iron–sulfur center; Q, coenzyme Q; a, a_3, b, C, C_1, cytochromes.

How Can Energy Failure Trigger Excitotoxic Brain Damage?

As soon as concentrations of mitochondrial toxins have reached appropriate (toxic) levels, the function of the mitochondrial respiratory chain are disturbed (see Figs. 2 and 3). The resulting intracellular energy deprivation causes reduction of ATP stores in mitochondria and consequently in the cytoplasm, which interferes with Na^+/K^+-ATPase activity and leads to disturbances in the maintenance of the membrane potential (Figs. 4B and 5). Defective function of Na^+/K^+-ATPase retards repolarization of the cell membrane, leading to inappropriate (prolonged) opening of voltage-dependent ion channels (Fig. 4B). These initial disturbances will cause mild and reversible increases of the Ca^{2+} concentration in the cytoplasm, lessening the voltage-dependent Mg^{2+} block of NMDA channels (Figs. 4B and 5). As the number of activated NMDA channels increases, increasing amounts of Na^+ and Ca^{2+} will enter the cell (Fig. 4B). Excessive elevation of intracellular Na^{2+} concentration critically disturbs Na^+/Ca^{2+}-exchange func-

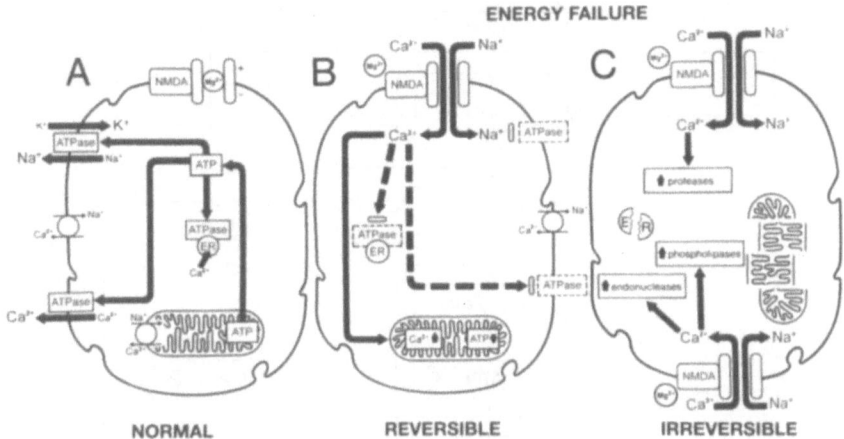

Figure 4. Schematic diagram of the excitotoxic mechanisms triggered by energy failure in neurons. **A:** Energy metabolism under physiological conditions. **B:** Reversible disturbances in the energy metabolism and cell function triggered by energy failure. **C:** Irreversible changes induced by sustained energy failure. Abbreviations: ER, endoplasmic reticulum; NMDA, N-methyl-D-aspartate; ATPase, phosphatase.

tion and leads to additional increase of intracellular Ca^{2+} concentration as a result of prevention of ATP-dependent Ca^{2+} extrusion. Further, the highly energy-dependent Ca^{2+} storage in the endoplasmic reticulum fails because of insufficient supply of the cell with ATP. Similarly, Ca^{2+}-ATPase activity fails and Ca^{2+} accumulation in the cell increases further. At that stage, sustained energy deprivation may rapidly cause membrane depolarization and opening of still inactive NMDA channels (Fig. 4C), thus exposing the neuron to the toxic action of endogenous glutamate. The resulting rapid increase in Ca^{2+} and Na^+ concentrations in the cell leads initially to the storage of Ca^{2+} in mitochondria, which further potentiates energy demand because Ca^{2+} overload of mitochondria inhibits ATP synthesis (Choi, 1992; Miller et al., 1989; Orrenius et al., 1992). The immediate consequence of Ca^{2+} overload of mitochondria is irreversible blockade of the respiratory chain and energy metabolism, leading to activation of mitochondrial phospholipases and mitochondrial damage. Such sequence of events leads rapidly to additional elevation of Ca^{2+} in the cytoplasm of energy-deprived neurons and consequently to activation of self-destructive processes including activation of phospholipases, endonucleases, and proteases (Figs 4C and 5). Intracellular influx of Cl^- and H_2O may also contribute to cell death at the final stage of metabolic disturbances (Olney, 1989; Rothman and Olney, 1987).

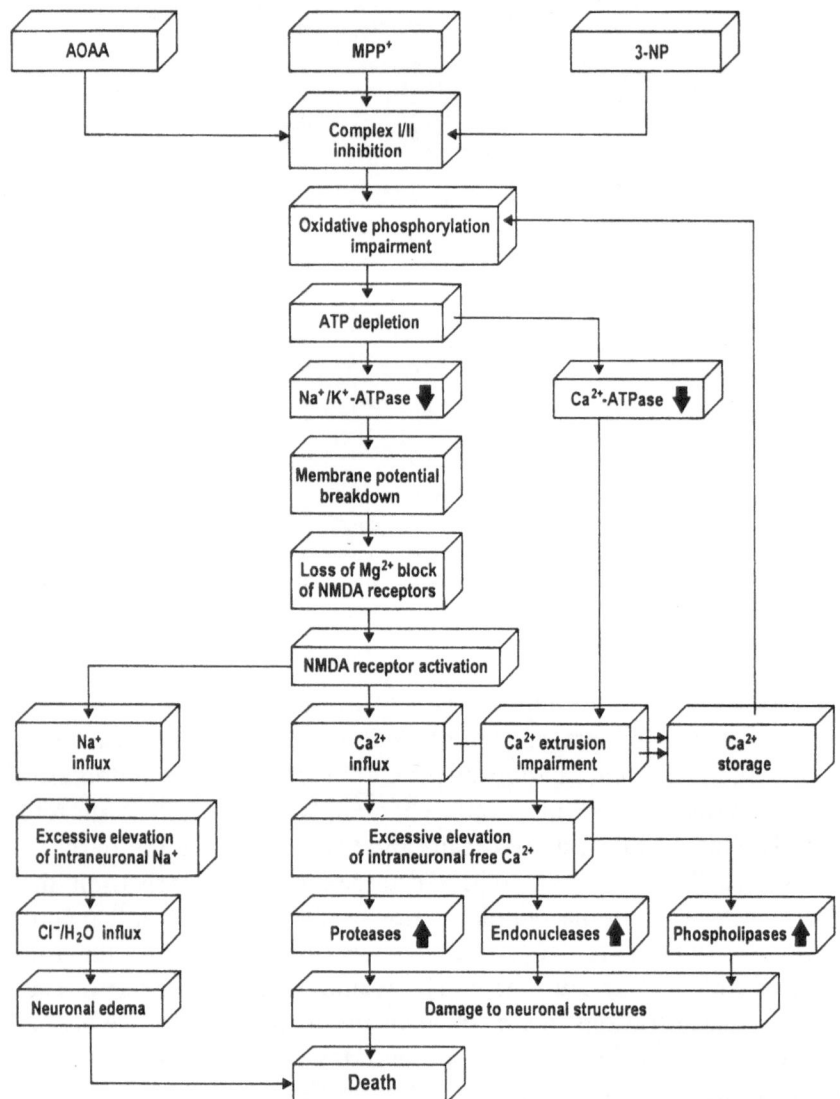

Figure 5. Schematic diagram illustrated possible sequence of events triggered in neurons by mitochondrial toxins.

Experimental Evidence

The question of whether Glutamate receptors are involved in neurotoxicity induced by mitochondrial has been addressed by Beal and his associates (Srivastava et al., 1993), who demonstrated that intrastriatal administration of MPP$^+$ in rats leads to nigral damage, which is sensitive to NMDA antagonists.

Another piece of evidence implying involvement of glutamate-dependent processes in toxicity of MPP$^+$ is represented by the data of Ikonomidou and Olney, who demonstrated that nigral damage following intrastriatal administration of MPP$^+$ in mice is of the axon-sparing type (unpublished observations). The nigral damage following intrastriatal administration of MPP$^+$ and its sensitivity to NMDA antagonists has been initially demonstrated in rats (Turski et al., 1991). We confirmed these observations in mice (Fig. 6) and also found that striatal damage induced by MPP$^+$ is not a prerequisite for the nigral destruction, because intrastriatal administration of toxic doses of AOAA or 3-NP does not result in subsequent damage in the substantia nigra pars compacta. These data demonstrate the crucial role of the NMDA receptor in neurotoxicity mediated by MPP$^+$in vivo and explain the observations that temporary protection against MPP$^+$/MPTP toxicity in rodents and primates can be provided by NMDA antagonists (Corsini et al., 1991; Lange et al., 1992; Srivastava et al., 1993; Storey et al., 1992; Turski 1991; Turski and Melamed, 1993; Turski et al., 1991; Zuddas et al., 1992).

Clinic

Clinical evidence suggests that such a scenario of events may be involved in cell death in chronic neurodegenerative disorders. In Parkinson's disease, complex I activity is significantly reduced in the substantia nigra but not in other brain regions (Jenner et al., 1992; Schapira et al., 1990). In Huntington's disease complex I activity is significantly reduced in platelets (Parker et al., 1990a) while basal ganglia and cortex show decreased metabolism (Brennan et al., 1985). In Alzheimer's disease reduced activity of cytochrome oxidase has been reported (Parker et al., 1990b). In degenerative ataxias reduced complex I activity is observed in muscles (Schöls et al., 1992). There are also a number of disorders associated with point mutations in mitochondrial DNA, energy metabolism disturbances, and several aspects of neurodegeneration (Wallace, 1992). Leber's optic atrophy, myoclonus epilepsy with ragged red fibers (MERRF), and mitochondrial encephalomyopathy with lactic acidosis and stroke-like episodes (MELAS) represent the most frequent examples of such disorders (Wallace, 1992).

Therapeutic Implications

Experimental data suggest that glutamate, acting preferentially via NMDA receptor gated channels, is engaged in the sequence of events leading to the neurotoxic action of compounds that disturb the function of

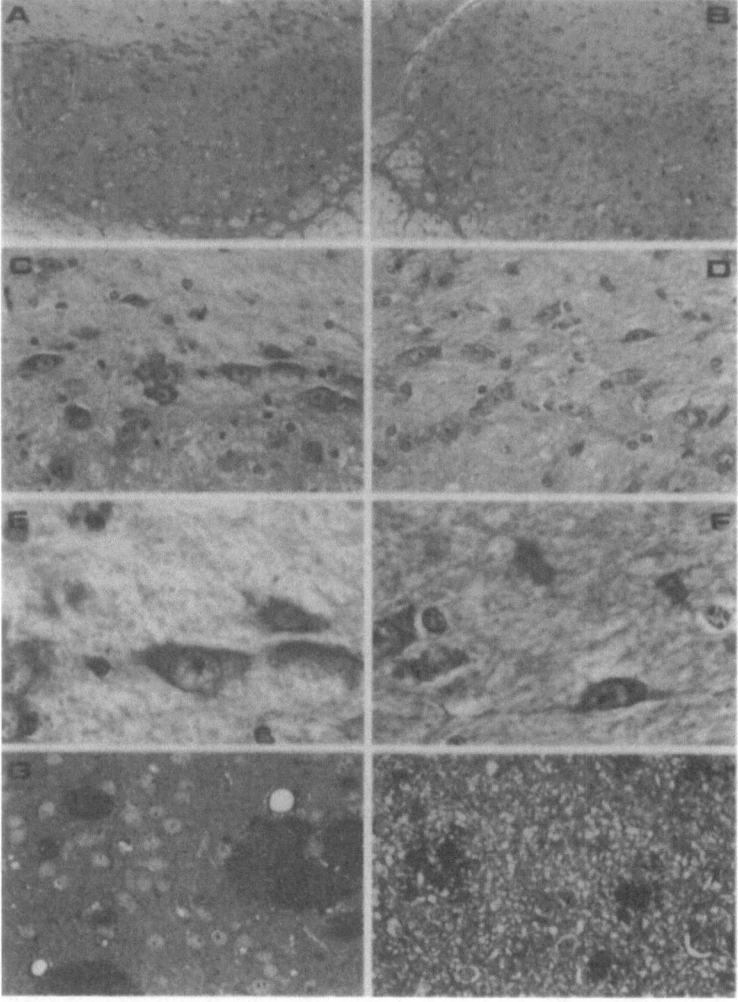

Figure 6. Neuropathological sequelae of 1-methyl-4-phenylpyridinium ion (MPP$^+$) in the mouse brain after unilateral (right) microinjection of 45 nmol into the striatum. **A:** Normal cytoarchitecture of the substantia nigra pars compacta 72 h after intrastriatal microinjection of vehicle on the same site. **B:** The substantia nigra pars compacta with apparent loss of its neuronal population 72 h after microinjection of 45 nmol of MPP$^+$ into the striatum on the same site. **C** and **E:** Higher magnification demonstrates normal morphology of dopaminergic cells in the substantia nigra pars compacta after treatment of the striatum with vehicle. Normal neurons possess typical nuclei with clear nucleoplasm and prominent nucleolus, surrounded by cytoplasm containing Nissl substance. **D** and **F:** Higher magnification shows early degenerative changes in nigral cells on the site of MPP$^+$ microinjection into the striatum. The degenerating neurons show typical narrowings, the nucleoplasm is less clear and the nucleolus less prominent, and the surrounding cytoplasm contains clumpings of Nissl substance. The neurons appear shrunken and are surrounded with dilated clear spaces. Cresyl violet stain, ×40 in **A, B;** ×100 in **C, D;** ×400 in **E, F. G:** No signs of neuronal degeneration are discernible in the striatum 72 h after microinjection of vehicle. **H:** Extensive disruption of the striatum in a mouse microinjected with 45 nmol of MPP$^+$ is observed 72 h after treatment. Methylene blue/azure II stain, ×40.

the mitochondrial respiratory chain. Accordingly, NMDA antagonists were found to protect temporarily against toxicity of several mitochondrial toxins. It is therefore attractive to speculate that NMDA receptor blockade will offer efficient protection against such toxicity. However, analysis of sequential changes in cells undergoing sustained energy deficits shows that activation of NMDA receptor gated channels represents only part of the complex processes leading to cell death, and imply that NMDA receptor antagonism might not represent a causal therapeutic approach to neurological diseases caused by deficient energy metabolism in mitochondria (see Fig. 5). What NMDA antagonism does is to prolong the life span of the cell undergoing energy failure. Such action might be expected to retard the transition between reversible and irreversible changes in the cell caused by sustained energy failure. Thus, it may also provide valuable time for therapeutic interventions that would prevent energy failure which appears to occur in the process of aging or in the course of abiotrophic (neurodegenerative) disorders. The antagonism at NMDA receptors will never establish normal function of the cell when deleterious factors persist. However, NMDA receptor blockade may efficiently prolong the time window during which causal factors can be eliminated. The causal factors are (1) mitochondrial toxins of the AOAA, MPP^+, and 3-NP types or related toxins working at different levels of the respiratory chain, such as nitric oxide (Stamler et al., 1992; Youdim, 1993), azides, cyanide, or possibly manganese (Brouillet et al., 1993) or (2) other metabolic processes that prevent a sufficient supply of respiratory chain enzymes with reducing equivalents necessary for oxidative phosphorylation such as those present in genetic disorders of mitochondrial energy metabolism.

The proposed action of NMDA antagonists on neurons undergoing pathological energy failure implies that the moment of therapeutic intervention has to be carefully selected in order to achieve protection. The NMDA antagonist will not interfere with the part of toxicity induced by mitochondrial poisons in the respiratory chain (see Fig. 3). Thus, if toxic action on mitochondrial respiratory enzymes persists, protective action of NMDA antagonists will not be seen. Further, if therapy with NMDA antagonists is introduced after transition of the cell into the irreversible stage, protective action with NMDA antagonists will not occur. In animal studies, NMDA antagonists were found to be beneficial only when their pharmacokinetic properties and the timing of therapy allowed for protective effect to take place. The half-life of such toxins as AOAA and malonic acid is short, ranging between 1 and 2 hours in rodents, while that of 3-NP and MPP^+ is long, ranging from several hours to days. For this reason, NMDA antagonists of sufficiently long half-life such as CPP, and to a lesser extent, MK-801, can protect against AOAA toxicity because they can efficiently block the transition between reversible and irreversible changes in cells undergoing energy failure and allow for the toxin to either disappear from the cell or for its concentration to decrease below a critical level. In the case of MPP^+, although its type of action does not differ from that of other mitochondrial toxins, the situation is much more complicated. Because the half-life of MPP^+ is much longer than that of available NMDA antagonists, it is necessary to continue administration of the antagonist for several hours or days to see any protective effect against *in vivo* toxicity of MPP^+. Such experiments are additionally complicated by the fact that in situations in which massive toxicity occurs within minutes, NMDA antagonists must be administered in almost toxic doses. In several cases, therefore, studies with subchronic or chronic administration of NMDA antagonists are impossible due to systemic toxicity.

References

Alston TA, Medla L, Bright HJ (1977): 3-Nitropropionate, the toxic substance of Indigofera, is a suicide inactivator of succinate dehydrogenase. *Proc Natl Acad Sci USA* 74:3767–3771

Beal MF, Swartz KJ, Hyman BT, Storey E, Finn SF, Koroshetz W (1991): Aminooxyacetic acid results in excitotoxin lesions by a novel indirect mechanisms. *J Neurochem* 57:1068–1073

Beal MF, Brouillet E, Jenkins BG, Ferrante RJ, Kowall NW, Miller JM, Storey E, Srivastava R, Rosen BR, Hyman BT (1993): Neurochemical and histologic characterization of striatal excitotoxic lesions produced by the mitochondrial toxin 3-nitropropionic acid. *J Neurosci* 13:4181–4192

Brennan WA, Bird ED, Aprillo VR (1985): Regional mitochondrial metabolism in Huntington's disease brain. *J Neurochem* 44:1448–1450

Brouillet E, Jenkins BG, Hyman BT, Ferrante RJ, Kowall NA, Srivastava R, Roy DS, Rosen BR, Beal MF (1993): Age-dependent vulnerability of the striatum to the mitochondrial toxin 3-nitropropionic acid. *J Neurochem* 60:356–359

Brouillet EP, Shinobu L, McGarvey U, Beal MF (1993): Manganese injection into the rat striatum produces excitotoxic lesions by impairing energy metabolism. *Exp Neurol* 120:89–94

Choi DW (1992): Excitotoxic cell death. *J Neurobiol* 23:1261–1276

Corsini GU, Vaglini F, Fornai F, Saginario A, Zuddas A (1991): (+)MK 801 prevents dopaminergic perikarya damage in MPTP and acetaldehyde-treated mice. *Posters Neurosci* 1:33–36

Di Monte D, Jewell SA, Ekstrom C, Sandy MS, Smith MT (1986): 1-Methyl-4-phenyl-1,2,3,6-tetrahydropyridine (MPTP) and 1-methyl-4-phenylpyridine (MPP^+) cause rapid ATP depletion in isolated hepatocytes. *Biochem Biophys Res Commun* 137:310–315

Gould DH, Gustine DL (1982): Basal ganglia degeneration, myelin alterations, and enzyme inhibition in mice by the plant toxin 3-nitropropanoic acid. *Neuropathol Appl Neurobiol* 8:377–393

Jenner P, Schapira AHV, Marsden CD (1992): New insights into the cause of Parkinson's disease. *Neurology* 42:2241–2250

Lange KW, Youdim MBH, Riederer P (1992): Neurotoxicity and neuroprotection in Parkinson's disease. *J Neural Transm* S38:27–44

Ludolph A, He F, Spencer PS, Hammerstad J, Sabri M (1991): 3-Nitropropionic acid – exogenous animal neurotoxin and possible human striatal toxin. *Can J Neurol Sci* 18:492–498

Miller RJ, Murphy SN, Glaum SR (1989): Neuronal Ca^{2+} channels and their regulation by excitatory amino acids. *Ann NY Acad Sci* 568:149–158

Mizuno Y, Suzuki K, Sone N, Saitoh T (1988): Inhibition of mitochondrial respiration by PTP in mouse brain in vivo. *Neurosci Lett* 91:349–353

Nicklas WJ, Vyas I, Heikkila RE (1985): Inhibition of NADH-linked oxidation in brain mitochondria by MPP^+, a metabolite of the neurotoxin MPTP. *Life Sci* 36:2503–2508

Novelli A, Reilly JA, Lysko PG, Henneberry RC (1988): Glutamate becomes neurotoxic via the *N*-methyl-D-aspartate receptor when intracellular energy levels are reduced. *Brain Res* 451:205–212

Olney JW (1989): Excitatory amino acids and neuropsychiatric disorders. *Biol Psychiatry* 26:505–525

Orrenius S, Burkitt MJ, Kass GEN, Dypbukt JM, Nicotera P (1992): Calcium ions and oxidative cell injury. *Ann Neurol* 32:533–534

Parker WD, Boyson SJ, Luder AS, Parks JK (1990a): Evidence for a defect in NADH: ubiquinone oxidoreductase (complex I) in Huntington's disease. *Neurology* 40: 1231–1234

Parker WD, Filley CM, Parks JG (1990b): Cytochrome oxidase deficiency in Alzheimer's disease. *Neurology* 40:1302–1303

Rothman SM, Olney JW (1987): Excitotoxicity and the NMDA receptor. *Trends Neurosci* 10:299–302

Schapira AHV, Cooper JM, Dexter D, Clark JB, Jenner P, Marsden CD (1990): Mitochondrial complex I deficiency in Parkinson's disease. *J Neurochem* 55:2142–2145

Schöls L, Reichmann H, Langkafel M, Kuhn W, Przuntek H (1992): Mitochondrial disorders in cerebellar ataxias. *Mov Disord* 7:S44

Schwarcz R, Speciale C, Turski WA (1990): Kynurenines, glia and the pathogenesis of neurodegenerative disorders. In: *Parkinsonism and Ageing*, Calne DB, Comi G, Crippa D, Horowski R, Trabucchi M, eds., pp. 97–105. New York: Raven Press

Stamler JS, Singel DJ, Loscalzo J (1992): Biochemistry of nitric oxide and its redox-activated forms. *Science* 258: 1898–1902

Storey E, Hyman BT, Jenkins B, Brouillet E, Miller JM, Rosen BR, Beal MF (1992): 1-Methyl-4-phenylpyridinium produces excitotoxic lesions in rat striatum as a result of impairment of oxidative metabolism. *J Neurochem* 58:1975–1978

Srivastava R, Brouillet E, Beal MF, Storey E, Hyman BT (1993): Blockade of 1-methyl-4-phenylpyridinium ion (MPP^+) nigral toxicity in the rat by prior decortication or MK-801 treatment a stereological estimate of neuronal loss. *Neurobial Aging* 14:295–301

Turski L (1991): Excitatory amino acid antagonists and Parkinsons's disease. In: *Parkinson's Disease – From Basic Research and Early Diagnosis to Long-Term Treatment*, Rinne UK, Nagatsu T, Horowski R, eds., pp. 97–114. Bussum: Medicom

Turski L, Melamed E (1993): Is there a role for excitatory amino acid antagonists? In: *Parkinson's Disease – Controversial Issues in therapy*, Marsden CD, Oertel WH, eds., pp. 44–53. Bussum: Medicom

Turski L, Bressler K, Rettig K-J, Löschmann P-A Wachtel H (1991): Protection of substantia nigra from MPP$^+$ neurotoxicity by *N*-methyl-D-aspartate antagonists. *Nature* 349:414–418

Turski WA (1991): Aminooxyacetic acid produces excitotoxic lesions in the rat substantia nigra. *Naunyn-Schmiedebergs Arch Pharmacol* 344:R67

Turski WA, Urbańska E, Sieklucka M, Ikonomidou C (1992): Quinolinate-like neurotoxicity produced by aminooxyacetic acid in rat striatum. *Amino Acids* 2:245–253

Urbańska E, Ikonomidou C, Sieklucka M, Turski WA (1989): Aminooxyacetic acid produces excitotoxic lesions in the rat striatum. *Soc Neurosci Abstr* 15:764

Urbańska E, Ikonomidou C, Sieklucka M, Turski WA (1991): Aminooxyacetic acid produces excitotoxic lesions in the rat striatum. *Synapse* 9:129–135

Wallace DC (1992): Diseases of the mitochondrial DNA. *Annu Rev Biochem* 61:1175–1212

Youdim MBH (1993): The biology of toxic events in Parkinson's disease. In: *Advances in Research on Neurodegeneration*, Vol. I, Calne DB, Horowski R, Mizuno Y, Poewe WH, Riederer P, Youdim MBH, eds., pp. 71–90. Boston: Birkhäuser

Zeevalk GD, Nicklas WJ (1990): Chemically induced hypoglycemia and anoxia: relationship to glutamate receptor-mediated toxicity in retina. *J Pharmacol Exp Ther* 253:1285–1292

Zeevalk GD, Nicklas WJ (1991): Mechanisms underlying initiation of excitotoxicity associated with metabolic inhibition. *J Pharmacol Exp Ther* 257: 870–878

Zuddas A, Oberto G, Vaglini F, Fascetti F, Fornai F, Corsini GU (1992): MK 801 prevents MPTP-induced parkinsonism in primates. *J Neurochem* 59:733–739

13

Proteases and Pathological Neurodegeneration

ROBERT SIMAN, MARY J. SAVAGE, AND JILL M. ROBERTS-LEWIS

An understanding of the biochemical processes that lead to neuronal damage is crucial to the development of therapies aimed at slowing the progression of neurodegenerative diseases. While brain proteases have long been recognized for their importance to neuropeptide metabolism and protein turnover (Loh et al., 1984; Pope and Nixon, 1984), it is becoming increasingly clear that proteolysis plays a role in pathological neuronal degeneration as well. This chapter briefly reviews the evidence relating proteolytic mechanisms to the neurodegeneration triggered by injury or disease. The focus is on a calcium-dependent protease, calpain 1, and its possible involvement in mediating structural damage produced by excessive accumulation of intracellular free calcium. Because the role of calpain 1 in neurodegenerative processes has been the subject of recent review (Seubert and Lynch, 1990; Siman, 1990; 1992), the present brief review is followed by a description of new studies directed at the localization, timing, and mode of activation of calpain 1 in animal models of neuronal damage.

The Calcium-Dependent Protease Calpain 1, and Ischemic and Traumatic Neuronal Damage

At rest, intraneuronal free calcium is buffered to submicromolar levels but, under conditions of extreme toxic neuronal excitation (termed "excitotoxicity"; Olney et al., 1971) or pathological injury, free calcium concentrations dramatically increase (Evans et al., 1984; Kudo and Ogura, 1986; Schlaepfer, 1979). Because an excessive elevation in intracellular calcium has been linked to degeneration of a large number of cell types (Schanne et al., 1979), the neuronal damage associated with extreme excitation or injury could be calcium mediated. A variety of enzymes and protein–protein associations are calcium dependent; thus, a challenge of recent research has been to identify particular calcium-dependent processes that may underlie excitotoxic or injury-induced neuronal death.

Pharmacological, biochemical, and neuroanatomical studies have linked activation of a calcium-dependent neutral cysteine protease, referred to as calpain 1 or μ-calpain (Mellgren and Murachi, 1990), to calcium-mediated neurodegeneration. Studies of axotomy-induced neurodegeneration were the first to associate calcium influx and a concomitant protease activation to delayed neuronal degeneration (Schlaepfer, 1979; Schlaepfer and Hasler, 1979). A more recent focus has been excitotoxicity. Excessive stimulation of excitatory amino acid receptors leads to a delayed neuronal death that is calcium dependent (Choi, 1985; Manev et al., 1989) and is accompanied by enhanced protein degradation (Seubert et al., 1988; Siman and Noszek, 1988; Siman et al., 1989). Several features of the protein breakdown suggest that it is caused by activation of calpain 1 (Siman and Noszek, 1988). Calpain 1 has an absolute requirement for calcium for its activation, is essentially inactive at the calcium levels found in resting neurons, and is activated by calcium in the 1-μm range, a concentration transiently reached in neurons undergoing extreme physiological or pharmacological excitation (Kudo and Ogura, 1986; Regehr et al., 1989). Moreover, several protease inhibitors that share the ability to block calpain are neuroprotective both in the hippocampal slice preparation (Siman, 1990), and in hippocampus *in vivo* following an episode of transient global cerebral ischemia (Lee et al., 1991; Lutz et al., 1991) that produces a delayed excitotoxic injury (Gill et al., 1988; Simon et al., 1984). Immunohistochemical observations have confirmed that calpain I is a component of the perikarya and dendrites of diverse neuronal populations, including several that are particularly vulnerable in neurodegenerative diseases (Siman et al., 1985; 1990). Taken together, the studies indicate that calpain I is present in neurons, that it may be activated under conditions that elicit excitotoxic neurodegeneration, and that its inhibition may be sufficient to at least partially spare neurons from death.

Localization and Timing of Calpain Activation Following Transient Cerebral Ischemia

While the studies just summarized present considerable evidence that protease activation may play a role in excitotoxic and ischemic neurodegeneration, a host of questions remain unanswered. Does the protease activation that follows transient ischemia occur before neurons have begun to degenerate, or is it merely a reflection of an already ensuing neuronal structural disintegration? Can calpain 1 be confirmed as the endogeneous protease that is activated? Is calpain 1 activation only associated with stimuli that produce neuronal injury, or could it have a role in normal physiological brain processes? What neurotransmitter receptors are responsible for the protease activation associated with ischemia? A neuroanatomical method capable of detecting calpain activation would provide a means of approaching these questions.

We have recently developed such a method, based on an antibody that selectively labels a protein on its degradation by calpain but which does not recognize either the intact protein or the protein that has been degraded by other proteases. The protein chosen is brain spectrin (also called fodrin), an actin-binding structural component of neurons that comprises about 1–2% of the total brain protein (Davis and Bennett, 1983). Brain spectrin is an excellent calpain substrate, and undergoes limited proteolysis ($K_m \sim 50$ nM; Siman et al., 1984), with the 240 kDa α-subunit being cleaved approximately in half to form fragments of about 145 and 150 kDa. The spectrin fragments are themselves relatively resistant to further degradation (Harris et al., 1988; Siman et al., 1984). Importantly for the present method, the site of calpain cleavage of the α-subunit of brain spectrin has been precisely located and sequenced (Harris et al., 1988). We raised antibodies to two hexapeptides corresponding to the newly exposed termini of the two α-spectrin fragments generated by calpain 1 hydrolysis: the NH_2-terminal domain of the COOH-terminal fragment (GMMPRD, using the one-letter amino acid code), and the COOH-terminal domain of the NH_2-terminal fragment (QQQEVY). If these antibodies only recognize calpain-degraded spectrin, and not either intact spectrin or spectrin fragments produced by other proteases cleaving at other sites in the α-subunit, they would be useful for immunohistochemical localization of calpain-degraded spectrin in the brain in animal models of neurodegeneration, as well as in the human diseases themselves.

Immunoblot analysis demonstrates that the antibodies indeed recognize calpain-degraded spectrin much more readily than intact spectrin or the spectrin degraded by a variety of other proteases. Both anti-GMMPRD and anti-QQQEVY label a single 145- to 150-kDa polypeptide on immunoblots of rodent brain membranes that had been incubated in the presence of calcium to activate the endogenous calpain. Intact α-spectrin of more 240-kDa is unstained. In contrast, a polyclonal antibody raised against purified brain spectrin (Siman and Noszek, 1988; Siman et al., 1984) labels both the intact α-subunit and two major proteolytic fragments of 145 to 150 kDa. Supporting the interpretation that the fragments are generated by calpain activation, they are present at nearly undetectable levels in membranes not treated with calcium, and their calcium-mediated appearance is blocked by calpain inhibitors. Our interpretation of these results is that calpain-mediated spectrin degradation uncovers epitopes which are hidden in the intact protein but become unmasked on cleavage by calpain. It is likely that the anti-GMMPRD and anti-QQQEVY antibodies each label one of the two major fragments detected by polyclonal antispectrin antibodies.

Having developed probes for the selective labeling of calpain-degraded spectrin, we next performed an immunohistochemical study to localize calpain-degraded spectrin following transient global cerebral ischemia in the gerbil. In this model, 5-minute bilateral carotid artery occlusion produces a delayed, selective excitotoxic lesion restricted primarily to the hippocampal area CA1 (Kirino and Sano, 1984). The neuronal degeneration is apparent by 24 hours using silver impregnation methods, and the neuronal loss is detectable with Nissl stains by 4 days. In control animals subjected to the surgical procedure but not the ischemia, only faint anti-QQQEVY immunoreactivity was observed in neuronal perikarya distributed throughout the brain (Fig. 1A). However, as early as 30 minutes after ischemia anti-QQQEVY immunoreactivity became intense in the perikarya and dendrites of circumscribed neuronal populations of the forebrain (Fig. 1B). Immunostaining was most apparent in parietal, frontal, and piriform cortex (especially in layers 3 and 5), hippocampus (areas CA3 and CA1), thalamus (several ventral and lateral nuclei), striatum (caudate and putamen), and olfactory tubercle. Thus, spectrin degradation occurs in a number of forebrain areas of the gerbil following a short period of global ischemia, including several regions that exhibit little or no neuronal loss days after the insult.

The regional pattern of anti-QQQEVY immunoreactivity changed dramatically at longer survival times. By 2 days post ischemia, immunoreactivity was virtually gone, with the notable exception of intense labeling of the perikarya, apical and basal dendrites of hippocampal pyramidal neurons of area CA1 (Fig. 1C and D). This immunostaining was also prominent at 3 days but largely disappeared by 5 days, by which time many CA1 neurons had degenerated and been cleared. Therefore, while spectrin degradation is stimulated in response to ischemia in a number of brain areas, a spectrin degradation that is sustained for at least 48 to 72 hours is restricted to those hippocampal neurons destined to degenerate.

The time course of spectrin degradation following transient global ischemia in the gerbil has been confirmed by immunoblot analysis. A marked increase in hippocampal anti-QQQEVY immunoreactivity occurs in as early as 30 minutes and persists for 3 days. Immunoreactivity for anti-GMMPDR, which detects the other α-spectrin fragment

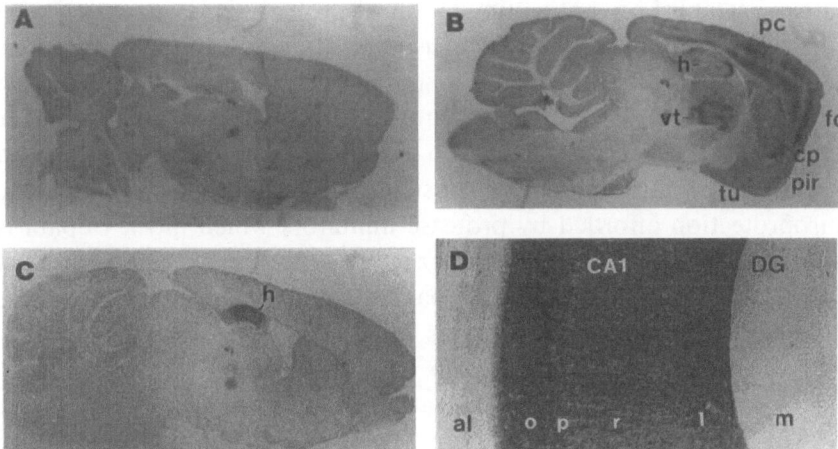

Figure 1. Immunohistochemical localization of degraded spectrin following transient global cerebral ischemia in the gerbil. **A:** Control, **B:** 30 min after a 5-min bilateral occlusion of the carotid arteries, **C, D:** 2 days. Sagittal sections were stained with anti-QQQEVY, an antibody that selectively recognizes calpain-degraded spectrin, but not the intact molecule. **A–C:** While sham-operated brain exhibits only faint immunoreactivity, by 30 min intense labeling is observed in several forebrain areas, including parietal (pc), frontal (fc), and piriform (pir) cortex, hippocampus (h), ventral thalamic nuclei (vt), and olfactory tubercle (tu). By 2 days, however, immunostaining persisted predominantly in the hippocampus. **D:** Higher magnification view of hippocampal immunoreactivity at 2 days post ischemia. Degraded spectrin immunoreactivity is restricted to area CA1 pyramidal cell bodies and their apical and basal dendrites. Thus, area CA1 is intensely stained in strata oriens (o), pyramidale (p), radiatum (r), and lacunosum moleculare (l). The overlying alveus (al) and underlying dentate gyrus (DG) stratum moleculare (m) are devoid of immunoreactivity.

generated by calpain cleavage, also increases in hippocampus in response to transient global ischemia. Because gerbil forebrain membrane fractions only exhibit immunoreactivity for these two antibodies in conditions which result in calpain activation (addition of calcium, in the absence of calpain inhibitors), and not on digestion with seven other cysteine or serine proteases, it is highly likely that the ischemia-induced increase in spectrin degradation is a result of the activation of calpain.

Summary and Concluding Remarks

Biochemical and pharmacological experiments have implicated activation of the calcium-dependent neutral cysteine protease calpain 1 in pathological excitotoxic neurodegeneration. Degradation of a preferred calpain substrate, brain spectrin, is markedly increased following a number of insults that lead to neuronal death, while protease inhibitors that block calpain are neuroprotective both *in vitro* and *in vivo*. Therefore, it is now established that a stimulation of proteolysis is associated with neurodegeneration. However, conclusive identification of the endogenous protease responsible for enhanced spectrin degradation is problematic. For example, while a number of features of increased spectrin turnover suggest that it is caused an activation of calpain 1 (discussed in Siman and Noszek, 1988), it has not been possible to determine this directly. The neuroprotection afforded by protease inhibitors which block calpain is also suggestive (Lee et al., 1991; Lutz et al., 1991; Siman, 1990) but must be considered inconclusive on the basis of the broad specificity of these inhibitors for a number of proteases.

To further evaluate the calpain hypothesis of excitotoxic neurodegeneration, the timing and localization of spectrin degradation were assessed using antibodies that are selective for spectrin degradation mediated by calpain. A sustained spectrin degradation was correlated with vulnerability of hippocampal pyramidal neurons of area CA1 to ischemic neuronal death, and was initiated before the neurons degenerated. This method is currently being used to identify the neuroreceptor classes whose activation leads to spectrin degradation, both in areas in which neurodegeneration ensues (hippocampal area CA1) and in regions in which a transient spectrin breakdown is not accompanied by neuronal death (parietal, frontal, and piriform cortex, striatum, thalamus, olfactory tubercle).

While a growing body of evidence has linked calpain activation to neurodegeneration, a definitive test of the calpain hypothesis may require the knockout of calpain, either with deliverable and highly selective inhibitors or by molecular genetic methods.

It is noteworthy that proteolysis has now been dissociated from neurodegeneration, because spectrin degradation can be stimulated without being accompanied by neuronal death. This supports the possibility that physiologically relevant changes in neuronal activity may regulate the breakdown of proteins of importance to neuronal function. Because spectrin is a prominent component of a membrane skeletal system that contributes to the structural integrity of neurons (Davis and Bennett, 1983), it is intriguing to consider that physiological control of its degradation may be a mechanism for producing neuronal structural change, for example, such as may occur during neural development or associated with synaptic plasticity (Seubert and Lynch, 1990; Siman et al., 1987).

Finally, in view of the increasing links between proteolysis and neurodegeneration, it is important to consider that proteolytic mechanisms other than the one described here may be involved in neuropathological processes. As one example, proteolysis is currently being intensively examined for its role in generating the β/A4 protein, the principal component of amyloid deposits that accumulate with aging and especially with Alzheimer's disease and Down's syndrome. Just as protein synthesis is under complex modulatory control, both by transcriptional and posttranscriptional factors, so too may alterations in protein degradation be a means of modifying the steady-state levels and hence the function of neurobiologically important proteins. A loss of control over protein degradation may have deleterious and pathological consequences for neurons.

Acknowledgements

We thank the Cephalon Chemistry group for preparing peptides for antibody production, Val Marcy and Leonard Pinsker for excellent technical assistance, and Drs. Frank Baldino and Jeffry Vaught for their continued support of this research.

References

Choi DW (1985): Glutamate neurotoxicity is cortical cell culture in calcium dependent. *Neurosci Lett* 58:293–297

Davis J, Bennett V (1983):Brain spectrin. Isolation of subunits and formation of hybrids with erythrocyte spectrin subunits. *J Biol Chem* 258:7757–7766

Evans MC, Griffiths T, Meldrum BS (1984): Kainic acid seizures and the reversibility of calcium loading in vulnerable neurons in the hippocampus. *Neuropathol Appl Neurobiol* 10:285–302

Gill R, Foster AC, Woodruff GN (1988): MK-801 is neuroprotective in gerbils when administered during the post-ischaemic period. *Neuroscience* 25:847–855

Harris AS, Croall DE, Morrow JS (1988): The calmodulin-binding site in α-fodrin is near the calcium-dependent protease-I cleavage site. *J Biol Chem* 263:15754–15761

Kirino T, Sano K (1984): Selective vulnerability in the gerbil hippocampus following transient ischemia. *Acta Neuropath (Berl)* 62:201–208

Kudo Y, Ogura A (1986): Glutamate-induced increase in intracellular Ca^{2+} concentration in isolated hippocampal neurones. *Br J Pharmacol* 89:191–198

Lee KS, Frank S, Vanderklish P, Arai A, Lynch G (1991): Inhibition of proteolysis protects hippocampal neurons from ischemia. *Proc Natl Acad Sci USA* 88:7233–7237

Loh YP, Brownstein MJ, Gainer H (1984): Proteolysis in neuropeptide processing and other neural functions. *Annu Rev Neurosci* 7:189–222

Lutz DL, Dean RL, Harris ME, Miotke JA, Ton HT, Miyazaki BK, Eveleth DD, Bartus RT (1991): Intracellular events related to the delayed neuronal death following transient global ischemia. *Neurosci Abstr* 17:1264

Manev H, Favaron M, Guidotti A, Costa E (1989): Delayed increase of Ca^{2+} influx elicited by glutamate: role in neuronal death. *Mol Pharmacol* 36:106–112

Mellgren RL, Murachi T (1990): *Intracellular Calcium-Dependent Proteolysis*. Boca Raton: CRC Press

Olney JW, Ho OL, Rhee V (1971): Cytotoxic effects of acidic and sulphur containing amino acids on the infant mouse central nervous system. *Exp Brain Res* 14:61–76

Pope A, Nixon RA (1984): Proteases of human brain. *Neurochem Res* 9:291–323

Regehr WG, Connor JA, Tank DW (1989): Optical imaging of calcium accumulation in hippocampal pyramidal cells during synaptic activation. *Nature* 341:533–536

Schanne FAX, Kane AB, Young EE, Farber JL (1979): Calcium dependence of toxic cell death: a final common pathway. *Science* 206:700–702

Schlaepfer WW (1979): Nature of mammalian neurofilaments and their breakdown by calcium. *Prog Neuropathol* 4:101–123

Schlaepfer WW, Hasler MB (1979): Characterization of the calcium-induced disruption of neurofilaments in rat peripheral nerve. *Brain Res* 168:299–309

Seubert P, Lynch G (1990): Plasticity to pathology: brain calpains as modifiers of synaptic structure. In: *Intracellular Calcium-Dependent Proteolysis*, Mellgren RL, Murachi, T, eds., pp. 251–263. Boca Raton: CRC Press

Seubert P, Larson J, Oliver M, Jung MW, Baudry M, Lynch G (1988): Stimulation of NMDA receptors induces proteolysis of spectrin in hippocampus. *Brain Res* 460:189–194

Siman R (1990): Role of calpain 1 in excitatory amino acid-induced degenerative structural changes. In: *Neurotoxicity of Excitatory Amino Acids*, Guidotti A, ed., pp. 145–161. New York: Raven Press

Siman R (1992): Proteolytic mechanism for the neurodegeneration of Alzheimer's disease. *Ann NY Acad Sci* 674:193–202

Siman R, Noszek JC (1988): Excitatory amino acids activate calpain 1 and induce structural protein breakdown *in vivo*. *Neuron* 1:279–287

Siman R, Baudry M, Lynch G (1984): Brain fodrin: substrate for calpain 1, an endogenous calcium-activated protease. *Proc Natl Acad Sci USA* 81:3572–3576

Siman R, Baudry M, Lynch G (1987): Calcium-activated proteases as possible mediators of synaptic plasticity. In: *Synaptic Function*, Edelman GM, Gall WE, Cowan WM, eds., pp. 519–548. New York: Wiley

Siman R, Card JP, Davis LG (1990): Proteolytic processing of β-amyloid precursor by calpain 1. *J Neurosci* 10:2400–2411

Siman R, Noszek JB, Kegerise C (1989): Calpain 1 activation is specifically related to excitatory amino acid induction of hippocampal damage. *J Neurosci* 9:1579–1590

Siman R, Gall C, Perlmutter LS, Christian C, Baudry M, Lynch G (1985): Distribution of calpain 1, an enzyme associated with degenerative activity, in rat brain. *Brain Res* 347:399–403

14

Endogenous MPTP-Like Amines in the Brain: Isoquinolines

Toshiharu Nagatsu, Makoto Naoi, Toshimitsu Niwa, and Mitsuo Yoshida

The discovery of N-methyl-4-phenyl-1,2,3,6-tetrahydropyridine (MPTP) as a parkinsonism-producing neurotoxin (Davis et al., 1979; Langston et al., 1983) has greatly contributed to the pathogenesis of Parkinson's disease. Efforts have been made to find MPTP-like neurotoxins in the brain of parkinsonian patients. MPTP is a precursor neurotoxin, and the oxidized form, by monoamine oxidase type B, N-methyl-4-phenylpyridinium ion (MPP^+), is the active neurotoxin (Chiba et al., 1984). It is assumed, therefore, that if any hypothetical MPTP-like neurotoxins exist in the parkinsonian brain they might be oxidized by monoamine oxidase to active neurotoxins.

Endogenous MPTP-Like Amines

Two groups of endogenous MPTP-like amines have been found in the human brain: isoquinolines (IQs) and β-carbolines (BCs). Tetrahydroisoquinolines (TIQs) were first found as *in vivo* metabolites of L-dopa in man (Sandler et al., 1973). TIQs subsequently were also found in normal and parkinsonian human brains (Figs. 1 and 2). 1,2,3,4-Tetrahydroisoquinoline (TIQ) (Niwa et al., 1987, 1989a; Ohta et al., 1987) and 1-methyl-tetrahydroisoquinoline (1-Me-TIQ) (Ohta et al., 1987) were found in control and parkinsonian human brains. TIQ and 1-Me-TIQ may be synthesized from phenylethylamine. 1-Methyl-6,7-dihydroxy-1,2,3,4-tetrahydroisoquinoline (1-Me-DH-TIQ, norsalsolinol NORSAL), and 1,2-dimethyl-6,7-dihydroxy-1,2,3,4-tetrahydroisoquinoline $(1,N(ME)_2\text{-}DH\text{-}TIQ$, salsolinol, SAL), their N-methylated compounds which are assumed to be synthesized from dopamine, were found in normal and parkinsonian human brains (Niwa et al., 1991). These isoquinolines were also found in various foods (Makino et al., 1988; Niwa et al., 1989b).

ADVANCES IN RESEARCH ON NEURODEGENERATION, II
Y. Mizuno et al.
© 1994 Birkhäuser Boston

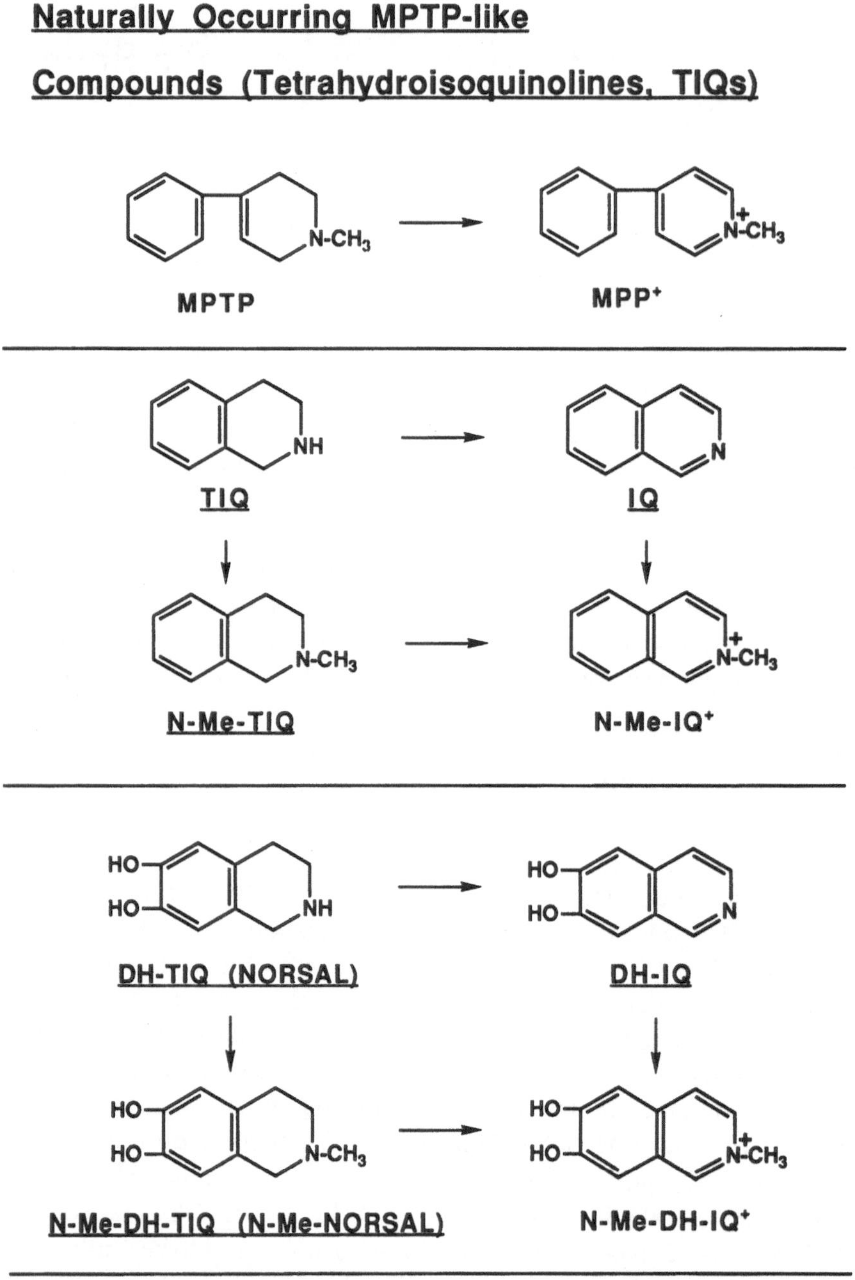

Naturally Occurring MPTP-like

Compounds (Tetrahydroisoquinolines, TIQs)

Figure 1. Structures of endogenous MPTP-like compounds, tetrahydroisoquinolines (TIQs), and the probable oxidized isoquinolinium ions (IQ⁺s).

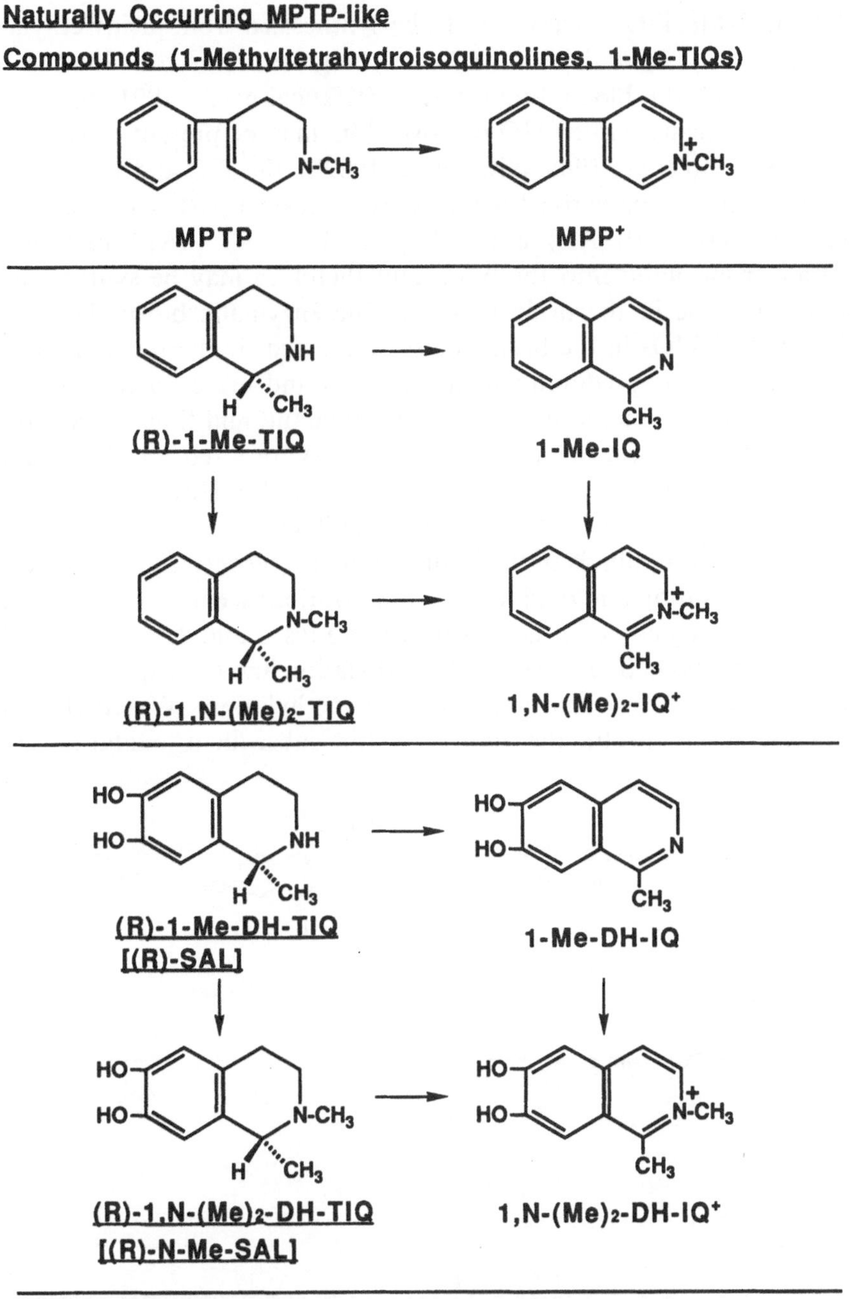

Naturally Occurring MPTP-like
Compounds (1-Methyltetrahydroisoquinolines, 1-Me-TIQs)

Figure 2. Structures of endogenous MPTP-like compounds, 1-methyl-tetrahydroisoquinolines (1-Me-TIQs), and the probable oxidized 1-methyl-isoquinolinium ions (1-Me-IQ$^+$s).

Biosynthesis of Endogenous MPTP-Like Isoquinolines

TIQ and 1-Me-TIQ are assumed to be synthesized from phenylethyla-mine (Fig. 3). TIQ and 1-Me-TIQ easily migrated from the blood into brain through the blood–brain barrier (Kikuchi et al., 1991; Niwa et al., 1988). Because either TIQ or 1-Me-TIQ may be present in various foods (Makino et al., 1988; Niwa et al., 1989b), the TIQ and 1-Me-TIQ in the brain may be derived from foods at least in part. However, N-Me-DH-TIQ (NORSAL) and 1,N-(Me)$_2$-DH-TIQ (SAL) may not migrate from blood into the brain and therefore may be synthesized from dopamine in the brain (Fig. 4). The enzymatic biosynthesis of TIQs or DH-TIQs in the brain is also supported by the fact that R-1-Me-TIQs may be predominant in the brain and urine, in contrast to foods in which the unnatural S form is abundant, and thus the R form may be the natural form enzymatically synthesized in the brain (Makino et al., 1990; Strolin-Benedetti et al., 1989). However, because both the R and S enantiomers of 1-Me-DH-TIQ may exist in the brain, a part of the compounds in the brain could also be derived from foods.

N-Methylation and oxidation (aromatization) seems to be essential for the neurotoxicity of TIQs. As shown in Figs. 1 and 2, there are two possible metabolic pathways: (1) N-methylation and subsequent oxidation, or (2) oxidation and subsequent N-methylation. N-Methylation of TIQs seems to be the first step for subsequent oxidation by

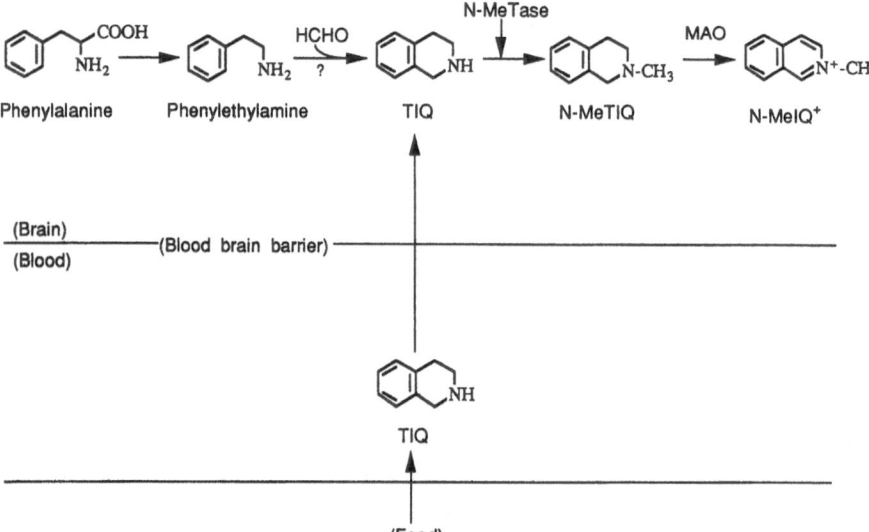

Figure 3. Possible pathway of formation of N-methyl-isoquinolinium ion (N-MeIQ$^+$) in the brain.

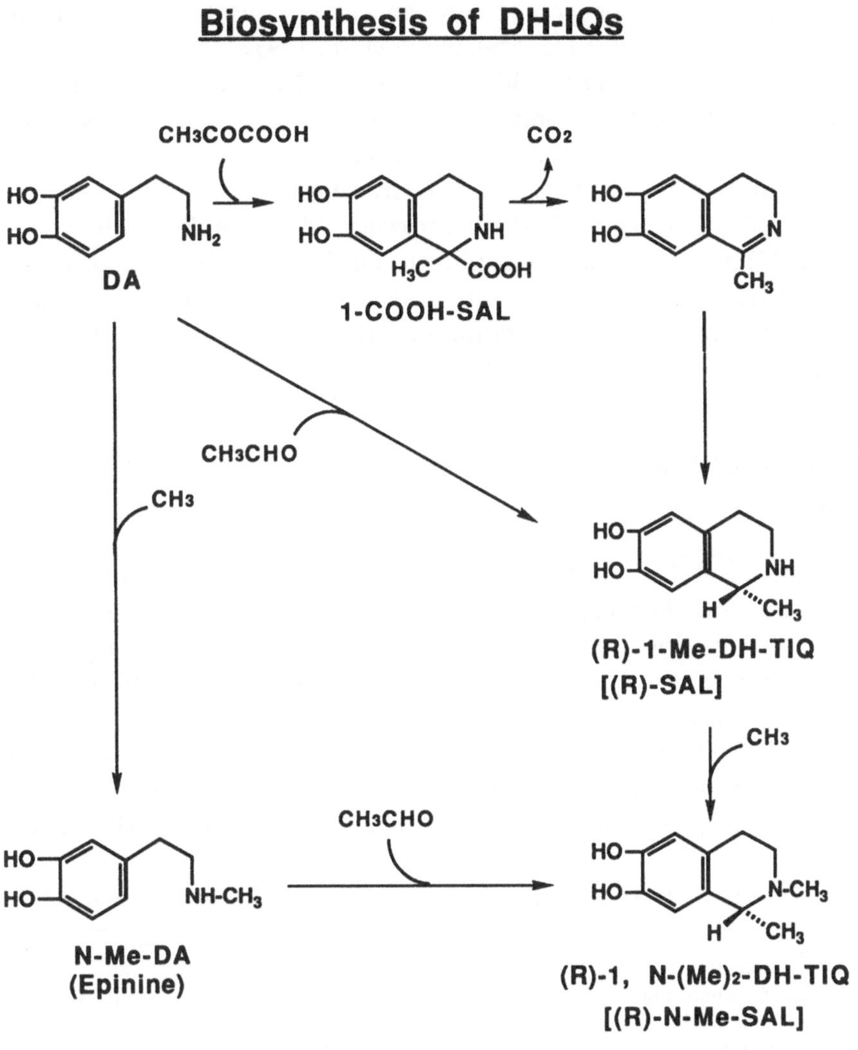

Biosynthesis of DH-IQs

Figure 4. Possible pathway of biosynthesis of dihydroxytetrahydroisoquinolines (DH-TIQs) in the brain.

monoamine oxidase to isoquinolinium ions (IQ^+s) (Naoi et al., 1989a, 1989b). *N*-Methylation of salsolinol is also confirmed *in vivo* by microdialysis (Maruyama et al., Niwa et al., 1992). Thus, *N*-methylation of TIQs to *N*-Me-TIQs and oxidation (aromatization) seems to be the main pathway to form *N*-Me-IQ^+s. However, 1,*N*-(Me)$_2$-DH-TIQ (N-Me-SAL) may also be formed via *N*-methyl-dopamine (epinine), which is found in either normal or parkinsonian brains (Kazita et al., 1993) (Fig. 4).

Like TIQs, β-carboline is also *N*-methylated, and *N*-methylated βcarbolinium ion is proposed to be an endogenous MPP$^+$-like amine (Collins and Neafsey, 1985; Matsubara et al., 1993).

The Parkinson's disease-like effects of S-adenoysl-L-methionine, the compound stimulating N-methylation reaction in the brain, may also suggest that N-methylation is an important reaction in the pathogenesis of Parkinson's disease (Charlton and Crowell, 1992).

4-Hydroxylation by P-450 hydroxylase (debrisoquine hydroxylase, CYP2D6) seems to be important for the metabolism of exogeneous TIQs derived from foods, and therefore a deficiency in debrisoquine hydroxylase may increase the migration of TIQs from blood into the brain (Makino et al., 1990).

Neurotoxic Effects of Endogenous MPTP-Like Amines in the Brain

TIQs or DH-TIQs may be first N-methylated into N-Me-TIQs or N-Me-DH-TIQs, and then may be oxidized into N-me-IQs$^+$ or N-Me-DH-IQs$^+$ to produce neurotoxicity (Naoi et al., 1989a, 1989b). TIQs or DH-TIQs have various acute effects on nigrostriatal dopaminergic neurons in the brain, similar to those of MPTP (Table 1).

TIQs inhibit tyrosine hydroxylase. R-DH-TIQ (R-SAL) inhibits tyrosine hydroxylase by reducing the affinity of the cofactor (6R)-L-*erythro*-tetrahydrobiopterin for the enzyme (Minami et al., 1992). R-SAL similarly

Table 1. Effects of MPTP (MPP$^+$) and TIQs (IQ$^+$s) on Dopaminergic (DA) Neurons[a]

Effect	MPTP	TIQs
Oxidation by monoamine oxidase (MAO)	Yes	Yes (weak)
MAO inhibition	Yes	Yes
Uptake into DA neurons	Yes	Yes
Uptake into synaptic vesicles	Yes	?
Release of DA	Yes	?
Tyrosine hydroxylase (TH) inhibition	Yes	Yes
TH protein decrease	Yes	Yes
TH mRNA decrease	Yes	Yes
Aromatic L-amino acid decarboxylase inhibition	Yes	Yes
Combination with neuromelanin	Yes	?
Accumulation in DA neurons	Yes	Yes (weak)
Accumulation into mitochondria	Yes	Yes (weak)
Mitochondrial complex I inhibition	Yes	Yes
Decrease in adenosine triphosphate (ATP) formation	Yes	Yes
Radical formation	Yes	Yes
Cell death	Yes	No

[a]MPTP 1-[N]-methyl-4-phenyl-1,2,3,6-tetrahydropyridine; MPP$^+$, 1-[N]-methyl-4-phenyl-pyridinium ion; TIQs, tetrahydroisoquinolines; IQs$^+$, isoquinolinium ions.

inhibits another pterin-dependent, serotonin-synthesizing monooxygenase, tryptophan hydroxylase (Ota et al., 1992).

After chronic administration in C57BL/6J mice, TIQ decreases tyrosine hydroxylase protein in mesencephalic dopamine neurons, as detected immunohistochemically, but does not cause cell death (Ogawa et al., 1989). TIQs are also the inhibitors of monoamine oxidase, which oxidizes dopamine (Strolin-Benedetti and Dostert, 1992). DH-TIQs and N-Me-DH-TIQs are poor substrates but inhibit monoamine oxidase type A and B (Minami et al., 1993). As compared to TIQs, N-Me-TIQs seem to be slowly but significantly oxidized by monoamine oxidase in vitro (Naoi et al., 1989a). The oxidation of TIQs and N-Me-TIQs in vivo by monoamine oxidase remains to be further confirmed.

The inhibition of complex I in the electron transport system of mitochondria and the resultant adenosine triphosphate (ATP) deficiency (energy crisis) are assumed to be the direct cause of neuronal cell death by MPP^+. As in the case of MPP^+, $N\text{-Me-IQ}^+$ and N-Me-TIQ selectively inhibit complex I in isolated mitochondria prepared from mouse brain (Suzuki et al., 1992). N-methylated β-carbolines also inhibit complex I (Fields et al., 1992). The reason that TIQs or N-Me-TIQs, which inhibit mitochondrial complex I like MPP^+, do not cause death of nigrostriatal dopamine neurons is not yet clear. It is likely that TIQs or N-Me-TIQs and the oxidized products may not accumulate selectively in the mitochondria of nigrostriatal dopaminergic neurons, and thus may not inhibit complex I strongly enough to reduce ATP formation and thus cause neuronal cell death.

Probable Relationship Between Endogenous MPTP-Like Amines and Parkinson's Disease

Although no immunohistochemical evidence has been found for the role of an endogenous neurotoxin related to MPTP (or MPP^+) in parkinsonian brains, IQs and BCs may be such endogenous compounds because the structures and the effects are similar to MPTP.

TIQs or N-Me-TIQs are similar to MPTP or MPP^+ in their acute effects on nigrostriatal dopaminergic neurons, inhibiting dopamine synthesis and decreasing dopamine. However, their acute effects are weaker than those of MPP^+. Further, TIQs, N-Me-TIQs, and their oxidized compounds may not produce cell death in vivo. $N\text{-Me-IQ}^+$, which is the most potent inhibitor of complex I among IQs, destroys dopaminergic mesencephalic neurons but not γ-amino butyric acid (GABA) neurons only in the cell culture system (Niijima et al., 1991). The concentrations of TIQs or N-Me-TIQs in the human brain are approximately 10 ng/g brain tissue, and there are no significant differences between normal and parkinsonian brains in these concentrations. Moreover, intracerebral regional distribution of TIQs or N-Me-TIQs is not specific for the nigrostriatal dopaminergic region. These observations are in contrast to MPTP and MPP$^+$, which specifically destroy nigrostriatal dopaminergic neurons (Michel et al., 1989).

TIQ acutely produces a parkinsonism-like motor disturbance that is reversed by L-dopa in monkeys, but the symptoms are transient and reversible (Nagatsu and Yoshida, 1988; Yoshida et al., 1990). This is consistent with the finding that TIQ decreases tyrosine hydroxylase (TH) activity and TH protein, but does not cause nigrostriatal dopamine cell death in mice (Ogawa et al., 1989). In contrast to TIQ, 1-Me-TIQs are relatively rich in nigrostriatal dopamine regions, and 1-Me-TIQ concentrations are lower in parkinsonian brains than in control brains (Ohta et al., 1987). An interesting finding is that 1-Me-TIQ prevents parkinsonism-like behavior abnormalities produced by either MPTP or TIQ (Tasaki et al., 1991). This fact could suggest the presence of some TIQ-like compounds that may be related to Parkinson's disease. A question is whether or not endogenous 1-Me-TIQs (1-Me-TIQ or SAL) can be protective against parkinsonism. Another suggestive piece of evidence indicating the relation of IQs and Parkinson's disease is that a person who is poor metabolizer of debrisoquine and has low activity of CYP2D6 metabolizing IQs may be susceptible to Parkinson's disease.

In conclusion, further studies are required on the biosynthesis and metabolism of endogenous IQs to elucidate their pathological role in relationships to Parkinson's disease.

Acknowledgments

This work was supported by grants-in-aid for Scientific Research from the Ministry of Education, Science and Culture of Japan.

References

Charlton CG, Crowell B Jr (1992): Parkinson's disease-like effects of S-adenosyl-L-methionine: effects of L-dopa. *Pharmacol Biochem Behav* 43:423–431

Chiba K, Trevor A, Castagnoli N Jr (1984): Metabolism of the neurotoxic tertiary amine, MPTP, by brain monoamine oxidase. *Biochem Biophys Res Commun* 120:574–578

Collins MA, Neafsey EJ (1985): Beta-carboline analogues of N-methyl-4-phenyltetrahydropyridine (MPTP): endogenous factors underlying idiopathic parkinsonism? *Neurosci Lett* 55:179–184

Davis GCB, Williams AC, Markey SP, Ebert MH, Caine ED, Reichert CM, Kopin IJ
(1979): Chronic parkinsonism secondary to intravenous injection of meperidine
analogues. *Psychiatry Res* 1:249–254

Fields JZ, Albore RR, Neafsey EJ, Collins MA (1992): Inhibition of mitochondrial
succinate oxidation – similarities and differences between *N*-methylated β-
carbolines and MPP[+]. *Arch Biochem Biophys* 294:539–543

Kazita M, Niwa T, Takeda N, Yoshizumi H, Tatematsu A, Watanabe K, Nagatsu T
(1993): Presence of N-methyldopamine in parkinsonian and normal human
brains. *J Chromatogr* 613:1–8

Kikuchi K, Nagatsu Y, Makino Y, Mashino T, Ohta S, Hirobe M (1991):
Metabolism and penetration through blood-brain barrier of parkinsonism-
related compounds. 1,2,3,4-tetrahydroisoquinoline and 1-methyl-1,2,3,4-tetra-
hydroisoquinoline. *Drug Metab Dispos* 19:257–262

Langston JW, Ballard P, Tetrud JW, Irwin I (1983): Chronic parkinsonism in humans
due to a product of meperidine-analog synthesis. *Science* 219:979–980

Makino Y, Ohta S, Tachikawa O, Hirobe M (1988): Presence of tetrahydroisoquinoline and 1-methyl-tetrahydroisoquinoline in foods: compounds related to
Parkinson's disease. *Life Sci* 43:373–378

Makino Y, Tasaki Y, Ohta S, Hirobe M (1990): Confirmation of the enantiomers of
1-methyl-1,2,3,4-tetrahydroisoquinoline in the mouse brain and foods applying
gas chromatography/mass spectrometry with negative ion chemical ionization.
Biomed Environ Mass Spectrom 19:415–419

Maruyama W, Nakahara D, Ota M, Takahashi T, Takahashi A, Nagatsu T, Naoi M
(1992): *N*-Methylation of dopamine-derived 6,7-dihydroxy-1,2,3,4-tetrahydroi-
soquinoline, (R)-salsolinol, in rat brains: in vivo microdialysis study. *J Neurochem* 59:395–400

Matsubara K, Collins MA, Akane A, Ikebuchi J, Neafsey EJ, Kagawa M, Shiono H
(1993): Potential bioactivated neurotoxicants, *N*-methylated β-carbonium ions,
are present in human brain. *Brain Res* 610:90–96

Michel PP, Dandapani BK, Sanchez-Ramos, J, Efange S, Pressman BC, Hefti F
(1989): Toxic effects of potential environmental neurotoxins related to 1-methyl-
4-phenylpyridium on cultured rat dopaminergic neurons. *J Pharmacol Exp
Therap* 248:842–850

Minami M, Maruyama W, Dostert P, Nagatsu T, Naoi M (1993): Inhibition of type A
and B monoamine oxidase by 6,7-dihydroxy-1,2,3,4-tetrahydroisoquinolines and
their N-methylated derivatives. *J Neural Transm* 92:125–135

Minami M, Takahashi T, Maruyama W, Takahashi A, Dostert P, Nagatsu T, Naoi
M (1992): Inhibition of tyrosine hydroxylase by R and S enantiometers of
salsolinol, 1-methyl-6,7-dihydroxy-1,2,3,4-tetrahydroisoquinoline. *J Neurochem*
58:2097–2101

Nagatsu T, Yoshida M (1988): An endogenous substance of the brain, tetrahydroisoquinoline, produces parkinsonism in primate with decreased dopamine,
tyrosine hydroxylase and biopterin in the nigrostriatal regions. *Neurosci Lett*
87:178–182

Naoi M, Matsuura S, Parvez H, Takahashi T, Hirata Y, Minami M, Nagatsu T
(1989a): Oxidation of *N*-methyl-1,2,3,4-tetrahydroisoquinoline into the *N*-
methylisoquinolinium ion by monoamine oxidase. *J Neurochem* 52:653–655

Naoi M, Matsuura S, Takahashi T, Nagatsu T (1989b): An N-methyl-transferase in
human brain catalyzes *N*-methylation of 1,2,3,4-tetrahydroisoquinoline, a pre-

cursor of a dopaminergic neurotoxin, *N*-methylisoquinolinium ion. *Biochem Biophys Res Commun* 161:1213–1219

Niijima K, Araki M, Ogawa M, Suzuki K, Mizuno Y, Nagatsu I, Kimura H, Yoshida M, Nagatsu T (1991): *N*-Methylisoquinolinium ion (NMIQ$^+$) destroys cultured mesencephalic dopamine neurons. *Biog Amines* 8:61–67

Niwa T, Takeda N, Kaneda N, Hashizume Y, Nagatsu T (1987): Presence of tetrahydroisoquinoline and 2-methyl-tetrahydoquinoline in parkinsonian and normal human brains. *Biochem Biophys Res Commun* 144:1084–1089

Niwa T, Takeda N, Tatematsu A, Matsuura S, Yoshida M, Nagatsu T (1988): Migration of tetrahydroisoquinoline, a possible parkinsonian neurotoxin, into monkey brain from blood as proved by gas chromatography-mass spectrometry. *J Chromatogr* 452:85–91

Niwa T, Takeda N, Sasaoka T, Kaneda N, Hashizume Y, Yoshizumi H, tatematsu A, Nagatsu T (1989a): Detection of tetrahydroisoquinoline in parkinsonian brain as an endogenous amine by use of gas chromatography-mass spectrometry. *J Chromatogr* 491:397–403

Niwa T, Yoshizumi H, Tatematsu A, Matsuura S, Nagatsu T (1989b): Presence of tetrahydroisoquinoline, a parkinsonism-related compound, in foods. *J Chromatogr* 493:347–352

Niwa T, Takeda N, Yoshizumi H, Tatematsu A, Yoshida M, Dostert P, Naoi M, Nagatsu T (1991): Presence of 2-methyl-6,7-dihydroxy-1,2,3,4-tetrahydroisoquinoline and 1,2-dimethyl-6,7-dihydroxy-1,2,3,4-tetrahydroisoquinoline, novel endogenous amines, in parkinsonian and normal human brains. *Biochem Biophys Res Commun* 177:603–609

Niwa T, Maruyama W, Nakahara D, Takeda N, Yoshizumi H, Tatematsu A, Takahashi A, Dostert P, Naoi M, Nagatsu T (1992): Endogenous synthesis of *N*-methylsalsolinol, an analogue of 1-methyl-4-phenyl-1,2,3,6-tetrahydropyridine, in rat brain during in vivo microdialysis with salsolinol as demonstrated by gas chromatography-mass spectrometry. *J Chromatogr* 578:109–115

Ogawa M, Araki M, Nagatsu I, Nagatsu T, Yoshida M (1989): The effect of 1,2,3,4-tetrahydroisoquinoline (TIQ) on mesencephalic dopaminergic neurons inC57BL/6J mice: immunohistochemical studies – tyrosine hydroxylase. *Biog Amines* 6:427–436

Ohta S, Kohno M, Makino Y, Tachikawa O, Hirobe M (1987): Tetrahydroisoquinoline and 1-methyl-tetrahydroisoquinoline are present in the human brain: relation to Parkinson's disease. *Biomed Res* 8:453–456

Ota M, Dostert P, Hamanaka T, Nagatsu T, Naoi M (1992): Inhibition of tryptophan hydroxylase by (R)- and (S)-1-methyl-6,7-dihydroxy-1,2,3,4-tetrahydroisoquinolines (salsolinols). *Neuropharmacology* 31:337–341

Sandler M, Bonham-Carter S, Hunter KR, Stern GM (1973): Tetrahydroisoquinoline alkaloids: in vivo metabolites of L-dopa in man. *Nature* 241:439–443

Strolin-Benedetti M, Dostert P (1992): Monoamine oxidase: from physiology and pathophysiology to the design and clinical application to reversible inhibitors. In: *Advances in Drug Research*, Vol. 23, Testa B, ed., pp. 65–125. San Diego: Academic Press

Strolin-Benedetti M, Bellotti V, Pianezzola E, Moro E, Carminati P, Dostert P (1989): Ratio of the R and S enantiomers of salsolinol in food and human urine. *J Neural Transm* 77:47–53

Suzuki K, Mizuno Y, Yamauchi Y, Nagatsu T, Yoshida M (1992): Selective inhibition of complex I by *N*-methylisoquinolinium ion and *N*-methyl-1,2,3,4-tetrahydroisoquinoline in isolated mitochondria prepared from mouse brain. *J Neural Sci* 109:219–223

Tasaki Y, Makino Y, Ohta S, Hirobe M (1991): 1-Methyl-1,2,3,4-tetrahydroisoquinoline, decreasing in 1-methyl-4-phenyl-1,2,3,6-tetrahydropyridine-treated mouse, prevents parkinsonism-like behavior abnormalities. *J Neurochem* 57:1940–1943

Yoshida M, Niwa T, Nagatsu T (1990): Parkinsonism in monkeys produced by chronic administration of an endogenous substance of the brain, tetrahydroisoquinolines: the behavioral and biochemical changes. *Neurosci Lett* 119: 109–113

15

Discussion: 8–11 A.M. – February 9, 1993

REPORTED BY YOSHIKUNI MIZUNO

After Beal's paper, Calne asked Beal to comment a little bit more about the distribution of the agent that Beal presented. Beal stated that the agent might be more widely distributed in the environment, and he further mentioned the disease in cattle called staffers which is found in the western part of North America and Canadian provinces and is caused by cattle being exposed to mildewed hay, or mildewed feed. Therefore, low-dose exposure may be possible under some circumstances.

Poewe introduced the story of bilateral striatal necrosis in the horse induced by star thistle, which might be another source of this strange compound. Then, he raised the question whether the selective vulnerability of striatum to noxious stimuli might be related to the high degree of age-dependent occurrence of mitochondrial DNA (mtDNA) deletions and defects in oxidative phosphorylation. The answer could be that a subtle defect in the basal ganglia might generate free radical oxidative damage that would further generate more extensive damage, or the initial damage might progress with normal aging leading to progressive degeneration.

Orrenius asked whether Beal had studied the correlation between the 5 kb deletion and oxidative damage to nuclear DNA. The answer was no.

Olanow asked whether the mtDNA deletion might be primary or secondary. Beal answered this question by introducing their experiment, in which they measured nuclear DNA after exposure for 1 month to 3-nitropropionic acid and saw an increase in oxidative damage to DNA, indicating that the mitochondrially generated defect produced oxidative damage to DNA. Another issue that Beal stressed was the importance of animal models, particularly transgenic animals with specific lesions, to answer this question, and he commented about human diseases with known mtDNA mutations associated with bilateral striatal necrosis such as a family with Leber's disease, both associated with progressive putamenal degeneration. In these families, mitochondrial defects appear to be primary.

ADVANCES IN RESEARCH ON NEURODEGENERATION, II
Y. Mizuno et al.
© 1994 Birkhäuser Boston

Mizuno stated that they found the same 5-kb deletion of mitochondrial DNA as reported in mitochondrial myopathies in patients with Parkinson's disease (PD); the deletion appeared at a younger age in PD patients than control subjects: he postulated that oxidative damage to mtDNA might induce point mutations. The question was on the mechanism of increase in mtDNA deletion that Beal had found. Beal mentioned recent articles by Hayakawa et al. reporting an increase in deleted mtDNA out of proportion in aged muscles, and, in another article, reporting age-dependent increase in mtDNA deletion that showed a direct correlation with the increase in 8-hydroxydeoxyguanosine (8-OHDG) in the aged human heart. As 8-OHDG has been considered a reliable measurement of oxidative damage, the mechanism of mtDNA deletion may well be the oxidative damage to DNA.

Following Turski's paper, Siman raised the issue regarding the limited sparing produced by NMDA antagonists against MPP^+ toxicity. The question was whether MPP^+ was long lived in the tissue or whether an alternative explanation might exist such as a non-NMDA-receptor-mediated process that would be initiated by the toxin. The answer was that among the three toxins discussed, MPP^+ survived much longer in the brain than two other toxins, but regarding the possible involvement of other types of receptors, Turski was not sure.

Beal commented that it would be easy to block the toxicity of aminooxyacetic acid using NMDA antagonists because aminooxyacetic acid had only transient metabolic effects, but after MPP^+ introduction, persisting ATP depletion could be observed in the striatum 48 hours after the injection of the toxin.

Calne stated that MPP^+ might be sequestrated for some 48 hours, but that human degenerative diseases would be progressive for 30 years, and he raised the question whether it would be appropriate to represent human diseases with those animal models. Then Calne introduced the story of lathyrism after exposure to aminooxyalylamino propionic acid (AOAA), and stated that those patients had pyramidal signs, mostly in the legs, but no extrapyramidal deficits, stressing the difference between the MPP^+ model and lathryism.

Eisen commented on another animal model induced by Kanzo that had a very similar story to lathyrism, mainly involving the legs. Calne raised the question whether a nonprogressive disorder after exposure could be a good model of neurodegenerative diseases. The answer was that it could not be a model for genetic defects.

Then Olanow stated that we did not know much about the real long-term consequences of a single exposure. Calne agreed with Olanow, and commented that neuromelanin might be a good indicator to see whether a time-limited event could lead to death of some cells or sickness of another cells so that they gradually would die. Then Calne suggested that postpolio syndrome might be another example of a single exposure leading to a progressive disorder. Eisen stated that postpolio syndrome had nothing to do with continuing virus or infection, and that it had been accepted as an overload phenomenon combined with the aging of remaining neurons.

Gajdusek raised the question whether there was any toxin in the world that could produce a fatal cascade of disease years after initial exposure with no continuing exposures. Calne stated that Von Economo's encephalitis might be an example of the delayed appearance of neurological manifestations after infection. Gajdusek mentioned that there were numbers of such examples in retroviral infections. Calne asked whether these were related to activation of viral infection again or was some other mechanism involved? Gajdusek answered that in a slow virus infection like CJD there was a continuous replication. Calne argued that there was no such evidence for Economo's encephalitis. Gajdusek responded that Economo's encephalitis was a late phenomenon. That would also be true of a lot of retrovirus infections such as the recently described HTL V1-associated Jamaican neuropathy, in which almost no viral particles or viral duplication could be demonstrated in the neurons, and massive neuron death would be the result of cascades of cytokine activities killing neurons.

Olanow then mentioned the result of two other physical examples with long latency and subsequent progressive disease or deficit; one was radiation, and another was lightning, in which people struck by lightning would begin to develop a gradual myelopathy 2 to 3 years later.

Then Mizuno commented on the temporary effect of NMDA receptor blockade. He stated that there were at least two channels for Ca entry into the cells, one relating to the NMDA receptor and the other not, once ATP was depleted within the cells, intracellular Na^+ concentration would increase, which had to be expelled from the cells; however, because the activity of Na-K ATPase would be decreased as a result of ATP depletion, Na^+ would have to be expelled by exchange with extracellular Ca^{2+}, because NMDA receptor blockers would not block non-NMDA Ca channels such as the Ca ATPase-related channel. The question was whether this might be a reason for the temporary effect of NMDA receptor blockage. Turski answered that that was absolutely correct, but his belief was that the NMDA receptor-gated Ca channel would be more important for that type of toxicity.

After Nagatsu's paper, Hornykiewicz presented his data on the effect of salsolinol, TIQ, and dopamine using the rat myoclonic model that showed spontaneous regular twitching activity in the neck muscles; levodopa 50 mg/kg IV had no effect on this twitch. TIQ showed a short-lived increase in twitch activity that was ascribed to the dopamine-releasing action of TIQ whereas on the contrary salsolinol 20 mg/kg injected in the intracarotid artery of rats abolished dopaminergic twitch activity. Hornykiewicz suggested that those compounds might accumulate from endogenous sources and that they might possibly damage or protect dopaminergic neurons.

Youdim asked whether alcoholics would be more likely to be protected from or exposed to Parkinson's disease, as those condensation products had been known to be increased in chronic alcoholic patients. The answer was that there were no statistical studies on that subject.

Following Siman's paper, Horowski asked about the role of calpain in the long-term potentiation (LTP). Siman answered that calpain did have a role in LTP, as well as a variety of other compounds that had been shown to interfere with LTP.

Nagatsu stated that in the brain calpain II would be more abundant than calpain I. Siman agreed with Nagatsu, and stated that it had been claimed that calpain I would be localized in the neuron and that calpain II would be restricted in the nonneuronal elements. Then Nagatsu asked whether neurons containing calpain I would be more vulnerable to noxious stimuli. The answer was yes, and Siman commented that calpain I was highest in the olfactory nerve, which undergoes continuous degeneration and regeneration in old animals.

Orrenius asked whether calpain I would be inactivated by oxidative stress. The answer was that there was no direct evidence that calpain would be inactivated under the conditions of oxidative stress.

Then Olanow asked whether calpain would be more sensitive to a subtle elevation in the calcium concentration, and whether calpain would be the major enzyme causing cellular damage. Siman answered that the answer to that question would hinge on just how neuroprotective calpain inhibitors would prove to be among a myriad of calcium-dependent processes that would necessarily be insufficient to produce damage. Siman thought that calpain inhibition would be insufficient to be neuroprotective.

Then there was a question whether calpain would undergo any autoproteolysis for its activation. The answer was yes, and Siman commented that a small portion of the extreme amino terminal catalytic subunit had to be removed for the enzyme to be activated, and then he mentioned data from his group that suggest autoproteolytic activation of calpain I by excitotoxins.

Calne asked whether calpain activation would solubilize cytoskeletel proteins and lead to the accumulation of cytoskeletal products. The answer was that there was no evidence to link calpain activation with accumulation of cytoskeletal proteins.

Horowski asked Siman to comment on endogenous calpain inhibitors. Siman stated that there were two classes of endogenous inhibitors, a large protein inhibitor, calpastatin, and a small protein inhibitor, cystatin, and that calpastatin seemed to be present in most of the places where calpain was located. Regarding the question as to how calpain could become activated in the face of coincident presence of endogenous inhibitor proteins, Siman stated that some speculated that the affinity and temporal association between calpain and the substrate proteins versus calpain and calpastatin might influence how calpastatin would regulate the calpain activity.

Then Eisen raised the question of whether the cellular mechanisms discussed would apply to animals, although degenerative diseases only occur in man. Calne responded that human degenerative diseases might be in some way related to the aging of the nervous system, and Calne thought that some animals would get naturally occurring disorders similar to human diseases if the animals could live long enough.

Bainbridge stated that calpain-specific damage might well be in the synaptic axon terminals without actually killing the cells. The reason for this comment was the finding that high concentrations of Ca^{2+} would be necessary to activate calpain. The question was whether such a high Ca^{2+} concentration could be obtained by transient increase in Ca^{2+} influx might induce long-lasting damage. The answer was that the first connection between calcium overload-mediated neuronal damage and calpain had been made in an axotomy model, and that calcium influx and calpain activation would play at least a part of the role in structural disintegration of cytoskeleton that would occur at the cut ending.

Olanow asked Siman whether calpain could convert xanthine dehydrogenase to axanthine oxidase in an ischemic state. The answer was yes, and Siman mentioned that it would be a challenge for researchers in the future to discern how these various pathways such as nitric oxide production, free radical-mediated damage, and calcium-mediated damage would interact.

Part IV

SPECIAL TOPICS IN NEURODEGENERATION

16

Mitochondrial Disturbances in Parkinson's Disease

HEINZ REICHMANN, BERND JANETZKY, AND PETER RIEDERER

In 1962, Luft defined mitochondrial myopathies to consist of typical morphological and biochemical abnormalities of the mitochondria in association with characteristic clinical symptoms (Luft et al., 1962). In 1981, Egger and co-workers introduced the term 'mitochondrial cytopathy' (Egger et al., 1981). In 1989, three groups independently reported on the possibility that Parkinson's disease (PD) might belong to the mitochondrial cytopathies (Mizuno et al., 1989; Reichmann and Riederer, 1989; Schapira et al., 1989).

Biochemical and Molecular Genetic Considerations

Mitochondrial cytopathies are mostly based on disturbances of the respiratory chain which consists of five complexes. Complex I [reduced nicotinamide adenine dinucleotide (NADH) CoQ reductase] is the largest of the five and contains iron–sulfur (Fe–S) clusters. Seven of the more than forty subunits are encoded by the mitochondrial genome. Complex II (succinate dehydrogenase) is solely encoded by the nuclear genome. Complex III (ubichinon cytochrome c reductase) also contains iron–sulfur clusters. One of its 11 subunits, cytochrome b, is mitochondrially encoded. Complex IV (cytochrome c oxidase) consists of 13 subunits, 3 of which are mitochondrially encoded. Finally, complex V [adenosine triphosphate (ATP) synthetase] contains 2 subunits encoded by the mitochondrial genome.

Mitochondria are the only cell constituents containing their own genome. The mitochondrial genome (Fig. 1) is formed by a circular light and a heavy strand and contains 16,569 base pairs. Special interest in the mitochondrial genome stems from observations that both deletions and point mutations lead to encephalopathies such as the Kearns–Sayre–

ADVANCES IN RESEARCH ON NEURODEGENERATION, II
Y. Mizuno et al.
© 1994 Birkhäuser Boston

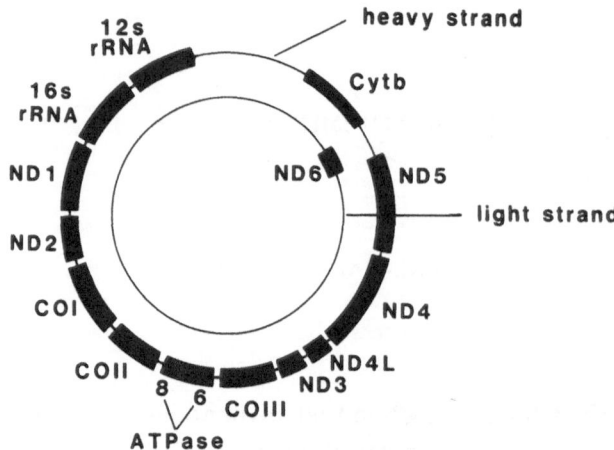

Figure 1. The mitochondrial genome consists of a light and a heavy strand and encodes for 13 proteins. Abbreviations: CO, cytochrome c oxidase subunit; ND, complex I subunit; ATPase, ATP synthetase subunit; cytb, cytochrome b subunit.

syndrome, MERRF (myoclonic epilepsy and ragged-red fibers syndrome), MELAS (mitochondrial encephalopathy, lactic acidosis, and stroke-like syndrome) or Leber's hereditary optic neuropathy (Goto et al., 1990; Hess et al., 1991; Holt et al., 1988; Moraes et al., 1988; Rotig et al., 1989; Shoffner et al., 1990; Wallace et al., 1988, 1990).

Why Should Parkinson's Disease Be a Mitochondrial Cytopathy?

There are several possibilities why Parkinson's disease might be associated with a mitochondrial dysfunction. It is well known that the exotoxin 1-methyl-4-phenyl-1,2,3,6-tetrahydropyridin (MPTP) induces Parkinson's disease. Glial monoamine oxidase (MAO-B) converts MPTP to its active metabolite 1-methyl-4-phenyl-pyridinium, which is preferentially stored in mitochondria from dopaminergic neurons in substantia nigra (SN) where it inhibits complex I (Mizuno et al., 1987; Nicklas et al., 1985). A second mechanism may come from iron disproportion in the SN where Fe^{3+} is significantly increased and may contribute to the "oxidative stress" phenomenon described in neurodegenerative diseases (Earle, 1968; Dexter et al., 1987; Götz et al., 1990; Sofic et al., 1988). Because Fe^{2+} is an important constituent in a number of respiratory chain complexes, its diminished levels may add to malfunction of the respiratory chain. A third factor is the reduction of glutathione in the substantia nigra from patients with PD (Jenner et al., 1992; Perry et al., 1982; Riederer et al., 1989) in association with free radicals that are generated during dopamine metabolism of which iron is a catalyst (Ben-Shachar et al., 1992). The increase in free radicals may well target the respiratory chain complexes. Finally, nitrous oxide from dopamine breakdown may lead to disturbances of the respiratory chain (Dawson et al., 1992).

For these reasons we analyzed, for the first time, complex I–IV in postmortem brain from patients with PD and compared these with age- and sex-matched controls (Reichmann and Riederer, 1989; Reichmann et al., 1990). The brains were obtained from 5 to 9.5 hours after death from patients with Hoehn and Yahr stage IV–V. Each patient had received L-dopa and other anti-Parkinson drugs. We analyzed NADH dehydrogenase (complex I), NADH cytochrome c reductase (complexes I and III), succinate dehydrogenase (complex II), succinate cytochrome c reductase (complex II and III), and cytochrome c oxidase (complex IV) from frontal cortex, substantia nigra, and putamen (Table 1). Only NADH cytochrome c reductase and succinate cytochrome c reductase showed a significant decrease in the substantia nigra. We interpreted these findings as a complex III defect. Meanwhile, Mizuno et al. (1989, 1990) underlined this finding but described in addition a complex I defect that was also favored by Schapira and co-workers (1989, 1990). Schapira's group stressed the fact that the complex I defect was a specific finding for

Table 1. Analyses of the Respiratory Chain in Postmortem Brain[a]

		SN	PUT	FC
NADH DH	Co	37.0 ± 3.8	30.2 ± 2.0	25.6 ± 10.3
	PD	36.5 ± 6.5	43.6 ± 9.4	31.3 ± 3.2
	%	-1.4	$+45$	$+22$
NADH Cyt c red	Co	5.4 ± 0.07	5.6 ± 0.5	3.9 ± 0.3
	PD	$3.5 \pm 0.5^*$	4.8 ± 1.9	4.0 ± 0.9
	%	-35	-14	$+3$
SDH	Co	2.3 ± 0.8	3.5 ± 1.0	2.5 ± 0.7
	PD	2.3 ± 0.8	3.8 ± 1.0	2.2 ± 0.7
	%	± 0	$+9$	-12
Succinate Cyt c red	Co	3.2 ± 0.3	4.9 ± 1.3	3.6 ± 1.1
	PD	$2.0 \pm 0.2^*$	5.1 ± 2.1	2.9 ± 0.8
	%	-38	$+4$	-19
COX	Co	3.0 ± 1.1	3.5 ± 1.4	3.3 ± 1.0
	PD	2.5 ± 0.9	4.2 ± 0.7	3.3 ± 0.7
	%	-17	$+20$	$+0$

[a]Enzyme activities are given in units/g brain (x ± SD), $n = 5$. $^*p < .05$. SN, substania nigra; PUT, putamen; FC, frontal cortex; DH, dehydrogenase; SDH, succinate dehydrogenase; Cyt c red, cytochrome c reductase; COX, cytochrome c oxidase; Co, controls; PD, Parkinson's disease.

Parkinson's disease because they did not find such changes in multisystem atrophy (MSA) (Schapira et al., 1990). The difference between SN from normals and from patients with PD reached 30%, although there was some overlap between the two groups.

The different findings among the three groups could have been caused by the time of storage of brain tissue. In a previous study we were able to show that the large complex I is extremely labile and that storage even at $-80°C$ may cause changes after 1 year (Pache and Reichmann, 1990). Second, the time interval between death and autopsy is critical. Finally, it seems to be most important to determine which test was used for the analysis of complex I. Because our first study used NADH dehydrogenase for the analysis of complex I, we may have missed a defect in the intramembrane part of the enzyme, which is built up by the subunits encoded by the mitochondrial genome. In our second series we also used CoQ1 to analyze NADH CoQ reductase as a marker for complex I, an assay with the advantage of covering the whole complex I. At this time, SN from PD patients showed a 13% reduction when compared to controls, which was not statistically significant. Thus, we believe that it is still uncertain whether PD is really associated with or even based on a specific complex I defect in the SN. This skepticism is corroborated by rather conflicting results in platelets from patients with various neurodegenerative disorders. In a pioneer study it was shown that mitochondria from platelets from patients with PD show a 50% reduction of complex I compared to platelets from controls (Parker et al., 1989). More recently (Krige et al., 1992), this dramatic difference could not be supported. A 14% or 16% reduction of complex I was reported (when corrected for the mitochondrial marker enzyme citrate synthetase) (Reichmann et al., 1985). Although both groups showed a huge overlap, these data were reported to reach statistical significance. In agreement with our own unpublished results from platelets, the authors stressed the fact that platelet analyses are not specific enough to allow diagnosis of PD in the peripheral blood.

Another tissue, skeletal muscle, has become associated with PD. Two groups reported on significant multicomplex diseases in muscles from patients with PD (Bindoff et al., 1989; Shoffner et al., 1991). Although the authors showed dramatic reductions of almost all complexes, they failed to show ragged-red fibers, a hallmark of mitochondrial myopathy, in any of their patients except one. Interestingly, such low levels of enzyme activity cause major muscle fatigue and patients are normally no longer ambulant, a finding that was not reported in their PD patients. Our own data (Table 2) did not support these findings. We analyzed five PD patients and one patient with MSA, and found no significant alterations; thus, we do not recommend muscle biopsy in PD.

Table 2. Respiratory Chain Activity^a in Skeletal Muscles from Patients with Parkinson's Disease

Enzyme	Pt 1	Pt 2	Pt 3	Pt 4	Pt 5	PtMSA	Controls: x ± SD (n)
NADH dehydrogenase	60.6	49.9	36.4	45.9	53.0	34.7	48 ± 9.4 (121)
NADH cytochrome c reductase/+rotenone	6.2/3.4	3.3/2.5	9.6/6.9	3.2/1.9	5.2/3.0	7.6/5.6	3.2 ± 1.5 (78)
Succinate dehydrogenase	3.4	1.8	1.4	2.1	2.3	1.8	2.4 ± 1.1 (160)
Succinate cytochrome c reductase	1.4	1.2	1.8	1.2	2.9	1.7	1.6 ± 0.6 (125)
Cytochrome c oxidase	7.3	4.2	4.7	4.2	6.0	2.4	2.8 ± 1.0 (113)

^{a}Enzyme activities are expressed in units/gram of muscle. Pt, patient; MSA, multisystem atrophy.

Because some subunits of complex I and III are encoded by the mitochondrial genome, we were the first to analyze the mitochondrial genome by the Southern blot technique (Lestienne et al., 1990). We isolated DNA from SN from six patients with PD and found no deletions. A study using the more sensitive polymerase chain reaction (PCR) described a 4977-base-pair deletion, the so-called common deletion that is found in mitochondrial encephalopathies (Ikebe et al., 1990). In a second study we also used PCR and found some deleted mt genomes (Lestienne et al., 1991). However, the control brains also contained deleted mt genomes, a fact that we described as representing aging.

Summary

In summary, our and others' data indicate that there might be a metabolic disturbance in mitochondria isolated from SN from PD. However, we do not support data that might suggest that PD could be diagnosed by means of muscle biopsy or analysis of mitochondria from platelets.

References

Ben-Shachar D, Eshel G, Riederer P, Youdim MBH (1992): Role of iron and iron chelation in dopaminergic-induced neurodegeneration: implication for Parkinson's disease. *Ann Neurol* 32:S105–S110
Bindoff LA, Birch Machin M, Cartlidge NEF, Parker WDJ, Turnbull DM (1989): Mitochondrial function in Parkinson's disease. *Lancet* 2:49
Dawson TM, Dawson VL, Snyder SH (1992): A novel messenger molecule in brain: the free radical, nitric oxide. *Ann Neurol* 32:297–311
Dexter DT, Wells FR, Agid F, Agid Y, Lees AJ, Jenner P, Marsden CD (1987): Increased nigral iron content in post mortem parkinsonian brain. *Lancet* ii:1219–1220
Earle KM (1968): Studies on Parkinson's disease including x-ray fluorescent spectroscopy of formalin fixed tissue. *J Neuropathol Exp Neurol* 27:1–14
Egger J, Lake BD, Wilson J (1981): Mitochondrial cytopathy. A multisystem disorder with ragged-red fibers on muscle biopsy. *Arch Dis Child* 56:741–752
Goto Y-I, Nonaka I, Horai S (1990): A mutation in the tRNA[Leu] (UUR) gene associated with the MELAS subgroup of mitochondrial encephalomyopathies. *Nature* 348:651–653
Götz ME, Freyberger A, Riederer P (1990): Oxidative stress: a role in the pathogenesis of Parkinson's disease. *J Neural Transm (Suppl)* 29:241–249
Hess JF, Parisi MA, Bennett JL, Clayton DA (1991): Impairment of mitochondrial transcription termination by a point mutation associated with the MELAS subgroup of mitochondrial encephalomyopathies. *Nature* 351:236–239
Holt IJ, Harding AE, Morgan-Hughes JA (1988): Deletions of muscle mitochondrial DNA in patients with mitochondrial myopathies. *Nature* 331:717–719
Ikebe S, Tanaka M, Ohno K, Sato W, Hattori K, Kondo T, Mizuno Y, Ozawa T

(1990): Increase of deleted mitochondrial DNA in the striatum in Parkinson's disease and senescence. *Biochem Biophys Res Commun* 170:1044–1048

Jenner P, Dexter DT, Sian J, Schapira AHV, Marsden CD (1992): Oxidative stress as a cause of nigral cell death in Parkinson's disease and incidental Lewy body disease. *Ann Neurol* 32:S82–S87

Krige D, Carroll MT, Cooper JM, Marsden CD, Schapira AHV (1992): Platelet mitochondrial function in Parkinson's disease. *Ann Neurol* 32:782–788

Lestienne P, Nelson J, Riederer P, Jellinger K, Reichmann H (1990): Normal mitochondrial genome in brain from patients with Parkinson's disease and complex I defect. *J Neuroimmunol* 55:1810–1812

Lestienne P, Nelson J, Riederer P, Reichmann H, Jellinger K (1991): Mitochondrial DNA in postmortem brain from patients with Parkinson's disease. *J Neurochem* 56:1819

Luft R, Ikkos D, Palmieri G, Ernster L, Afzelius B (1962): A case of severe hypermetabolism of nonthyroid origin with a defect in the maintenance of mitochondrial respiratory control. A correlated clinical, biochemical and morphological study. *J Clin Invest* 41:1776–1804

Mizuno Y, Sone N, Saitoh T (1987): Effects of 1-methyl-4-phenyl-1,2,3,6-tetrahydropyridine and 1-methyl-4-phenylpyridinium ion on activities of the enzymes in the electron transport system in mouse brain. *J Neurochem* 48:1787–1793

Mizuno Y, Suzuki K, Ohta S (1990): Postmortem changes in mitochondrial respiratory enzymes in brain and a preliminary observation in Parkinson's disease. *J Neurol Sci* 96:49–57

Mizuno Y, Ohta S, Tanaka M, Takamiya S, Suzuki K, Sato T, Oya H, Ozawa T, Kagawa Y (1989): Deficiencies in complex I subunits of the respiratory chain in Parkinson's disease. *Biochem Biophys Res Commun* 163:1450–1455

Moraes CT, DiMauro S, Zeviani M, Lombes A, Shanske S, Miranda A, Nakase H, Bonilla E, Werneck LC, Servidei S, Nonaka I, Koga Y, Spiro AJ, Brownell KW, Schmidt B, Schotland DL, Zupanc M, DeVivo DC, Schon E, Rowland LP (1989): Mitochondrial DNA deletions in progressive external ophthalmoplegia and Kearns–Sayre syndrome. *N Engl J Med* 320:1293–1299

Nicklas WJ, Vyas I, Heikkila RE (1985): Inhibition of NADH-linked oxidation in brain mitochondria by 1-methyl-4-phenylpyridine, a metabolite of the neurotoxic 1-methyl-4-phenyl-1,2,3,6-tetrahydropyridine. *Life Sci* 36:2503–2508

Pache T, Reichmann H (1990): On the stability of key enzymes of energy metabolism in muscle biopsies. *Enzyme* 43:183–187

Parker WD, Boyson SJ, Parks JK (1989): Abnormalities of the electron transport chain in idiopathic Parkinson's disease. *Ann Neurol* 26:719–723

Perry TL, Godin DV, Hansen S (1982): Parkinson's disease: a disorder due to nigral glutathione deficiency. *Neurosci Lett* 33:305–310

Reichmann H, Riederer P (1989): Biochemische Analyse der Atmungskettenkomplexe verschiedener Hirnregionen von Patienten mit Morbus Parkinson. In: *Symposium des BMFT Morbus Parkinson und andere Basalganglienerkrankungen*, S. 44 (abstr.)

Reichmann H, Riederer P, Seufert S (1990): Disturbances of the respiratory chain in brain from patients with Parkinson's disease. *Mov Disord* 5:28

Reichmann H, Hoppeler H, Mathieu-Costello O, von Bergen F, Pette D (1985): Biochemical and ultrastructural changes of skeletal muscle mitochondria after chronic electrical stimulation in rabbits. *Eur J Physiol (Pflüger's Arch)* 404:1–9

Riederer P, Sofic E, Rausch WD, Schmidt B, Reynolds GP, Jellinger K, Youdim MBH (1989): Transition metals, ferritin, glutathione, and ascorbic acid in parkinsonian brains. *J Neurochem* 52:515–520

Rotig A, Colonna M, Bonnefont JP, Blanche S, Fischer A, Sandubray JM, Munnich A (1989): Mitochondrial DNA deletion in Pearson's marrow/pancreas syndrome. *Lancet* 1:902–903

Schapira AVH, Cooper JM, Dexter D, Jenner P, Clark JB, Marsden CD (1989): Mitochondrial complex I deficiency in Parkinson's disease (letter). *Lancet* i:1269

Schapira AHV, Cooper JM, Dexter D, Clark JB, Jenner P, Marsden CD (1990): Mitochondrial complex I deficiency in Parkinson's disease. *J Neurochem* 54:823–827

Shoffner JM, Watts RL, Juncos JL, Torroni A, Wallace DC (1991): Mitochondrial oxidative phosphorylation defects in Parkinson's disease. *Ann Neurol* 30:332–339

Shoffner JM, Lott MT, Lezza AMS, Seibel P, Ballinger SW, Wallace DC (1990): Myoclonic epilepsy and ragged-red fiber disease (MERRF) is associated with a mitochondrial DNA tRNA[Lys] mutation. *Cell* 61:931–937

Sofic E, Riederer P, Heinsen H, Beckmann H, Reynolds GP, Hebenstreit G, Youdim MBH (1988): Increased iron (III) and total iron content in post mortem substantia nigra of parkinsonian brain. *J Neural Transm* 74:199–205

Wallace DC, Singh G, Lott MT, Hodge JA, Schurr TG, Lezza AMS, Elsas LJ, Nikoskelainen EK (1988): Mitochondrial DNA mutation associated with Leber's hereditary optic neuropathy. *Science* 242:1427–1430

Wallace DC, Zheng X, Lott MT, Shoffner JM, Hodge JA, Kelley RI, Epstein CM, Hopkins LC (1990): Myoclonic epilepsy and ragged-red fiber disease (MERRF): genetic, pathophysiological and biochemical characterization of a mitochondrial DNA disease. *Cell* 55:601–610

17

Trophic Factors and Parkinson's Disease

W.H. Oertel and A. Kupsch

During the development period, neurons are abundantly generated in the vertebrate nervous system. Following the arrival of their axons in the target areas, only a proportion of these neurons will survive. These neurons are thought to have successfully competed for a target-derived, retrogradely transported neurotrophic factor, present in limited amounts in the target fields. Such a neurotrophic factor, in its narrow definition, is a survival factor for embryonic neurons in either the peripheral or central nervous system. This definition is derived from research on nerve growth factor (NGF) (Levi-Montalcini and Booker, 1960). NGF belongs to the family of "neurotrophins," which subsumes brain-derived neurotrophic factor (BDNF; for reviews, see Barde, 1989; Levi-Montalcini, 1987; Thoenen et al., 1987), neurotrophin-3/neurotrophin 4 (NT-3/NT-4; see Glass et al., 1991; Hohn et al, 1990), and neurotrophin 5 (NT-5; see Berkemeier et al., 1991). In addition, a number of other nontarget-derived molecules are known to influence survival and differentiation of certain neurons and nonneuronal cells. These factors include ciliary neurotrophic factor (CNTF), acidic and basic fibroblast growth factor (FG F-1 and FGF-2, respectively), epidermal growth factor (EGF), insulin-like growth factors I and II (IGF-I, IGF-II), and muscle-derived differentiation factor (MDF).

Indirect Evidence for a Trophic Factor for Dopaminergic Neurons

Several observations in experimental and clinical research suggest the existence of a trophic factor or factors for dopaminergic neurons. When mice received an implant of adult adrenal medullary tissue 1 week after subcutaneous treatment with 1-methyl-4-phenyl-1,2,3,6-tetrahydropyridine (MPTP), a protoxin for dopaminergic nigral neurons, tyrosine hydroxylase- (TH-) immunoreactive fibers were reported to have a higher density on the implanted than the nonimplanted side (Bohn et al., 1987). In MPTP-treated parkinsonian primates, TH-immunoreactive fibers were enhanced around an empty cavity formed in the caudate nucleus. A similar finding was seen after tissue implantation into the cavity. This observation was independent of the type of tissue grafted and suggests a lesion-induced sprouting of remaining endogenous dopaminergic fibers (Bankiewicz et al., 1990).

Following transplantation of autologous adrenal medulla into the striatum of patients with Parkinson's disease (PD), a transient improvement of clinical symptoms was observed despite poor survival of chromaffin cells. One postmortem analysis of the striatum of a Parkinson patient, who had received an intrastriatal adrenal medullary implant, revealed TH-immunoreactive fibers around the grafted tissue, which itself contained very few TH-immunoreactive staining (Hirsch et al., 1990).

Neurotrophin: Nerve Growth Factor

Topical application of NGF or other members of the neurotrophin family can prevent the dysfunction of axotomized central cholinergic neurons in the normal adult rat brain (Hefti, 1986). Thus, the mammalian nervous system not only requires neurotrophic factors for its development but needs trophic support for maintenance and function of at least some (limbic/septohippocampal) cholinergic adult central nervous system (CNS) neurons. Whether cholinergic neurons affected by an unknown etiology in a neurodegenerative disorder may be rescued by increased trophic support is unknown.

The finding that adult cholinergic forebrain neurons utilize NGF for survival and normal function stimulated hopes that a trophic factor for adult dopaminergic neurons may be found. One may further speculate that in PD dopaminergic neurons degenerate because of lack in neurotrophic support. NGF supports survival of sympathetic ganglion cells. Catecholamine-containing cells of the adrenal medulla survive in culture and exhibit characteristics of sympathetic ganglion cells following the addition of NGF to the culture medium (Anderson and Axel, 1986). In studies on the 6-hydroxydopamine (6-OHDA) rat model, adult adrenal medullary tissue was transplanted into the dopamine deficient striatum and showed improved survival on coadministration of intraventricular NGF (Strömberg et al., 1985). Subsequently one PD patient received an autologous adrenal medullary intraputaminal transplant with a concomitant intraputaminal infusion of NGF (Olson et al., 1991). At 7 months post transplantation, a moderate improvement of clinical symptoms was described. Long-term follow-up data remain to be evaluated. NGF neither promotes the survival of embryonic mesencephalic dopaminergic neurons in culture (Dreyfus, 1989; Knüsel, 1990) nor does it rescue adult nigral dopaminergic neurons in the rat substantia nigra following hemitransection of the median forebrain bundle (Knüsel et al., 1992).

Neurotrophin: Brain Derived Neurotrophic Factor

Similar to NGF, BDNF increases the survival and differentiation of cholinergic neurons of the basal forebrain in culture (Alderson et al., 1990; Knüsel et al., 1991). Further, BDNF enhanced the number of TH-immunoreactive neurons in embryonic mesencephalic cultures and attenuated the effect of MPP^+, the metabolite of MPTP presumably toxic for dopaminergic neurons (Beck et al., 1992; Hyman et al., 1991). mRNA for BDNF has been demonstrated to be present in substantia nigra neurons in low amounts. Following intrastriatal injections BDNF was reported to be retrogradely transported to neurons in the substantia nigra (Wiegand et al., 1992).

However, a neuroprotective effect of BDNF on dopaminergic neurons has not been demonstrated *in vivo*. The loss of TH-immunoreactive nigral cells in rats following selective hemitransection of the nigrostriatal pathway was not prevented by intraventricular infusion of BDNF (Knüsel et al., 1992). In the MPTP mouse model, daily prenigral injection of $2\,\mu g$ of BDNF rostrally to the substantia nigra for 4 days (with MPTP administered once on day 2) failed to ameliorate the MPTP-induced loss of striatal dopamine 4 days after MPTP exposure (Kupsch et al., unpublished data). Similarly, chronic intraventricular infusion or daily intrastriatal injection of BDNF did not increase survival of grafted *fetal* nigral neurons in the 6-OHDA model of the rat, although functional graft effects were enhanced as assessed by an early reduction of amphetamine-induced rotations 3 weeks after transplantation (Sauer et al., 1993). It was recently reported that unilateral, intranigral infusions of BDNF for 2 weeks in normal rats increased amphetamine-induced, but not apomorphine-induced, rotations and enhanced striatal dopamine metabolism (increased dopamine/homo-vanillic acid ratios). This observation was interpreted as a presynaptic effect of BDNF (Altar et al., 1992).

Ciliary Neurotrophic Factor

CNTF does not fulfill the criteria of a neurotrophin, because, for example, the site of its production and the time course of its developmental expression do not correspond to the projection fields of CNTF-responsive neurons. Further, in contrast to receptors for other known neurotrophic factors, which predominantly belong to the family of receptor tyrosine kinases (Squinto et al., 1991), the CNTF receptor belongs to the family of cytokine receptors and shares subunits with the receptor complexes for interleukin 6 (for review, see Davis and Yancopoulos, 1993). The wide range of activities of CNTF includes peripheral effects, most prominent on developing ciliary ganglion cells. In culture CNTF enhanced the survival of certain classes of embryonic hippocampal neurons (Ip et al., 1991) and of spinal motoneurons. *In vivo* CNTF prevents the lesion-induced degeneration of (facial) motoneurons after axotomy in newborn rats (Sendtner et al., 1990) and prevents neurodegeneration in a genetic mouse model of progressive motor neuronopathy (Sendtner et al., 1992). The sensitivity of motoneurons to lesions rapidly decreases in the first 3 post natal weeks, and this decrease closely correlates with the increase of CNTF expression in the Schwann cells of the rat sciatic nerve (Stöckli et al., 1989). CNTF has, therefore, been suggested to be released after damage by the producing cell and may act as a "lesion factor." Interestingly, in a recent report CNTF was shown to prevent axotomy-induced nigral cell death, as assessed by Nissl-staining, but not axotomy-induced loss of immunocytochemical TH staining in the substantia nigra of rats (Hagg and Varon, 1993).

Fibroblast Growth Factors

FGF-2 (formerly called basic fibroblast growth factor, bFGF) exhibits a trophic effect on central embryonic dopaminergic and γ-aminobutyric acid- (GABA-) ergic neurons in culture that is mediated by mesencephalic glia (Engele and Bohn, 1991; Knüsel et al., 1990). Both FGF-2 and FGF-1 (formerly called acidic fibroblast growth factor) have been shown to be present in dopaminergic neurons of the ventral mesencephalon in rats, monkeys, and humans (Bean et al., 1991; Cintra et al., 1991).

In *in vivo* studies, infusions of FGF-2 into the striatal parenchyma failed to increase striatal dopamine concentrations or to consistently improve motor performance in the 6-OHDA rat model (Otto and Unsicker, 1992). In the MPTP mouse model, FGF-2 was administered in a gel foam into the striatum either simultaneously with the intraperitoneal application of MPTP or 3 days later than the toxin and was reported to partially attenuate MPTP-induced decreases in striatal dopamine content, TH activity, and TH immunoreactivity (Otto and Unsicker, 1990). No effect, however, was observed when FGF-2 was applied 7 days after systemic injection. Comparable studies on primates have not been published.

Epidermal Growth Factor

EGF immunoreactivity has been visualized in forebrain and midbrain structures, particularly in the substantia nigra and globus pallidus (Fallon, 1984). EGF increases the level of mRNA coding for tyrosine hydroxylase, the rate-limiting step in the synthesis of dopamine and other catecholamines (Lewis and Chikaraishi, 1987). *In vitro* EGF supports the survival of embryonic dopaminergic mesencephalic neurons, but also of cholinergic forebrain neurons. This effect is likely mediated by glial cells present in culture (Knüsel et al., 1990). In *in vivo* studies, intraventricular infusions of EGF were performed 5 weeks after a mechanical hemitransection of rat nigrostriatal pathway for another 4 weeks. EGF infusions were reported to result in an increase by 20% in the number of TH-positive substantia nigra neurons in comparison to lesioned control animals. In addition, a partial compensation of rotation behavior was seen following EGF infusion (Pezzoli et al., 1991). Likewise, intraventricular infusion of EGF promoted recovery of striatal dopamine concentrations in the MPTP mouse model. However, EGF also enhanced striatal dopaminergic parameters in untreated animals (Hadjiconstantinou et al., 1991). Corresponding studies on primates have not been published.

Muscle-Derived Differentiation Factor

Proteins directing phenotypic choices in peripheral neurons without influencing proliferation or viability are termed differentiation factors. Recently, muscle-derived differentiation factor (MDF), partially purified from muscle cells, has been shown to induce *in vitro* the appearance of the TH enzyme in neurons (striatum, collicular plate, cerebellum, cortex) that normally do not express this rate-limiting enzyme in catecholamine synthesis (Iacovitti, 1991). TH expression depended on the continuous presence of MDF. During development neurons appear to be responsive to MDF for only a limited time period. This time window corresponds to withdrawal from mitosis and to the period preceding the development of the blood–brain barrier (Iacovitti et al., 1992), suggesting that vascular smooth muscle might be a source of MDF. In cultures containing fetal mesencephalic dopaminergic neurons, MDF enhanced TH mRNA and TH enzyme activity up to 40 fold (Iacovitti et al., 1992). According to Jin et al. (1991), infusion of partially purified MDF was able to increase the TH activity in the dopamine-depleted striatum in the rat 6-OHDA model. Likewise, an increase of dopamine and DOPAC concentration and a partial compensation of motor asymmetry have been reported. No effect on striatal parameters, however, was found when partially purified MDF was infused into the intact striatum. These observations suggest that the genome of adult nerve cells regains its receptivity to embryonic (differentiation) factors after injury.

Conclusion and Open Questions

The factors BDNF, NT-4, FGF-2, EGF, and MDF have been shown to improve survival of mesencephalic dopaminergic neurons in culture. *In vivo* application of selected trophic factors has so far failed to provide evidence for a striking protective or restorative action on adult dopaminergic neurons in acute animal models of PD. Chronic animal models with delayed neuronal cell death may be necessary for testing the effects of trophic factors on dopaminergic neurons (Ichitani et al., 1991). In addition, a combination of trophic factors may be needed for a direct or glia-mediated effect on lesioned dopaminergic neurons.

As in Parkinson's disease, differentiated dopaminergic nigral neurons degenerate. The trophic factors or molecules used by adult dopaminergic neurons for survival and normal function are to be identified, and their physiological regulation is to be investigated. In respect to the known trophic molecules, the full range of responsive neurons needs to be elucidated and the dose–response relationship to be established *in vitro* and *in vivo* (Thoenen, 1991). For optimizing the direct application of known trophic molecules, the pharmacokinetics of these molecules administered into the ventricle or the CNS parenchyma must be studied. In parallel to these basic *in vivo* investigations in normal animals and in animal models of Parkinson's disease, several lines of research are likely to continue. (1) The intracerebral application of a trophic factor before, simultaneously with, or after the administration of a neurotoxin (such as MPTP or 6-OHDA) will investigate a potential protective or restorative role of trophic molecules by biochemical, anatomical, and behavioral methods. (2) The application of trophic factors will be combined with the neuronal transplantation technique of fetal dopaminergic neurons. This approach would mimic tissue culture experiments in the adult brain and has already been employed for FGF-2 and BDNF (Sauer et al., 1993; Steinbusch et al., 1990). (3) The transplantation of (preferably autologous) engineered cells that locally release the suitable trophic molecule into the appropriate area, and (4) the modification of the effects of endogenous neurotrophic molecules by pharmacological procedures (Nistico et al., 1992; Zafra et al., 1991) will be attempted. In this respect, deprenyl has been reported to promote survival of dopaminergic nigral neurons in the MPTP mouse model in concentrations too low to influence monoamino oxidase B (MAO-B) activity and administered with a delay of 3 days, suggesting that deprenyl may augment yet to be determined trophic responses (Tatton and Greenwood, 1991).

It is still not clear, however, if neurons in the substantia nigra disappear because of apoptosis (contraction of cytoplasm and nucleus; subsequent phagocytosis by adjacent cells) or pathological cell death or cell necrosis where the cell swells and bursts (Ffrench-Constant, 1992). Similarly, it is not known whether the degeneration of nigrostriatal dopaminergic neurons is partly attributable to a reduced trophic support or whether additional trophic support may counteract the degeneration of adult dopaminergic SN neurons in PD. It is conceivable that experimental efforts in this field will eventually allow us to go beyond the present stage of symptomatic therapy for Parkinson's disease.

References

Alderson RF, Alterman AL, Barde, YA, Lindsay RM (1990): Brain-derived neurotrophic factor increases survival and differentiated functions of rat septal cholinergic neurons in culture. *Neuron* 5:297–306

Altar CA, Boylan CB, Jackson C, Hershensson S, Miller J, Wiegand SJ, Lindsay RM, Hyman C (1992): Brain-derived neurotrophic factor augments rotational behavior and nigrostriatal dopamine turnover. *Proc Natl Acad Sci (USA)* 89:11347–11351

Anderson DJ, Axel R (1986): A bipotential neuroendocrine precursor whose choice of cell fate is determined by NGF and glucocorticoids. *Cell* 47:1079–1090

Bankiewicz KS, Plunkett RJ, Jacobowitz DM, Porrino L, Di Porzio U, London WT, Kopin IJ, Oldwin EH (1990): The effect of fetal mesencephalic implants on primate MPTP-induced parkinsonism. Histochemical and behavioural studies. *Neurosurgery* 72:231–244

Barde YA (1989): Trophic factors and neuronal survival. *Neuron* 2:1525–1534

Bean AJ, Elde R, Cao YH, Oellig C, Tamminga C, Goldstein M, Pettersson RF, Hökfelt T (1991): Expression of acidic and basic fibroblast growth factors in the substantia nigra of rat, monkey, and human. *Proc Natl Acad Sci (USA)* 88:10237–10241

Beck KD, Knüsel B, Winslow JW, Rosenthal A, Burton LE, Nikolics K, Hefti F (1992): Pretreatment of dopaminergic neurons in culture with brain-derived neurotrophic factor attenuates toxicity of 1-methyl-4-phenylpyridinium. *Neurodegeneration* 1:27–36

Berkemeier LR, Winslow JW, Kaplan DR, Nikolics K, Goeddel DV, Rosenthal A (1991): Neurotrophin 5, a novel neurotrophic factor that activates trk and trkB. *Neuron* 7:857–866

Bohn MC, Cupit L, Marciano F, Gash DM (1987): Adrenal medulla grafts enhance recovery of striatal dopaminergic fibers. *Science* 237:913–916

Cintra A, Cao YH, Oellig C, Tinner B, Bortolotti F, Goldstein M, Pettersson RF,

Fuxe K (1991): Basic FGF is present in dopaminergic neurons of the ventral midbrain of the rat. *Neuroreport* 2:597–600

Davis S, Yancopoulos GD (1993): The molecular biology of the CNTF receptor. *Curr Opin Neurobiol* 3:20–24

Dreyfus CF (1989): Effects of nerve growth factor on cholinergic brain neurons. *Trends Pharmacol Sci* 10:145–149

Engele J, Bohn MC (1991): The neurotrophic effects of fibroblast growth factor in vitro are mediated by mesencephalic glia. *J Neurosci* 11:3070–3078

Fallon (1984): Epidermal growth factor immunoreactive material in the central nervous system: location and development. *Science* 224:1107–1109

Ffrench-Constant C (1992): Cell death: a division too far? *Curr Opin Biol* 2:577–579

Glass DJ, Nye SH, Hantzopoulos P, Macchi MJ, Squinto SP, Goldfarb M, Yanco-poulos GD (1991): TrkB mediates BDNF/NT-3-dependent survival and prolif-eration in fibroblasts lacking the low affinity NGF receptor. *Cell* 66:405–413

Hadjiconstantinou M, Fitkin JG, Dalia A, Neff NH (1991): Epidermal growth factor enhances striatal dopaminergic parameters in the 1-methyl-4-phenyl-1,2,3,6-tetrahydropyridine-treated mouse. *J Neurochem* 57:479–482

Hagg T, Varon S (1993): Ciliary neurotrophic factor (CNTF) prevents axotomy-induced degeneration of adult rat substantia dopaminergic neurons. *Proc Natl Acad Sci USA* 90:6315–6319

Hefti F (1986): Nerve growth factor promotes survival of septal cholinergic neurons after fimbrial transections. *J Neurosci* 6:2155–2162

Hirsch EC, Duychaerts C, Javoy-Agid F, Hauw I-J, Agid Y (1990): Does adrenal graft enhance recovery of dopaminergic fibres in Parkinson's disease? *Ann Neurol* 27:676–682

Hohn A, Leibrock J, Bailey K, Barde Y-A (1990): Identification and characterization of a novel member of the nerve growth factor/brain derived neurotrophic factor family. *Nature* 344:339–341

Hyman C, Hofer M, Barde Y-A, Juhasz M, Yancopoulos GD, Squinto SP, Lindsay RM (1991): BDNF is a neurotrophic factor for dopaminergic neurons of the substantia nigra. *Nature* 350:230–232

Iacovitti L (1991): Effects of a novel differentiation factor on the development of catecholamine traits in noncatecholamine neurons from various regions of the rat brain: studies in tissue culture. *J Neurosci* 11:2403–2409

Iacovitti L, Evinger MJ, Stull ND (1992): Muscle-derived differentiation factor increases expression of the tyrosine hydroxylase gene and enzyme activity in cultured dopamine neurons from the rat midbrain. *Mol Brain Res* 16:215–222

Ichitani A, Okumara H, Matsumoto A, Nagatsu I, Iabata Y (1991): Degeneration of the nigral dopamine neurons after 6-hydroxydopamine injection in the rat striatum. *Brain Res* 549:350–353

Ip NY, Li Y, von de Stadt I, Panayotatos N, Alderson RF, Lindsay RM (1991): Ciliary neurotrophic factor enhances neuronal survival in embryonic rat hippocampal cultures. *J Neurosci* 11:3124–3134

Jin BK, Schneider JS, Du YY, Iacovitti L (1991): MDF, a muscle factor, produces partial motor recovery in 6-hydroxydopamine lesioned rats by increasing tyrosine hydroxylase activity and catechol levels. *Soc Neurosci Abstr* 18:1296

Knüsel B (1990): Trophic actions of recombinant human nerve growth factor on cultured rat embryonic CNS cells. *Exp Neurol* 110:274–283

Knüsel B, Michel PP, Schwaber JS, Hefti F (1990): Selective and nonselective stimulation of central cholinergic and dopaminergic development in vitro by nerve growth factor, basic fibroblast factor, epidermal growth factor, insulin and insulin-like growth factors I and II. *J Neurosci* 10:558–570

Knüsel B, Winslow JW, Rosenthal A, Burton LE, Seid DP, Nikolics K, Hefti F (1991): Promotion of central cholinergic and dopaminergic neuron differentiation by brain-derived neurotrophic factor but not neurotrophin 3. *Proc Natl Acad Sci (USA)* 88:961–965

Knüsel B, Beck KD, Winslow JW, Rosenthal A, Burton LE, Widmer HR, Nikolics K, Hefti F (1992): Brain-derived neurotrophic factor administration protects basal forebrain cholinergic but not nigral dopaminergic neurons from degenerative changes after axotomy in the adult rat brain. *J Neurosci* 12:4391–4402

Levi-Montalcini R (1987): The nerve growth factor: thirty-five years later. *EMBO J* 6:1145–1154

Levi-Montalcini R, Booker R (1960): Destruction of the sympathetic ganglia in mammals by an anti-serum to the nerve growth factor. *Proc Natl Acad Sci (USA)* 46:364–391

Lewis EJ, Chikaraishi DM (1987): Regulated expression of the tyrosine hydroxylase gene by epidermal growth factor. *Mol Cell Biol* 7:3332–3336

Nistico G, Ciriolo MR, Fiskin K, Iannone M, De-Martino A, Rotilio G (1992): NGF restores decrease in catalase activity and increases superoxide dismutase and glutathione peroxidase activity in the brain of aged rats. *Free Radical Biol Med* 12:177–181

Olson L, Backlund EO, Ebendal T, Freedman R, Hamberger B, Hansson P, Hoffer B, Lindblom U, Meyerson B, Strömberg I, Sydow O, Seiger A (1991): Intraputaminal infusion of nerve growth factor to support adrenal medullary autografts in Parkinson's disease. *Arch Neurol* 48:373–381

Otto D, Unsicker K (1990): Basic FGF reverses chemical and morphological deficits in the nigrostriatal system of MPTP-treated mice. *J Neurosci* 10:1912–1921

Otto D, Unsicker K (1992): Effects of FGF-2 on dopamine neurons. *Neurosci Facts* 3:882–883

Pezzoli G, Zecchinelli A, Ricciardi S, Burke RE, Fahn S, Scarlato G, Carenzi A (1991): Intraventricular infusion of epidermal growth factor restores dopaminergic pathway in hemiparkinsonian rats. *Mov Disord* 6:281–287

Sauer H, Fischer W, Nikkah G, Brundin P, Lindsay RM, Björklund A (1993): Brain-derived neurotrophic factor enhances function rather than survival of intrastriatal ventral mesencephalic grafts. *Brain Res* 626:37–44

Sendtner M, Kreutzberg GW, Thoenen H (1990): Ciliary neurotrophic factor prevents the degeneration of motor neurons after axotomy. *Nature* 345:440–441

Sendtner M, Schmalbruch H, Stöckli KA, Caroll P, Kreutzberg G, Thoenen H (1992): Ciliary neurotrophic factor prevents degeneration of motor neurons in mouse mutant progressive motor neuronopathy. *Nature* 358:502–504

Squinto SP, Stitt TN, Aldrich TH, Davis S, Bianco SM, Radziejewski C, Glass DJ, Masiakowski P, Furth ME, Valenzuela DM (1991): TrkB encodes a functional receptor for brain-derived neurotrophic factor and neurotrophin-3 but not nerve growth factor. *Cell* 65:885–893

Steinbusch HW, Vermeulen RJ, Tonnaer JA (1990): Basic fibroblast growth factor enhances survival and sprouting of fetal dopaminergic cells implanted in the denervated rat caudate-putamen: preliminary observations. *Prog Brain Res* 82:81–86

Stöckli KA, Lottspeich F, Sendtner M, Masiakowski P, Carroll P, Götz R, Lindholm D, Thoenen H (1989): Molecular cloning, expression and regional distribution of rat ciliary neurotrophic factor. *Nature* 342:920–923

Strömberg I, Herrera-Marschitz M, Ungerstedt U, Ebendal T, Olson L (1985): Chronic implants of chromaffin tissue into the dopamine-denervated striatum. Effects of NGF on graft survival, fiber growth and rotational behaviour. *Exp Brain Res* 60:335–349

Tatton WG, Greenwood CE (1991): Rescue of dying neurons: a new action of deprenyl in MPTP parkinsonism. *J Neurosci Res* 30:666–672

Thoenen H (1991): The changing scene of neurotrophic factors. *Trends Neurosci* 14:165–170

Thoenen H, Bandtlow C, Heumann R (1987): The physiological function of nerve growth factor in the central nervous system: comparison with the periphery. *Rev Physiol Biochem Pharmacol* 109:145–178

Wiegand SJ, Anderson K, Alexander C, Criden M, Altar CA, Lindsay RM, Distefano PS (1992): Receptor binding and axonal transport of [^{125}I]-labeled neurotrophins in the basal ganglia and related brain regions. *Mov Disord* 7, Suppl. 1, Abstr. P147B, p. 63

Zafra F, Castrén E, Thoenen H, Lindholm D (1991): Interplay between glutamate and gamma-aminobutyric acid transmitter systems in the physiological regulation of brain-derived neurotrophic factor and nerve growth factor synthesis in hippocampal neurons. *Proc Natl Acad Sci (USA)* 88:10027–10041

18

Spontaneous Generation of Infectious Amyloid Nucleants in the Transmissible and Nontransmissible Brain Amyloidoses

D. Carleton Gajdusek

In recent years we have become aware that the unconventional or atypical slow virus diseases of kuru–Creutzfeldt–Jacob syndrome (CJD) – Gerstmann Sträussler syndrome (GSS) and scrapie-bovine spongiform encephalopathy (BSE) are cerebral amyloidoses (Gajdusek, 1986, 1988a, 1988b, 1989, 1990, 1991a, 1991b, 1991c; Gajdusek and Gibbs, 1990; Gajdusek et al., 1991). As with most amyloidoses, the spontaneous *de novo* generation of amyloid fibrils is under genetic control, although in many susceptible hosts all individuals are susceptible to even a minimal intracerebral infective dose; thus, for such inoculation there is no genetic control other than the species barrier.

Transmissible and infectious amyloidoses of brain, as with all amyloidoses, require three stages of fibrillar polymerization of the amyloid subunit into insoluble semisolid arrays or microfibrils, which coalesce or agglutinate (aggregate) into structures of diverse morphology: scrapie-associated fibrils (SAFs) and kuru plaques. The first is preliminary processing of the precursor into the amyloid subunit or monomer (C-terminal truncation, N-terminal removal of the 22-amino-acid signal peptide, and release from the inositol-stearic acid membrane anchor); the second is nucleation-induced configurational change in the subunit into a cross β-pleated conformation; and the third is the formation of oligomers or polymers, usually dimers, tetramers, octamers, or hexadecamers, which may polymerize to produce fibrils visible under electron microscopy (SAFs) and coalesce into kuru plaques.

All β-pleated proteins can also form vitreous-like solid arrays that display extensive periodicity but which are not true three-dimensional crystals. They are, rather, semisolid, amorphous, vitreous, or mucilaginous pseudocrystals, thick emulsions, or gels that are insoluble precipitates in the

ADVANCES IN RESEARCH ON NEURODEGENERATION, II
Y. Mizuno et al.
© 1994 Birkhäuser Boston

hydrophilic media of the *milieu interieur*. On heating, drying, annealing, or aging, these arrays may increase their hydrogen bonding and decrease their hydration to assume increasingly a β-pleated structure, even in the case of some proteins with α-helical structure (Safar et al., 1993a, b). This is the heart of amyloidology and the basis of much of the biochemical alteration of proteins of cuisine and of aging of leather, parchment, rubber, natural fabrics, and even of cartilage and the lens of the eye.

Genetic Control of Generation of Infectious Amyloids in Creutzfeldt–Jakob Disease Syndromes

Eight point mutations, each changing an amino acid, have been found to cause familial CJD or its GSS and familial fatal insomnia (FFI) variants. Most GSS families display an amino acid replacement of proline by leucine at codon 102 (Goldgaber et al., 1989; Hsaio et al., 1989, 1990c; Kretzschmar et al., 1992). Two Japanese GSS families have the same proline to leucine change but at codon 105 (Kitamoto et al., 1993a). In two families with atypical GSS there is instead a replacement of alanine by valine at codon 117 (Doh-ura et al., 1989; Hsaio et al., 1990b). One GSS family has a codon 198 mutation replacing phenylalanine by serine (Hsaio et al., 1990a); and one other GSS family has a codon 217 mutation replacing glutamine by arginine (Dloughy et al., 1992; Hsaio et al., 1992a). The more common type of familial CJD has a codon 200 mutation that replaces glutamic acid with lysine (Goldfarb et al., 1990a, 1990b, 1990c, 1990d; Goldgaber et al., 1989). This has now been found in more than 60 families with more than 100 cases of CJD (Brown et al., 1992; Goldfarb et al., 1991c). However, in a large Finnish kindred with CJD (Haltia et al., 1979) aspartic acid is replaced by asparagine at codon 178 (Goldfarb et al., 1991a; Haltia et al., 1991), and there are Dutch, French, Hungarian, English, and American CJD families also with a codon 178 point mutation: 8 families in all with 97 CJD cases (Brown et al., 1991a, 1991b, 1991c, 1992a; Goldfarb et al., 1991c, 1992a; Nieto et al., 1991) (Fig. 1).

There is a Japanese family with a mutation in codon 145 that changes the codon to a stop codon. This so-called amber mutation produces a disease with a clinical course resembling Alzheimer's disease (Kitamoto et al., 1993, b).

Seven different insert mutations that are insertions of additional copies of an octapeptide repeat in the region normally containing five repeating octapeptide-coding sequences between codons 51 and 90 of the precursor gene also cause CJD in various modified clinical expressions.

There are twofold, fourfold, fivefold, sixfold, sevenfold, eightfold, and ninefold octapeptide repeats in different families (Brown et al., 1992b; Goldfarb et al., 1991b, 1992b, 1993b; Owen et al., 1989, 1990a, 1990b). Two families with five repeats have been identified; all others have been found in only one family. Thus, we know seven different insertional mutations in eight families that are responsible for the alteration of the normal precursor protein into the infectious amyloid form (see Fig. 1).

At codon 129 we have a nonpathogenic point mutation with substitution of valine for methionine, which is a silent polymorphism in the general population (Goldfarb et al., 1990a). Another silent polymorphism is a point mutation at codon 117 of GCA to GCG that causes no amino acid change. Finally, we find some normal subjects carry four instead of five copies of the octapeptide, normally at codon 41 to 91 (Goldfarb et al., 1991b). Two amino acid-changing point mutations have been found in sporadic cases of CJD in Japan (Kitamoto et al., 1993a). No mutations have been found in several other sporadic CJD cases and several kuru cases that have been fully sequenced.

Familial forms of CJD account for only about 5% of all cases. More than 90% are truly sporadic, and only about 1% have been shown to be iatrogenic, that is, from direct inoculation of the patient with infected material from a CJD patient. For all other cases, no chain of infection can be established nor do they appear to be familial. At present the best explanation for the regular incidence of sporadic nonfamilial CJD around the world is the *de novo* creation of the CJD amyloid infectious agent by a rare, spontaneous event occurring at a frequency of 1 per million population per annum, the surprisingly uniform worldwide incidence of CJD (Gajdusek, 1990). If one of the point mutations of familial CJD is present, this configurational change occurs with about a millionfold higher likelihood.

One corollary of this paradigm is that the replication of the infectious amyloid caused by inoculations of a different species does not 'breed true.' The point mutation is not copied in the amyloid formed in the new host, although it in turn is also infectious. The new CJD amyloid has the amino acid sequence of the precursor protein in the newly inoculated host. CJD from patients with the 102, 117, 178, 200, and 210 codon mutations have all been transmitted to monkeys and chimpanzees that do not carry these point mutations, nor do the infectious proteins made in these experimentally infected hosts contain those point mutations. The process of conformational change may well be an induced nucleation and homotaxic pattern setting for crystalline or fibril growth. The further elucidation of this transformation to β-pleated insoluble, protease-resistant, and infectious configuration will require the full structural comparison of infectious

Infectious Amyloidoses of Brain

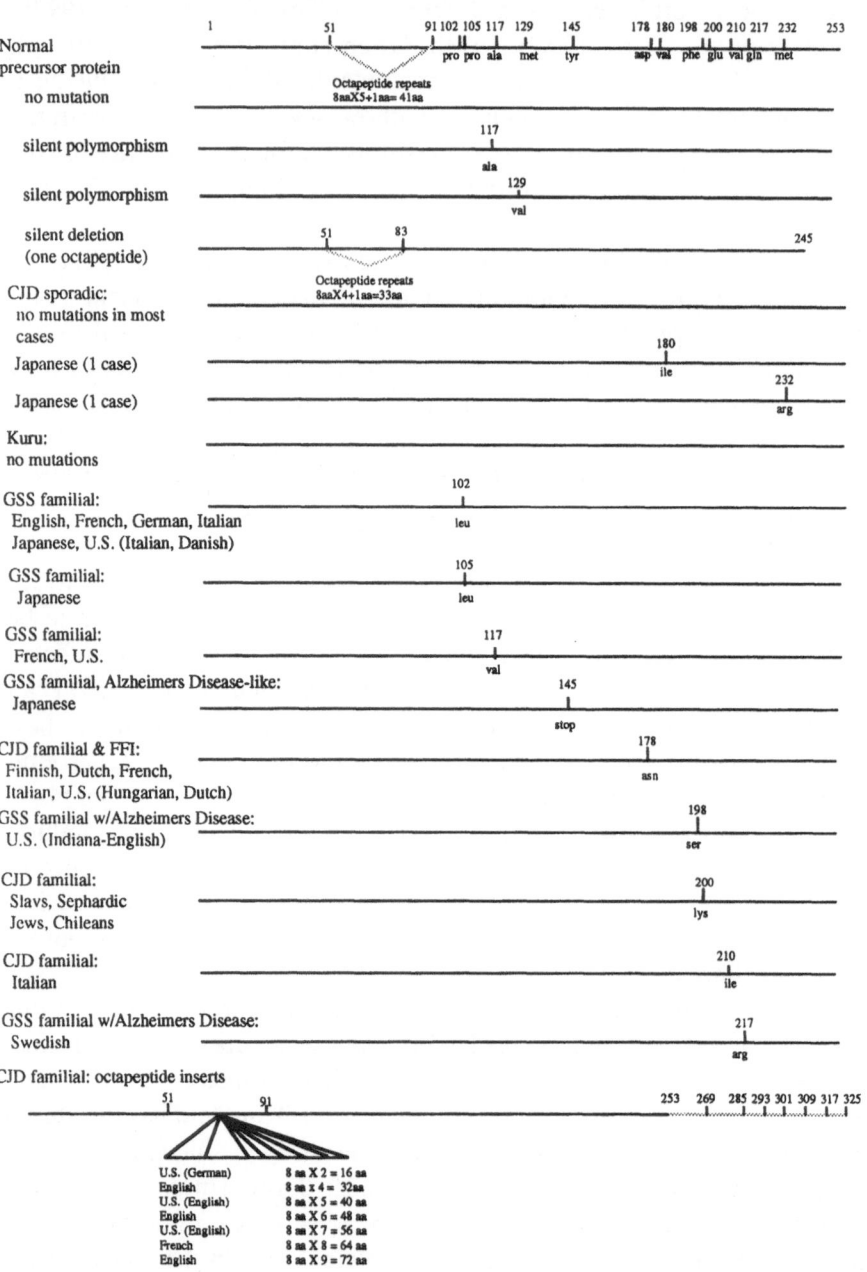

Figure 1. Twenty-one mutations in the gene specifying the host precursor molecule of CJD amyloid: 11 cause amino acid (aa) changes, 1 produces a stop codon, 1 a base change in the codon with no amino acid change, 7 are octapeptide inserts, 1 is an octapeptide deletion. Eight causing an amino acid change (102, 105, 117, 178, 198, 200, 210, 211) and 1 a stop codon (145) are found in families of diverse ethnic origins with familial CJD and its GSS and FFI variants. Three are silent polymorphisms: the codon 129 substitution of valine for methionine (which is

and noninfectious forms of the molecule, using nuclear magnetic resonance (NMR), the synchrocyclotron, circular dichroism spectroscopy, infrared spectroscopy, and high-resolution electron microscopy.

De novo (spontaneous) generation of the infectious form from the full-length CJD amyloid precursor may account for most sporadic CJD. It occurs to cause sporadic CJD as a rare stochastic event in 1 individual per million population base per annum (the worldwide incidence rate of CJD). In familial CJD, GSS, and FFI, these many point mutations (amino acid substitutions, a new stop codon, or octapeptide inserts) have increased the likelihood of this spontaneous conformational change about 10^6 fold.

It appears likely that a coordinate-covalent or covalent alteration in the precursor may be induced that endows the infectious nucleant with great stability (Safar et al., 1990, 1993b). We thus have reason to anticipate that the infectious form of the scrapie amyloid precursor may eventually be induced *in vitro*, even from synthetic polypeptides. These studies are under way, and monkeys and other animals inoculated with fibrils formed *in vitro* from synthetic peptides homologous to CJD pathogenic, mutation-containing regions of the CJD amyloid precursor gene are under observation.

Autonucleation with induction of conformational change in the full-length infectious amyloid precursor protein is the basic process of scrapie replication. We have suggested that fibril amyloid-enhancing factor is a scrapie-like infectious agent (Gajdusek, 1990), operating by an analogous self-induction of conformational change, much as small fibrils of tropo-collagen nucleate and pattern set the polymerization of collagen monomers into specific fibril networks (Guiroy and Gajdusek, 1988).

Oravske Kuru

Mitrová (1990), who has been following the high incidence of CJD throughout Slovakia for more than two decades, has identified a new

Figure 1 – *continued.* found in about 20% of the normal population); a base mutation in codon 117, causing no amino acid change; and an octapeptide deletion (in about 20% of the population). Seven additional mutations in families with CJD are insertions of octapeptide repeats into a region where there are already five copies of the same repeat. In a U.S. family, there are 2 copies of the octapeptide (8aa × 2 = 16aa) inserted, bringing the total to 7 copies; in an English family, there are 4 copies of the octapeptide (8aa × 4 = 32aa) inserted, bringing the total to 9 copies; in a second U.S. family there are 5 copies of the octapeptide (8aa × 5 = 40aa) inserted, bringing the total to 10 copies; in another English family, there are 6 copies (8aa × 7 = 56aa) inserted, bringing the total to 12 copies; in a French family there are 8 copies (8aa × 8 = 64aa) inserted, bringing the total to 13 copies; in another English family, there are 9 copies (8aa × 9 = 72aa) inserted, bringing the total to 14 copies.

focus of CJD in high incidences in several villages of Orava in the western foothills of the High Tatra mountains near the Polish border. In 1980, she identified an unusually high incidence of CJD in the rural Lucenec area of south-central Slovakia with many cases also occurring across the border in Hungary (Mitrová, 1980). During the past decade cases have been found in increasing frequency from the most sparsely populated rural sheep-raising area of Slovakia (Mitrová, 1990; Mitrová et al., 1991). Here an epidemic of CJD developed during the 1980s with some 30 cases occurring in patients born and reared in a dozen small villages with a total population of fewer than 15,000. This yields an incidence of more than 1,000 per million population per year in contrast to the worldwide incidence of 1 per million per year.

The most intensely involved villages of Zuberec and Habovka, with a total population of fewer than 2,000, have shown more than 20 cases of CJD in the past 3 years. The incidence in the villages has thus become more than 3,000 times higher than in the rest of the world, in such cities as Paris, London, New York, Sidney, Santiago, or Shanghai, or any other large cities, and it is yet 100 fold higher than that among the Sephardic Jews in Israel. Members of the same family with 20 to 30 years difference in age become sick at nearly the same time. This suggested a common source of infection rather than genetically determined etiology, as also did the new 'epidemic' of appearance of CJD in the 1980s. We suspected an accident of massive contamination of the population with sheep scrapie, which the Orava farmers have long recognized in their sheep as *klusavka*. For these reasons at first we believed that this outbreak might not be explained genetically.

However, we have now sequenced DNA from 9 of the Orava and 6 of the Lucenec CJD brains, and all have shown the substitution of lysine for glutamic acid at codon 200. Four of the 11 healthy, adult, first-order relatives studied have the same mutation (Goldgaber et al., 1989). CJD had not been known in Orava before the 1970s (Mitrová, 1990). The epidemic started with a few cases in the late 1970s and has developed into an escalating epidemic in the late 1980s. We have found some family members with the mutation although they are healthy and over 70 years of age. We are now looking for the cofactor that turns on the expression of the mutation, or a factor which in the past inhibited the posttranslational configuration change of the precursor to amyloid. Thus, the new question is not what has caused the Orava outbreak, which is known to be the codon 200 glutamic-acid-to-lysine point mutation, but rather what has prevented its expression in previous generations so that it has accumulated as a frequent silent nonpathogenic polymorphism, only expressing itself as a pathogenic mutation in these people in the past 15 years.

The CJD Genetic Marker for the Wandering Jews of the Diaspora

On discovering the codon 200 glutamine-to-lysine point mutation responsible for the high-incidence foci of CJD in both Lucenec and Orava regions of Slovakia and widely disseminated in Slavic peoples of Eastern Europe, we screened a large number of sporadic and familial CJD brain specimens from our archive of frozen brain accumulated during the past 30 years (Goldfarb et al., 1990c). This led us to discover the mutation in Greek CJD patients who were Sephardic Jews, and we quickly found the mutation in Sephardic Jews who had some diagnosis of CJD in France from Tunisia and in Sephardic Jews with CJD in Israel, both Libyan born and Israeli born. Ashkenazic Jewish CJD patients did not have the codon 200 glutamic-to-lysine point mutation (Goldfarb et al., 1990c).

We are thus now investigating other circum-Mediterranean Sephardic Jews with CJD and with particular attention to the Iberian Peninsula, particularly Spain where in 1492 the Catholic monarchs, Ferdinand and Isabella forced the quick conversion of large numbers of Sephardic Jews to Catholicism. Many of the remainder fled and gave rise to the large Sephardic Jewish group in Greece where we have found the mutation. Of those remaining in Spain and converted to Catholicism, many emigrated in the fifteenth century to the New World. We have now found that in Chile the proportion of familial cases among the CJD patients is several fold higher than elsewhere, and these patients and their family members have the 200 codon glutamine-to-lysine substitution (Brown et al., 1991c, 1992a; Goldfarb et al., 1991c).

The CJD Point Mutation for the Large Finnish Pedigree of Familial CJD

One of the largest familial CJD pedigrees is that published by Haltia et al. in Finland (1979), which we have now investigated and found therein none of the point mutations previously known in familial CJD or GSS, but instead a codon 178 replacement of aspartic acid by asparagine (Goldfarb et al., 1991a). We have now found this codon 178 mutation in Dutch, French, Hungarian, and American cases of familial CJD (Brown et al., 1992b; Nieto et al., 1991). Furthermore, in Italian, French, and

U.S. families the mutation causes a clinical variant of CJD, familial fatal insomnia (FFI).

Thus the paradigm from the amyloidosis literature, which states that any one of several amino acid substitutions in the precursor molecule causes an enormously increased likelihood of its posttranslational conversion to an amyloid conformation and its polymerization and deposition in the form of amyloid fibrils in various tissues, has proved amazingly predictive in unraveling the pathogenesis of familial CJD and GSS and also of β-amyloid deposition in normal aging, Alzheimer's disease, and Down's syndrome.

Varieties of Phenotypic Expression Determined by Different Mutations in the CJD Amyloid Precursor Gene

The pattern of clinical disease produced by the different mutations in different families is extremely uniform in some and quite variable in other families. It ranges from classical GSS in most families with codon 102, 105, and 117, and mutations to classical CJD with codon 178 and codon 200 mutations and the various insertions of 2, 4, 5, 6, 7, 8, or 9 octapeptide repeats. However, familial fatal insomnia (FFI) has been the clinical form of the disease in several families with codon 178 mutations whereas the clinical form of CJD without insomnia in other families with the same mutation. However, we have reported that presence of the valine polymorphism at codon 129 together with the 178 mutation on the same chromosome causes FFI, whereas the classical CJD-type disease appears in families with the more common methionine pleomorphism at codon 129 on the codon 178 mutated chromosome.

The age of onset is earlier and the duration of clinical disease is longer in codon 178 CJD than in codon 200 CJD, and in codon 200 disease the electroencephalograph (EEG) usually shows the characteristic CJD spike and slow-wave periodicity. No such EEG change is found in the codon 178 CJD patients. Even the incubation period for clinical disease in intracerebrally inoculated squirrel, spider, and capuchin monkeys differs for codon 178 and codon 200 cases of CJD, being considerably longer in codon 200 than for codon 178 cases.

Many other distinguishing phenotypical expressions of the pathogenic mutations have now been recorded. These include an Alzheimer's disease-type clinical course in the 145 stop codon mutation with no βA4 amyloid deposits in the amyloid plaques. On the other hand, the codon 198 and 217 have produced an Alzheimer's disease-like clinical course and also a combined CJD and Alzheimer's disease-type neuropathology with both the CJD amyloid and the βA4 amyloid plaques.

Transthyretin Amyloidoses of Familial Amyloidotic Polyneuropathy (FAP) as a Paradigm for the Genetic Control of Transmissible and Nontransmissible Brain Amyloidoses

Of most pertinence to our problem of the unconventional viruses, which are infectious amyloids, have been the transthyretin amyloidoses of familial amyloidotic polyneuropathies (FAP) (Costa et al., 1990; Gajdusek, 1991a, 1991b; Gajdusek et al., 1991). Patients are members of several hundred families scattered around the world in which the disease is an autosomal dominant trait. The onset of the clinical disease may occur at different ages, and leads to the destruction of peripheral nerves by progressive deposition of amyloid in the perineurium. The human transthyretin gene has been cloned and its full sequence of 6.9 kb composed of four exons and three introns is known. Its encoding gene is located on chromosome 18 (Sasaki et al., 1985; Tsuzuki et al., 1985). Transthyretin in its pure and crystalline form is a soluble prealbumin of 14-kDa with 127 amino acids. Its secondary, tertiary, and quaternary structures have been determined by x-ray crystallography. It is a symmetrical tetramer of 55 kDa made of four subunits showing extensive β-pleated sheet structure (Blake and Oatley, 1977; Blake et al., 1971, 1974, 1978). Thus, it is amyloidogenic by structural chemical considerations.

Members of different affected families have a mutation resulting in a 1-amino-acid substitution in the precursor that increase the statistical mechanical likelihood of the molecule falling into the amyloid conformation by a factor of about 10^4 to 10^6. There is no one specific mutation causing the disease in all families. Thus, in more than 100 investigated families more than 30 different mutations have been detected (Fig. 2). The transthyretin amyloid may be deposited in the anterior chamber of the eye to cause familial amyloidotic blindness, in the heart to cause amyloidotic cardiopathy, or asymptomatically in the intestinal wall, as well as around peripheral nerves to cause FAP. Different amino acid-changing mutations cause different clinical pictures ranging from disease in which several different organs are targeted by amyloid deposition to pure single organ-targeted amyloidosis. The FAP is thus caused by precipitation of amyloid formed from the transthyretin precursor, with any of a set of point mutation each causing a single amino acid replacement that increases the likelihood of amyloid formation.

This amyloid is not a replicating infectious molecule. Without one of these point mutations it is difficult to change the transthyretin polypeptide by concentration and nucleation into the amyloid configuration. With these single amino acid substitutions amyloid formation occurs spontaneously as a much more likely stochastic event, even extracellularly and *in vitro*.

In spite of the amyloidogenicity of the normal transthyretin by structural and chemical considerations, spontaneous amyloid formation does not occur in the absence of a facilitating mutation causing an amino acid substitution until the ninth decade, with the rare sporadic appearance of senile cardiac decompensation with cardiac amyloidosis. In these patients in their eighties, the full-length molecule without any mutation is the amyloid subunit. There are also several silent polymorphisms in the population with point mutations causing nonpathogenic single amino acid substitutions (see Fig. 2).

The codon 30 point mutation with proline replaced by methionine has been expressed in transgenic mice, which develop deposits of human amyloid containing the methionine-30 mutation similar to depositions in FAP, but also in the intestine and other tissues, and they pass this trait to their offspring (Wakasugi et al., 1988; Yi et al., 1990).

Analogies with Transmissible Dementias (CJD, GSS) Suggest That Transthyretin Amyloidoses of FAP and Other Amyloidoses May Also Be Transmissible and Infectious

The close parallel between multiple amino acid-changing mutations [each enormously facilitating the conversion to amyloid of the precursor protein, which usually fails to spontaneously fall into amyloid configuration, except as a rare event (1 per million population per annum, the world-wide incidence of sporadic CJD)] in the absence of any mutation in the precursor, and the transthyretin amyloidoses of FAP determined by any one of many different point mutations, strongly suggests that FAP may also be transmissible. It will be difficult to demonstrate this in experimental animals because long-term observation will be essential and because subtle clinical signs, rather than flagrant, fatal disease should be expected. This will also have to be controlled by histopathological search for amyloid deposits in the perineurium and in other tissues. Amyloidoses based on other precursors may likewise be transmissible under the proper experimental conditions. This might be demonstrated using transgenic mice expressing the human precursors.

TRANSTHYRETIN AMYLOIDOSES OF FAMILIAL AMYLOIDOTIC POLYNEUROPATHY (FAP)
Mutations Increasing Likelihood of Host Precursor Falling Into Amyloid Configuration

NORMAL	6	10		30	33	36		42	45	49	50	58	60		77	84	90		111	114	116		122	127
	gly	cys		val	phe	ala		glu	ala	thr	ser	leu	thr		ser	ile	his		leu	tyr	tyr		val	

FAMILIAL AMYLOIDOTIC POLYNEUROPATHY

Dutch, German, Greek, Italian, Japanese, Portuguese, Spanish, Swedish, Turkish	30 met	
Jewish	33 ile	
Greek USA	36 pro	
Japanese family KA	42 gly	
Italian- Irish	45 thr	
Italian	49 ala	
Jewish	49 gly	
Japanese family HY	50 arg	
German USA:MD	58 his	
Appalachian USA:WVA	60 ala	
German USA:IL	77 tyr	
Swiss USA:IN	84 ser	
Italian- Sicilian	90 asn	
Danish	111 met	
Japanese family TK	114 cys	

NORMAL: SILENT POLYMORPHISM

British	6 ser	
German- Portuguese	90 asn	
French- Canadian	116 val	
USA: Scandinavian	122 ile	

Figure 2. Sixteen different amino acid substitutions caused by point mutations in the gene specifying the transthyretin prealbumin precursor molecule in more than 20 families of various ethnic origins are shown. In 4 of these families, normal without FAP, the mutation is a silent nonpathogenic polymorphism. On codon 49 are two different amino acid substitutions, in a Jewish and Italian family, respectively. Codon 90 (asparagine replaces histamine) mutation has apparently caused FAP in the Italian Sicilian family, but not in the German and Portuguese families. There are more than 20 additional such point mutations reported in the recent literature as responsible for different symphonies of pleomorphic clinical expression of familial amyloidotic polyneuropathy, familial amyloidotic blindness, and familial amyloidotic cardiopathy.

Nucleating Induction of Configurational Change in Host Precursors and Polymerization to Fibrils as a General Phenomenon in Amyloidogenesis

We have demonstrated spontaneous generation of congophilic amyloid fibrils using synthetic polypeptides corresponding to sequences encoded by normal and mutant familial CJD alleles in the regions of codon 178 and codon 200. The 178 mutant and normal peptides formed fibrils with distinct morphological characteristics and differing aggregation tendencies from fibrils formed from the 200 mutant or normal peptides. The mutant peptides produce more filaments and denser masses of aggregate filaments than the unmutated peptides. Further mixtures of the normal with the mutant peptides for either codon region produce denser masses of fibrils than either peptide alone (Goldfarb et al., 1993a).

The amyloid deposits of FAP contain both the mutated and the unmutated molecules, the mutated having nucleated and induced the β-pleating and copolymerization of the unmutated molecules in the heterozygous patients (A.F. de Frietas, University of Oporto, personal communications).

Frangione has shown that the amyloid deposits in the vascular wall in hereditary cerebral hemorrhage with amyloidosis, Dutch type (HCHWA-D), contain both the codon 695 (glutamine substituted for glutamic acid), mutated amyloid βA4 protein, and the unmutated molecule with the normal βA4 sequence. The heterozygous patients are apparently polymerizing both the amyloid βA4 protein derived from the normal brain amyloid precursor protein (APP) and the mutated βA4 protein. Frangione and colleagues have synthesized polypeptides of the first 28 amino acids of the βA4 protein with and without the codon 695 mutation of HCHWA-D and studied the dynamics of fibril polymerization with each. The synthetic 28-amino-acid polypeptide with the mutation forms amyloids much faster than the polypeptide without the mutation. However, if both synthetic polypeptides are placed together in solution, the mutated polypeptide accelerates amyloid fibril formation by the unmutated polypeptide. Frangione uses the phrase accelerated instructive fibrillogenesis for this nucleating phenomenon of facilitation or induction of amyloidogenesis by a different amyloid (Frangione et al., 1992).

We are probably seeing the same phenomenon in the conversion of insulin-associated proteins to an amyloid in insulin-amyloid deposits in the amyloidosis of late diabetes. The same amyloid induction may also be occurring in the simultaneous appearance of βA4 amyloid and τ-amyloid in the neurofibrillary tangles of Alzheimer's disease, Down's syndrome, and normal aging brain.

Fibril Amyloid-Enhancing Factor in Experimental AA Amyloidosis May Be a Scrapie-Like Nucleating Infectious Protein

Amyloid-enhancing factor (Axelrad and Kisilevsky, 1980; Axelrad et al., 1982; Hol et al., 1985; Janigan, 1969; Janigan and Druet, 1968; Niewold et al., 1987; Ranlov, 1967) is a low molecular weight glycoprotein found in tissues containing AA amyloid, which accelerates the laying down of AA amyloid in tissues in experimentally induced AA amyloidosis in mice and hamsters, shortening the lag time to 2 days from several weeks. It apparently serves as a nucleus for fibril formation and deposition (Niewold et al., 1987) in animals with high serum level of acute-phase reactant AA amyloid precursor produced by the nonspecific activation of inflammatory response with injections of casein, silver nitrate, or lipopolysaccharide (Cohen, 1965; Janigan, 1965).

Fibril amyloid-enhancing factor (Niewold et al., 1987) is an example of pattern-setting induction of amyloid formation and polymerization, which is basically a nucleation process such as is required in all fibril polymerization. Such configurational change in the host precursor protein to the β-pleated infectious amyloid form occurs in the case of the transmissible agents of kuru-CJD-GSS-scrapie-transmissible mink encephalopathy-BSE. In these infections with infectious amyloid proteins a pattern-setting conformational change is induced in the host precursor. Thus, we suggest that the fibril amyloid-enhancing factor is a scrapie- (or kuru-CJD-GSS-) like agent, which induces a change in its own precursor to produce more of itself by copying its altered configuration. This pattern-setting nucleation we have mistaken for viral replication. It may be that we need to broaden our concept of a virus as have the computer virologists (Gajdusek, 1990; Guiroy and Gajdusek, 1988).

Alzheimer's Disease

The universal brain amyloidoses that everyone begins to get in old age and which are neuropathologically evident in all human brains from the ninth decade through the century are caused by amyloid deposits formed from a 42- or 43-amino-acid peptide (βA4) proteolytically cleaved from the 80-kDa brain amyloid precursor protein (APP). This precursor is a transmembrane protein, the amyloid subunit from which extends from the center of the transmembrane region to the fifteenth extracellular amino acid. It is normally processed with a high rate of turnover with cleavage in the extracellular segment, thereby preventing the formation of the amyloidogenetic 42- to 43-amino-acid βA4 peptide. All metabolic interferences, environmental or genetic, with the high rate of turnover lead to the possibility of cleavage resulting in this amyloidogenic peptide. This is the same process that when accelerated from environmental factors or from point mutations on the precursor or on other chromosomes, specifying still unidentified proteins which must be either enzymes, chaperonins, or binding proteins or other rate-influencing molecules, is the cause of Alzheimer's disease. In Down's syndrome, overproduction of the precursor appears to be enough to lead to formation of the βA4 peptide.

Familial Alzheimer's disease (FAD) families with pathological mutants of the APP gene account for only 3% to 5% of the FAD families, whereas FAD accounts for 10% to 20% of all Alzheimer's disease, 80% to 90% of Alzheimer's disease being sporadic. The majority of FAD families with early onset appear to have a point mutation now localized on chromosome 14, whereas the late-onset FAD families appear to have a mutation less firmly localized on chromosome 19.

Figure 3 presents the mutations thus far identified on the βA4 amyloid precursor protein (APP) and shows clearly the mounting parallel with the infectious brain amyloids of the spongiform encephalopathies (see Fig. 1). Both these transmissible and nontransmissible brain amyloidoses now demonstrate close similarities to the paradigm of the transthyretin amyloidoses of familial amyloidotic polyneuropathy (see Fig. 2) in which some 40 pathogenic point mutations have now been found.

The Semantic Word Wars of Slow Virologists and Amyloidologists

The amyloidologists assiduously avoid the terminology of microbiology in their discipline. We, from microbiology, have entered their field through the infectious amyloids of the subacute spongiform viral encephalopathies (SSVEs) of kuru-CJD-GSS-scrapie-BSE. Thus, we have used the term replication, and the concepts of virulence and host range and incubation period, in describing phenomena for which they use other words and phrases. Various authors have exhausted the thesaurus to find terminology different from that used by their competing colleagues to describe the production of conformational change of host precursor proteins to β-pleated structure and the polymerization of amyloid fibrillogenesis:

Brain Amyloid of Aging (ßA4)

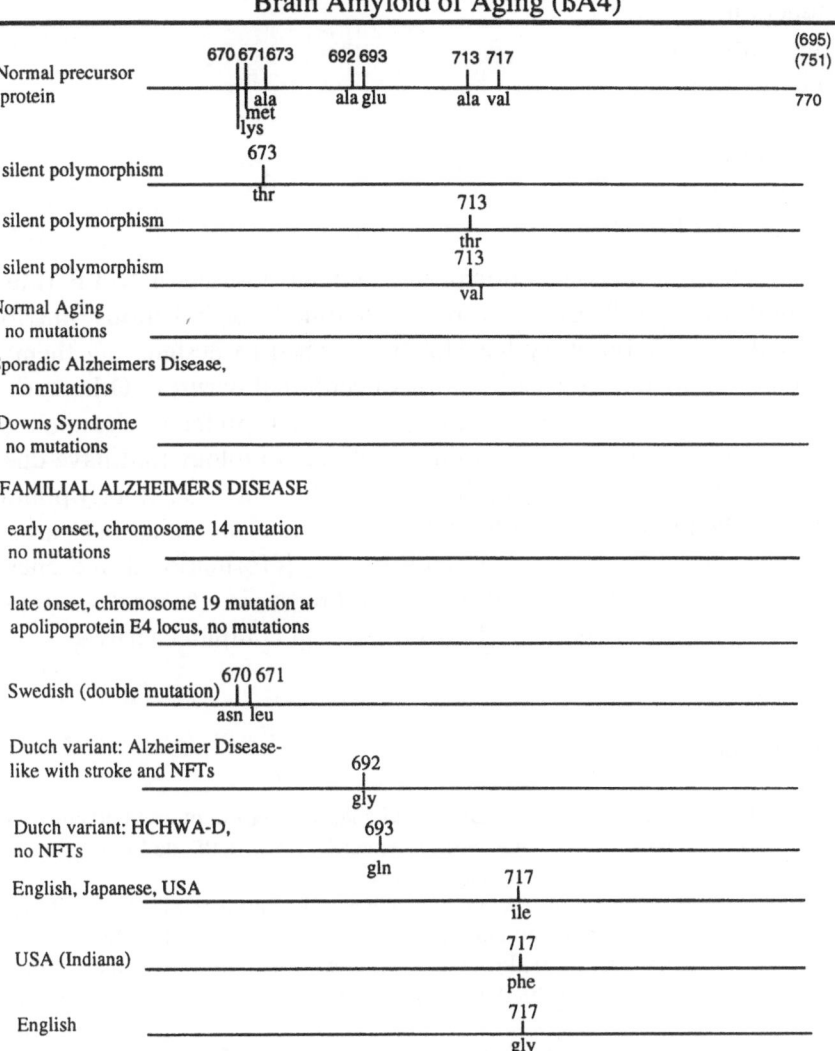

Figure 3. Eleven point mutations on the βA4 amyloid precursor protein of normal aging and Alzheimer's disease: three different amino acid substitutions at the same codon 717 all cause familial Alzheimer's disease (FAD) in rare British, Japanese, and US families. A double mutation at codon 670 and 671 causes FAD in a Swedish family. Two adjacent mutations on codons 692 and 693 each cause hereditary cerebral hemorrhage with amyloidosis, Dutch type (HCHWA-D), in a different Dutch family. A mutation on codon 673 and two different amino acid changes on codon 713 are silent polymorphisms. Sporadic Alzheimer's precursor protein. Only 3% of FAD have one of the 5 mutations causing the disease in rare families. Most of the early-onset FAD families have a mutation on chromosome 14, and late-onset FAD families appear to have a mutation on chromosome 19, but neither of these is associated with any mutation on the βA4 amyloid precursor protein gene.

Nucleation
Induction
Augmentation
Enhancement
Facilitation
Acceleration
Instruction
Heterodimer formation

Because the unconventional and atypical viruses of SSVE (kuru-CJD-GSS-scrapie-BSE) have been identified as infections amyloid molecules, our laboratory has slowly switched to designating them to infectious amyloids instead of unconventional viruses. Others have accepted the term prions for these agents. We prefer to draw on the important and informative paradigms of amyloidology that have directed much of our thinking over the past decade. I have facetiously pointed out that the founders of virology define a virus as an obligatory parasite of submicroscopic dimensions requiring the informational and energy systems of the host for replication: this embraces viroids, virules, virettes, nucleating agents of industrial infections, and computer viruses.

References

Axelrad MA, Kisilevsky R (1980): Biological characterization of amyloid enhancing factor. In: *Amyloid and Amyloidosis*, Glenner GG, Costa PP, de Freitas AF, eds., pp. 527–533. Amsterdam: Excerpta Medica

Axelrad MA, Kisilevsky R, Wilmer J, Chen SJ, Skinner M (1982): Further characterization of amyloid-enhancing factor. *Lab Invest* 47:139–146

Blake CCF, Oatley SJ (1977): Protein-DNA and protein-hormone interactions in prealbumin: a model of the thyroid hormone nuclear receptor? *Nature* 268:115–120

Blake CCF, Geisow MJ, Oatley, SJ, Rerat B, Rerat C (1978): Structure of prealbumin: secondary, tertiary and quaternary interactions determined by Fourier refinement at 1.8 Å. *J Mol Biol* 121:339–356

Blake CCF, Geisow MJ, Swan IDA, Rerat C, Rerat B (1974): Structure of human plasma prealbumin at 2.6 Å resolution: a preliminary report on the polypeptide chain conformation, quaternary structure and thyroxine binding. *J Mol Biol* 88:1–12

Blake CCF, Swan IDA, Rerat C, Berthou J, Laurent A, Rerat B (1971): An X-ray study of the subunit structure of prealbumin. *J Mol Biol* 61:217–224

Brown P, Gálvez S, Goldfarb LG, Nieto A, Cartier L, Gibbs CJ Jr, Gajdusek DC (1992): Familial Creutzfeldt-Jakob disease in Chile is associated with the codon 200[Asn] mutation of the chromosome 20 amyloid precursor gene. *J Neurol Sci* 112:65–67

Brown P, Goldfarb LG, Cathala F, Vrbovská A, Sulima M, Nieto A, Gibbs CJ Jr, Gajdusek DC (1991a): The molecular genetics of familial Creutzfeldt-Jakob disease in France. *J Neurol Sci* 105:240–246

Brown P, Goldfarb LG, Gajdusek DC (1991b): The new biology of spongiform encephalopathy: infectious amyloidoses with a genetic twist. *Lancet* 337:1019–1022

Brown P, Goldfarb LG, Gibbs CJ Jr, Gajdusek DC (1991c): The phenotypic expression of different mutations in transmissible familial Creutzfeldt-Jakob disease. *Eur J Epidemiol* 7(5):469–476

Brown P, Goldfarb LG, Kovanen J, Haltia M, Cathala F, Sulima M, Gibbs CJ Jr, Gajdusek DC (1992a): Phenotypic characteristics of familial Creutzfeldt-Jakob disease associated with the codon 178^{Asn} PPNP mutation. *Ann Neurol* 31:282–285

Brown P, Goldfarb LG, McCombie WR, Nieto A, Squillacote D, Sheremata W, Little BW, Godec MS, Gibbs CJ Jr, Gajdusek DC (1992b): Atypical Creutzfeldt-Jakob disease in an American family with an insert mutation in the PRNP amyloid precursor gene. *Neurology* 42:422–427

Cohen AS (1965): The constitution and genesis of amyloid. *Int Rev Exp Pathol* 4:159–243

Costa PP, de Freitas AF, Saraiva MJM, eds. (1990): *Familial Amyloidotic Polyneuropathy and Other Transthyretin Related Disorders*. Porto: Archives de Medicina

Dloughy SI, Hsiao K, Farlow MR, Foroud T, Conneally PM, Johnson P, Prusiner SB, Hodes ME, Ghetti B (1992): Linkage of the Indiana kindred of Gerstmann-Sträussler-Scheinker disease to the prion protein gene. *Nature Genet* 1:64–67

Doh-ura K, Tateishi J, Sasaki H, Kitamoto T, Sakaki Y (1989): Protein change at position 102 of prion gene is the most common but not the sole mutation related to Gerstmann-Sträussler syndrome. *Biochem Biophys Res Commun* 163:974–979

Frangione B, Wisniewski T, Ghiso J (1992): Accelerated instructive fibrillogenesis. *J Cell Biochem Suppl* 16E:200 (abstr.).

Gajdusek DC (1986): Unconventional virus infections as cerebral amyloidoses. In: *Unconventional Virus Diseases of the Central Nervous System*, Court LA, Dormont D, Brown P, eds. [Proceedings of Conference, Paris, December 2–6, 1986], pp. 641–659. Fontenay-aux-Roses, France: Commissariat a l'Energie Atomique (CEA), Service de Documentation

Gajdusek DC (1988a): Transmissible and non-transmissible amyloidoses: autocatalytic post-translational conversion of host precursor to β-pleated configurations. *J Neuroimmunol* 20:95–110

Gajdusek DC (1988b): Etiology versus pathogenesis: the causes of post-translational modifications of host specified brain proteins to amyloid configuration. In: *Genetics and Alzheimer's Disease*, Proceedings of a meeting held by the Foundation IPSEN pour la Recherche Thérapeutique, Paris, March 25, Sinet PM, Lamour Y, Christen Y, eds., pp. 174–176. Berlin: Springer-Verlag

Gajdusek DC (1989): Fantasy of a "virus" from the inorganic world: pathogenesis of cerebral amyloidoses by polymer nucleating agents and/or 'viruses." In: *Modern Trends in Human Leukemia, Vol VIII*, Neth R, Gallo RC, Greaves M, Gaedicke G, Gohla S, Mannweiller K, Ritter J., eds., pp. 481–499. New York: Springer-Verlag

Gajdusek DC (1990): Subacute spongiform encephalopathies: transmissible cerebral amyloidoses caused by unconventional viruses. In: *Virology*, 2nd Ed., Fields BN, Knipe DM, Chanock RM, Hirsch MS, Melnick JL, Monath TP, Roizman B, eds., pp. 2289–2324. New York: Raven Press

Gajdusek DC (1991a): Genetic control of *de novo* conversion to infectious amyloids of host precursor proteins: Kuru-CJD-scrape. In: *Concepts in Biomedical Research*, Proceedings of paul Ehrlich Institute Scientific Conference. New York: Springer-Verlag

Gajdusek DC (1991b): Transthyretin amyloidoses of familial amyloidotic polyneuropathy as a paradigm for the genetic control of *de novo* generation of Creutzfeldt-Jakob disease infectious amyloid by a spontaneous change in the configuration of the host precursor protein. In: *Sub-Acute Spongiform Encephalopathies, Current Topics of Veterinary and Animal Science, Vol. 55*, Bradley R, Savey M, Marchant BA, eds., pp. 91–114. Kluwer Academic Publishers

Gajdusek DC (1991c): The transmissible amyloidoses: genetic control of spontaneous generation of infectious amyloid proteins by nucleation of configurational change in host precursors kuru-CJD-Scrapie-BSE. *Eur J Epidemiol* 7:567–577

Gajdusek DC, Gibbs CJ Jr, (1991): Brain amyloidoses: precursor proteins and the amyloids of transmissible and nontransmissible dementias: scrapie-kuru-CJD viruses as infectious polypeptides or amyloid-enhancing factors. In: *Biomedical Advances in Aging*, Goldstein AL, ed., pp. 3–24. New York: Plenum Publishing

Gajdusek DC, Beyreuther K, Brown P, Cork LC, Cunningham DD, Frangione B, Gibbs CJ Jr, Goldfarb LG, Goldgaber D, Hsiao KK, Koo EH, Martin LJ, Masters CL, Odenwald WF, Price DL, Prusiner SB, Ruddle FH, Safar J, Scangos G, Schmechel DE, Shashikant CS, Shlichta PJ, Sisodia SS, Trapp BD, Unterbeck A, Van Nostrand WE, Violette SM, Walker LC, Wirak D (1991): Regulation and genetic control of brain amyloid. *Brain Res Rev* 16:83–114

Goldfarb LG, Brown P, Goldgaber D, Asher D, Rubenstein R, Brown WT, Piccardo P, Kasasak J, Boellaard JW, Gajdusek DC (1990c): Creutzfeldt-Jakob disease and kuru patients lack a mutation consistently found in Gerstmann-Sträussler-Scheinker syndrome. *Exp Neurol* 108:247–250

Goldfarb LG, Brown P, Goldgaber D, Garruto RM, Yanagihara R, Asher DM, Gajdusek DC 91990b): Identical mutation in unrelated patients with Creutzfeldt-Jakob disease. *Lancet* 336:174–175

Goldfarb LG, Korczyn AO, Brown P, Chapman J, Gajdusek DC (1990c): Mutation in codon 200 of scrapie amyloid precursor gene linked to CJD in Sephardic Jews. *Lancet* 336:637

Goldfarb LG, Mitrová E, Brown P, Toh BH, Gajdusek DC (1990d): Mutation in codon 200 of scrapie amyloid protein gene in two clusters of Creutzfeldt-Jakob disease in Slovakia. *Lancet* 336:514–515

Goldfarb LG, Brown P, Mitrová E, Cervenakova L, Goldin L, Korczyn AD, Chapman I, Gálvez S, Cartier L, Rubenstein R, Gajdusek DC (1991a): Creutzfeldt-Jakob disease associated with the PRNP codon 200[lys] mutation: an analysis of 45 families. *Eur J Epidemiol* 7:477–486

Goldfarb LG, Haltia M, Brown P, Nieto A, Kovanen J, McCombie WR, Trapp S, Gajdusek DC (1991b): New mutation in scrapie amyloid precursor gene (at codon 178) in Finnish Creutzfeldt-Jakob kindred. *Lancet* 337:425

Goldfarb LG, Brown P, McCombie WR, Goldgaber D, Swergold GD, Wills PR, Cervenakova L, Baron H, Gibbs CJ Jr, Gajdusek DC (1991c): Transmissible familial Creutzfeldt-Jakob disease associated with five, seven, and eight extra octapeptide coding repeats in the PRNP gene. *Proc Natl Acad Sci USA* 88:10926–10930

Goldfarb LG, Brown P, Haltia M, Cathala F, McCombie WR, Kovanen J,

Cervenakova L, Goldin L, Nieto A, Godec M, Asher DM, Gajdusek DC (1992a): Creutzfeldt-Jakob disease associated with the codon 178^{ASN} PRNP mutation in families of European origin. *Ann Neurol* 31(3):274–281

Goldfarb LG, Brown P, Vrbovska A, Baron H, McCombie WR, Cathala F, Gibbs CJ Jr, Gajdusek DC (1992b): An insert mutation in the chromosome 20 amyloid precursor gene in a Gerstmann-Sträussler-Scheinker family. *J Neurol Sci* 111:189–194

Goldfarb LG, Brown P, Haltia M, Ghiso J, Frangione B, Gajdusek DC (1993a): Synthetic peptides corresponding to different mutated regions of the amyloid gene in familial Creutzfeldt-Jakob disease show enhanced *in vitro* formation of morphologically distinct amyloid fibrils. *Proc Natl Acad Sci USA* 90:4451–4454

Goldfarb LG, Brown P, Little BW, Cervenáková L, Kenney K, Gibbs CJ Jr, Gajdusek DC (1993b): A new (2-repeat) octapeptide coding insert mutation in Creutzfeldt-Jakob disease. *Neurology* 43:2392–2394

Goldgaber D, Goldfarb LG, Brown P, Asher DM, Brown WT, Lin S, Teener JW, Feinstone SM, Rubenstein B, Kascsak R, Boellaard JW, Gajdusek DC (1989): Mutations in familial Creutzfeldt-Jakob disease and Gerstmann-Sträussler syndrome. *Exp Neurol* 106:204–206

Guiroy DC, Gajdusek DC (1988): Fibril-derived amyloid enhancing factors as nucleating agents in Alzheimer's disease and transmissible virus dementia. In: *Molecular Genetic Mechanisms in Neurodegenerative Disorders*, Brown P, Bolis L, Gajdusek DC, eds., *Discussions in Neuroscience*, Geneva: FESN Vol. 5, pp. 69–73

Haltia M, Kovanen J, van Crevel H, Bots GTAM, Stefanko S (1979): Familial Creutzfeldt-Jakob disease. *J Neurol Sci* 42:381–389

Haltia M, Kovanen J, Goldfarb LG, Brown P, Gajdusek DC (1991): Familial Creutzfeldt-Jakob disease in Finland: epidemiological, clinical, pathological and molecular genetic studies. *Eur J Epidemiol* 7(5):494–500

Hol PR, van Andel ACJ, van Ederen AM, Draäyer J, Gruys E (1985): Amyloid enhancing factor in hamster. *Br J Exp Pathol* 66:689–697

Hsiao K, Baker HF, Crow TJ, Poulter M, Owen E, Terwilliger JD, Westaway D, Ott J, Prusiner SB (1989): Linkage of prion protein missense variant to Gerstmann-Sträussler syndrome. *Nature* 338:342–345

Hsiao K, Cass C, Conneally PM, Dloughy SR, Hodes ME, Farlow MR, Ghetti B, Prusiner SB (1990a): Atypical Gerstmann-Sträussler-Scheinker syndrome with neurofibrillary tangles: no mutations in the prion protein open-reading-frame in a portion of the Indiana kindred. *Neurobiol Aging* 11:3, 302

Hsiao K, Cass C, Schellenberg G, Bird T, Devine-Gage E, Wisniewski M, Prusiner SB (1990b): A prion protein variant in a family with a telencephalic form of Gerstmann-Sträussler-Scheinker syndrome. *Neurology* 41:681–684

Hsiao K, Dloughy SR, Farlow MR, Cass C, Da Costa M, Conneally PM, Hodes ME, Ghetti B, Prusiner SB (1992a): Mutant prion proteins in Gerstmann-Sträussler-Scheinker disease with neurofibrillary tangles. *Nature Genet* 1:68–71

Hsiao KK, Doh-ura K, Kitamoto T, Tateishi J, Prusiner SB (1990c): A prion protein amino acid substitution in ataxic Gerstmann-Sträussler syndrome. *Ann Neurol* 26:137

Janigan DT (1965): Experimental amyloidoses. *Am J Pathol* 47:159–171

Janigan DT (1969): Pathogenetic mechanisms in protein-induced amyloidosis. *Am J Pathol* 55:379–393

Janigan DT, Druet RL (1968): Experimental murine amyloidosis in X-irradiated recipients of spleen homogenates or serum from sensitized donors. *Am J Pathol* 52:381–390

Kitamoto T, Ohta M, Doh-ura K, Hitash S, Tarao Y, Tateishi J (1993a): Novel missvariants of prion protein in Creutzfeldt-Jakob disease or Gertsmann-Sträussler syndrome. *Biochem Biophys Res Commun* 191:709

Kitamoto T, Iizuka R, Tateishi J (1993b): An amber mutation of prion protein in Gertsmann-Sträussler syndrome with mutant PrP plaques. *Biochem Biophys Res Commun* 192:525–531

Kretzschmar HA, Kufer P, Riethmüller G, DeArmond S, Prusiner SB, Schiffer D (1992): Prion protein mutation at codon 102 in an Italian family with Gerstmann-Sträussler-Scheinker syndrome. *Neurology* 42:809–810

Mitrová E (1980): Focal accumulation of Creutzfeldt-Jakob disease in Slovakia. In: *Search for the Cause of Multiple Sclerosis and Other Chronic Disease of the Central Nervous System*, Boese A, ed., pp. 356–366. Weinheim: Verlag Chemie

Mitrová E (1990): Analytical epidemiology and risk factors of CJD. In *Unconventional Virus Diseases of the Central Nervous System*, Court LA, Dormont D, Brown P, Kingsbury DT, eds. Paris: Commissanat á l'Energie Atomique, Service de Documentation

Mitrová E, Brown P, Hroncová D, Tatara M, Zilák J (1991): Focal accumulation of CJD in Slovakia: retrospective investigation of a new rural familial cluster. *Eur J Epidemiol* 7:487–489

Nieto A, Goldfarb LG, Brown P, Wexler P, Chodosh HL, McCombie WR, Trapp S (1991): Mutation in codon 178 of amyloid precursor gene occurs in Creutzfeldt-Jakob disease families of diverse ethnic origins. *Lancet* 337:622–623

Niewold TA, Hol PR, van Andel ACJ, Lutz ETG, Gruys E (1987): Enhancement of amyloid induction by amyloid fibril fragments in hamster. *Lab Invest* 56:544–549

Owen F, Poulter M, Collinge J, Crow T (1990a): Codon 129 changes in the prion protein gene in Caucasians. *Am J Hum Genet* 46:1215–1216

Owen F, Poulter M, Lofthouse R, Collinge J, Crow TJ, Risby D, Baker HF, Ridley RM, Hsiao K, Prusiner SB (1989): Insertion in prion protein gene in familial Creutzfeldt-Jakob disease. *Lancet* i:51–52

Owen F, Poulter M, Shah T, Collinge J, Lofthaus R, Baker H, Ridley R, McVey J, Crow TJ (1990b): An in-frame insertion in the prion protein gene in familial Creutzfeldt-Jakob disease. *Mol Brain Res* 7:273–276

Ranlov P (1967): The adoptive transfer of experimental mouse amyloidosis by intravenous injection of spleen cell extracts from casein-treated syngeneic donor mice. *Acta Pathol Microbiol Scand* 70:321–335

Safar J: Infectious amyloid, prions, unconventional viruses and disease, review. *Neurobiol Aging* (in press, a)

Safar J, Wang W, Padgett MP, Ceroni M, Piccardo P, Zopf D, Gajdusek DC, Gibbs CJ Jr (1990): Molecular mass, biochemical composition and physicochemical behavior of the infectious form of the scrapie precursor protein monomer. *Proc Natl Acad Sci USA* 87:6373–6377

Safar J, Roller PP, Ruben GC, Gajdusek DC, Gibbs CJ Jr (1993a): Secondary structure of proteins associated in thin films. *Biopolymers* 33:1461–1476

Safar J, Roller PP, Gajdusek DC, Gibbs CJ Jr (1993b): Confirmational transitions, dissociation, and unfolding of scrapie amyloid (prion) proteins. *J Biol Chem* 268:20276–20284

Sasaki H, Yoshioka N, Takagi Y, Sakaki Y (1985): Structure of the chromosomal gene for human serum prealbumin. *Gene* 37:191–197

Tsuzuki T, Mita S, Maede S, Araki S, Shimada KJ (1985): Structure of the human prealbumin gene. *Biol Chem* 260:12224–12227

Wakasugi S, Inomoto T, Yi S, Naito M, Ushira M, Iwanaga T, Maeda S, Araki K, Miyasaki J, Takahashi K, Shimada K, Yamamure K (1988): A potential animal model for familial amyloidotic polyneuropathy through introduction of human mutant transthyretin gene into mice. In: *Amyloid and Amyloidoses*, Takashi I, Shakuro A, Fumike O, Shozo K, Eiro T, eds., pp. 393–398. New York: Plenum Press

Yi S, Tadahashi K, Tashiro F, Wakasugi S, Yamamura K, Araki S (1990): Pathological similarity to human familial amyloidotic polyneuropathy (FAP) type 1 in transgenic mice carrying the human mutant transthyretin gene. In: *Program and Abstracts of the VIth International Symposium on Amyloidosis*, Oslo, Norway, August 5–9, 1990, p. 58, Abstr. 07/5

19

Amyotrophic Lateral Sclerosis/Parkinsonism-Dementia Complex of Guam: Two Distinct Clinical Entities or a Single Disease Process with a Spectrum of Neuropathological and Clinical Expression?

DANIEL P. PERL

Guam is the largest of the Marianas islands, an archipelago in the western pacific that lies approximately 3800 miles west of Hawaii and 1500 miles south of Tokyo. Guam has a total land area of 225 square miles and measures approximately 30 miles long and 4 to 9 miles wide. Of the total civilian population of 110,000, approximately 55,000 of the island's inhabitants are an indigenous native people referred to as Chamorros, with 25,000 inhabitants being migrants from the Philippines while an additional 20,000 inhabitants originate from other ethnic backgrounds (predominantly Caucasian, Carolinian, Hawaiian, and other Asian immigrants). Finally, there are several large military bases on the island with approximately 25,000 military personnel and dependents assigned to these facilities. The assignments of these military personnel are rotated frequently, and they typically do not reside on the island for longer than a year or two.

Guam has been recognized as the site of a remarkable concentration of cases of neurodegenerative diseases. The diseases are referred to as the amyotrophic lateral sclerosis/parkinsonism dementia complex of Guam and were initially characterized both clinically and neuropathologically in a series of papers by Mulder, Kurland, Hirano, and colleagues. Initial medical recognition of the high incidence of neurological disease among the native population of Guam was made in 1944 by Dr. Harry Zimmerman, a pathologist assigned to Guam by the U.S. Navy. He identified several cases of amyotrophic lateral sclerosis in natives being cared for in the local civilian hospital.

The initial reports of a focus of neurological disease on Guam stimulated numerous epidemiologic, clinical, neuropathological, and etio-

ADVANCES IN RESEARCH ON NEURODEGENERATION, II
Y. Mizuno et al.
© 1994 Birkhäuser Boston

logical studies to better characterize the at-risk population and the neurodegenerative disorders with which the natives were plagued. An important
aspect of these studies was to identify the underlying cause(s) of the problem.
Initially, only amyotrophic lateral sclerosis was recognized to be highly
prevalent among the Guamanian Chamorro population (Hirano et al.,
1961a) but neurological surveys of the island quickly revealed a large
number of cases who showed predominantly parkinsonian symptoms
accompanied by dementia, and this became known as the parkinsonism
dementia complex of Guam (Hirano et al., 1961b). Door-to-door surveys
demonstrated that although affected natives were widely distributed on
Guam, the greatest prevalence of neurological disease was found in several
small villages on the southern end of the island and on the adjacent smaller
island of Rota (Reed et al., 1966, 1987). In a study performed in 1953–1954,
Kurland and Mulder (1954) estimated that the prevalence of amyotrophic
lateral sclerosis among the Chamorro population of Guam was approximately 420 per 100,000 population (versus 6 per 100,000 in the continental
United States). Except for rare cases among the Filipino migrants to the
island, the disease is confined to the local Chamorro population.

Studies of amyotrophic lateral sclerosis (ALS) among Guamanians
revealed that the clinical features of their illness were virtually indistinguishable from those of ALS patients encountered elsewhere in the
world (Mulder and Espinosa, 1969). Neuropathological changes in the
spinal cord were also virtually identical to those classically ascribed to the
disease (Hirano et al., 1967). However, Malamud et al. (1961) identified
large numbers of neurofibrillary tangles in the brains of affected individuals. The appearance of numerous neurofibrillary tangles in the
hippocampus, entorhinal cortex, and neocortex clearly distinguishes the
Guamanian form of ALS from that seen elsewhere in the world (Hirano
et al., 1967). Nevertheless, the Marianas form of ALS was considered to
be a valid model of motor neuron disease, and research programs to
identify the underlying cause of ALS among the Chamorros of Guam
carried the clear implication that findings among this high-incidence
focus would "surely contribute to a better understanding of the disease
[ALS] elsewhere" (Gajdusek, 1982).

The identification of a form of parkinsonism associated with severe
dementia in high prevalence among Guamanian Chamorros added to the
complexity of the problem. Most of the parkinsonism cases encountered
on the island also showed signs of rather profound cognitive dysfunction,
even in the early phases of the disease. Although cognitive impairment
can be encountered in association with classic idiopathic Parkinson's
disease, dementia is generally considered to be a rather late feature of the
disease. While James Parkinson's (1817) admonition that in paralysis

agitans the "intellect remains uninjured" is no longer considered to be correct, in the earlier phases of Parkinson's disease this remains an accurate description. Neuropathological investigations of the Guamanian form of parkinsonism revealed the presence of extensive neurofibrillary tangle formation in the hippocampus, the neocortex, and in the substantia nigra, locus ceruleus, and periaqueductal gray matter with an absence of Lewy bodies, the inclusion bodies that have traditionally been considered to be a neuropathological hallmark of idiopathic Parkinson's disease. These neuropathological features, particularly those in the brain stem, were rather similar to that described in post encephalitic parkinsonism (Oppenheimer and Esiri, 1992; Torvik and Meen, 1966). From these observations, it was suggested that the parkinsonism-dementia complex of Guam might well represent a form of postencephalitic parkinsonism similar to that which followed the epidemic of encephalitis lethargica described by von Ecconomo. Clinically, postencephalitic parkinsonism is difficult to distinguish from the idiopathic form, although oculogyric crises are said to be prominently seen in the former (Adams and Victor, 1993). Clinical investigations of Guamanian cases failed to identify such oculogyric features (Elizan et al. 1966), although the specificity of this negative finding is difficult to weigh.

Could repeated epidemics of encephalitis produce a continuous record of subsequent disease and yet have been unrecognized by survivors and unaffected individuals on Guam? Studies of serum and postmortem brain tissues from affected individuals have failed to show any reproducible evidence of the presence, either active or preceding, of any potentially neurotrophic infection (Gibbs and Gajdusek, 1982). It is clear that a high incidence of neurological disease had existed for many years before Zimmerman's initial observations in 1944. Archival death certificate records available from around 1900 document numerous diagnoses of ALS and of presenile dementia among Guam natives, and folklore accounts suggest that the problem existed before this. Nevertheless, the natives have not recalled past episodes of encephalitis although epidemics of Japanese B encephalitis and mumps did occur on the island in December 1947 and April 1948 (Elizan et al., 1966). Although the neighboring small island of Rota also shows evidence of a high prevalence of identical neurological disorders, the nearby Marianas islands of Tinian and Saipan, readily accessible to Guam's native population as well as to potential vectors for spreading viral infections, have never shown any propensity for these diseases. It seems rather implausible that a viral infection with the propensity for neural invasion and latency could be uniquely restricted with such high prevalence to Guam and Rota yet not appear, even to a small degree, in the other inhabited neighboring islands of the archipelago. Finally, a link of postencephalitic neurodegeneration with parkinsonian features to cases of ALS has little precedence in the medical literature. Nevertheless, the concept of the neurodegeneration related to a postencephalitic process continues to be raised (Hudson and Rice, 1990).

It has therefore been important to evaluate whether the Marianas form of ALS and parkinsonism-dementia of Guam represent two separate distinct entities or the two extremes of a spectrum of clinical manifestations of a single neurodegenerative disorder. Resolution of this critical question would have important implications for approaches to concepts of etiology and pathogenesis of these diseases as encountered on Guam as well as elsewhere in the world.

In this chapter, I will examine the evidence suggesting overlap between the two forms of neurological disease encountered among the Guamanian Chamorros. As I review, on both clinical and neuropathological grounds there is considerable evidence of overlap between the two, suggesting that they do indeed represent the extremes of a broad spectrum of neurodegenerative disease reflecting either common etiological mechanisms or underlying pathogenetic processes.

Evidence of Parkinsonism-Dementia Among Guamanian Patients with ALS

Clinical

The manifestations of cases of amyotrophic lateral sclerosis among Guamanian Chamorros are said to be clinically indistinguishable from the disease as seen elsewhere in the world (Mulder and Espinosa, 1969). Although the age of onset is somewhat earlier in the Guamanian patients, the duration of illness, male predominance, and presenting signs and symptoms consisting of weakness, atrophy, and fasciculations are virtually identical. It is rare for superimposed overt parkinsonian signs and symptoms to be noted in Guamanian ALS patients. Elizan et al. (1966) reported that only 5 of 104 Guam ALS cases subsequently developed a definite clinical picture of parkinsonism-dementia complex while an additional 5 patients showed parkinsonian features in the absence of organic mental symptoms. In a further review of clinical presentation, Rodgers-Johnson and colleagues (1986) reported that of 279 Guam patients who had been clinically diagnosed as ALS, minimal extrapyramidal signs were found in 15 patients (5%) and mild dementia in only 12 (4%).

However, evidence of extrapyramidal system involvement in Guamanian ALS patients has been obtained from positron emission tomography

(PET) studies. Striatal dopamine metabolism was recently reported in a group of patients from Guam using PET scanning of $[^{18}F]$6-fluorodopa uptake (Snow et al., 1990). As a group, the four Guamanian ALS patients showed decreased striatal fluorodopa uptake that was intermediate between that encountered in Guam parkinsonism-dementia cases and controls. This important study provides important functional data supporting the notion that these cases also demonstrate pathology in the nigrostriatal dopamine pathway despite classic ALS symptomatology.

Neuropathology

The initial classic neuropathological descriptions of the Guamanian form of ALS documented evidence of widespread pathological involvement of neuronal populations outside the usual involvement of the pyramidal motor system (Malamud et al., 1961). In the initial report by Malamud and co-workers, neurofibrillary tangles were identified in all 22 cases (Malamud et al., 1961). In such cases prominent neurofibrillary tangle formation was identified in the hippocampus and brain stem, including the substantia nigra (Hirano et al., 1967; Malamud et al., 1961). In the review by Rodgers-Johnson and colleagues (1986) of neuropathological findings of 209 autopsies performed on Guamanian ALS cases, 63 (46%) showed evidence of neuronal loss and depigmentation in the substantia nigra. This later study must be viewed with some caution because it was derived from review of the neuropathology findings incorporated in neuropathology reports from a number of different neuropathologists and, over the years, no specific protocol for brain sampling and neuropathology data collection was adopted or followed. Despite these limitations, extensive examples of substantia nigra degeneration were clearly identified by numerous independent observers.

Evidence of ALS Among Cases of Parkinsonism-Dementia Complex of Guam

Clinical

Many cases of parkinsonism-dementia complex show prominent clinical evidence of superimposed amyotrophy. In Elizan's series (1966) of 72 PDC patients, 38% subsequently went on to develop a clinical picture of superimposed ALS. Further, 12 cases of what was considered 'pure' parkinsonism-dementia showed electromyographic evidence of a lower motor neuron lesion, despite the absence of any clinically observable evidence of focal muscular wasting. Rodgers-Johnson et al. (1986), reviewing a large series of patients, reported that of 328 patients considered clinically to have parkinsonism-dementia 34% also showed a positive Babinski sign and 32% demonstrated fasciculations or muscular atrophy.

Neuropathology

In the initial neuropathological descriptions of parkinsonism-dementia complex, 17 of 45 (38%) cases were reported to show typical changes of ALS in the spinal cord (Hirano et al., 1961b). The retrospective review of Rodgers-Johnson et al (1986) indicated that lateral column demyelination and loss of anterior horn cells were also included in the neuropathological reports in 35% of 113 PDC autopsies for whom spinal cord specimens were available. It is unclear whether the availability of spinal cord samples in these parkinsonism-dementia cases were more likely to occur in cases with superimposed amyotrophy or whether this constitutes a representative sample. The comparability of the extent of involvement of the spinal cord in the neuropathology studies with the clinical observations suggests the latter.

Clinicopathological Correlation

Review of neuropathological findings of large numbers of cases of ALS/parkinsonism-dementia complex of Guam indicates that the distribution of neuropathological involvement is widespread and that far more cases with superimposed neuropathological changes (overlap) exist than would be appreciated simply by clinical evaluation. It appears that the extent of superimposition of upper and lower motor neuron pathology in cases with primary substantia nigral degeneration can eventually be properly appreciated by clinical observation. In general, amyotrophic features in cases of parkinsonism-dementia tend to be observable in the later stages of disease and are documented in clinical reports in approximately 40% of cases. This is in good accord with neuropathological studies in which spinal cord lesions associated with ALS were recognized in 35% of cases where spinal cord specimens were available.

It should be recognized that in most cases of ALS, whether seen among the Guamanian Chamorro or in populations elsewhere in the world, the neuropathological features encountered in the spinal cord are definitive and rather easily recognized by the neuropathologists when an appropriate specimen is made available. However, in my experience milder forms of involvement in the spinal cord may be present and are difficult to document with certainty. This generally takes the form of mild loss of anterior horn cells with mild focal shrinkage and pyknosis of remaining neurons. Lateral column myelin pallor can be difficult to document without good histological preparations. Mishandling of the spinal cord can produce a wide range of artifacts which may preclude the identification of these changes. This suggests that in many additional cases of parkinsonism-dementia a more subtle degree of upper and lower motor neuron pathology might well have been present but has not been specifically identified or documented neuropathologically.

The experience with clinicopathological correlation of extrapyramidal features superimposed on Guamanian cases of ALS indicates that correlation of pathology with clinical manifestations is rather poor. Published neuropathological studies agree that approximately 45% of Guamanian ALS cases also show significant evidence of neuronal loss in the substantia nigra. This is in contradistinction to only 5% of ALS cases manifesting extrapyramidal features on clinical examination. It is possible that the neuronal reserve in the extrapyramidal system is greater than that of the pyramidal motor system and that sufficient numbers of substantia nigral neurons have not been lost for symptoms to be clinically apparent. It is clear that one must lose a significant proportion of nigral neurons before one begins to manifest clinically apparent parkinsonian features, and the lack of sufficient degenerative changes may account for the lack of overt symptomatology. On the other hand, it is possible that loss of extrapyramidal control of voluntary muscles that have undergone partial denervation related to ALS may not have the degree of recognizable clinical effects as those on normally innervated skeletal muscular system.

From the perspective of the neuropathologist, it is clear from a review of these data that relatively few cases of neurodegenerative disease among Guamanian Chamorros are "pure" in the sense that either the upper and lower motor neurons are affected while the extrapyramidal system remains completely spared. In a similar fashion, if looked at with care, few parkinsonism-dementia complex cases fail to show evidence of pathology in the lateral columns and anterior horn cells of the spinal cord. The clinical features tend to be misleading, particularly in evaluating cases in which the initiating symptoms were marked by amyotrophy. In such cases, any evidence of superimposed extrapryamidal involvement will rarely be appreciated. When the early course of illness is marked by either extrapyramidal symptomatology or dementia, then a substantial proportion of cases will reveal the presence of amyotrophic pathology as manifested by the presence of fasciculations or wasting. Studies suggest that in additional cases, despite an entirely negative clinical examination, electromyographic approaches will uncover the presence of significant motor neuron pathology. At autopsy, the full extent of overlapping pathology becomes clearer, although in my opinion even here some of the more subtle pathological manifestations can be missed. In general, with respect to upper and lower motor neuron involvement, losses have to be fairly substantial before a diagnosis of amyotrophic lateral sclerosis is reached by morphological criteria.

On the basis of the foregoing discussion, I believe that it can be argued that amyotrophic lateral sclerosis/parkinsonism dementia complex of Guam represents a spectrum of clinical manifestations of a single neurodegenerative disorder rather than two distinct and separate clinical entities. Whether an individual patient is considered to have the amyotrophic lateral sclerosis or the parkinsonian form of the disease is guided by the initiating clinical manifestations, which presumably reflect the site of earliest and most severe neuronal degeneration. In general, cases presenting with ALS are younger and endure a shorter clinical course, when compared to those who initiate with parkinsonian features. These concepts have a number of important implications, particularly with respect to the observations of Garruto and co-workers (1985) on changes in the epidemiology of the epidemic of neurological diseases on Guam. Examining trends in incidence rates of ALS and parkinsonism-dementia among the Chamorro population on Guam, they reported a dramatic drop in cases of ALS along with a rise in their age of onset. Decreases in rates of parkinsonism dementia were also observed but these were not nearly as dramatic. The incidence figures they reported were derived by examining the numbers of cases presenting at the National Institute of Neurological and Communicative Disorders and Stroke (NINCDS) research station on Guam and by employing the clinical impression based on the predominant neurological symptomatology in the early phases of the illness. Considering the lack of specificity of the individual clinical manifestations of the disease, the more important change appears to be an increase in the age of onset with a concomitant tendency to manifest parkinsonism or even dementia in its earliest clinical manifestations. Considering the earlier discussion, it is quite possible that over the past 35 years the overall extent of the problem may not have changed at all, except that fewer cases begin as ALS before the age of 45 and more initiate after age 60 with features of parkinsonism or dementia.

Finally, what are the implications of these observations with regard to an understanding of comparable diseases encountered elsewhere in the world? For many years approaches to neurological disease in the Marianas has been viewed as an opportunity to explore etiopathogenetic concepts related to ALS. Similar concepts regarding Parkinson's disease are less frequently articulated, perhaps resulting from confusion related to characterizing and understanding pathogenetic forces that might underlie the numerous and diverse forms of parkinsonism. Finally, as we have recently argued, the natives of Guam demonstrate neurofibrillary tangles as well as most of the other histopathological features of Alzheimer's disease and thus represent an important model for this important neurodegenerative disease. The observations on affected Guam natives imply that ALS, Parkinson's disease, and even Alzheimer's disease share common pathogenetic pathways and that similar evidence of overlap might be anticipated among affected non-Guamanian patients. A review of comparable evidence in non-Guamanian populations is not in order in this chapter, except to note that evidence is accumulating that parkinsonian features are encountered in both clinical and neuropathological studies of cases of Alzheimer's disease, that Alzheimer's disease-related features are encountered in many cases of Parkinson's disease, and that similar overlap with ALS is also been observed in non-Guamanian cases.

With this in mind, one begins to appreciate that the opportunities offered through the study of affected Guam natives are much broader than originally recognized. It has been my view that the cases of neurological disease encountered in the Guamanian Chamorro represents the "Rosetta Stone" of the neurodegenerative diseases common to the elderly. (The Rosetta Stone is a slab of black basalt, discovered in Egypt in 1799, on which text was written in three ancient languages, Greek, the demotic language, and Egyptian hieroglyphics. Through an understanding of the Greek passage the other two major ancient languages could finally be decoded and numerous other passages could then be understood.) It is our hope that through the deciphering of the clues available through the study of Guam, its people, and its environment, we may one day be able to understand etiological and pathogenetic issues with respect to the three major neurodegenerative diseases encountered among the elderly worldwide, namely amyotrophic lateral sclerosis, Parkinson's disease, and Alzheimer's disease.

References

Adams RD, Victor M (1993): *Principles of Neurology* 5th Ed. New York: McGraw-Hill

Elizan TS, Hirano A, Abrams BM, Need RL, Van Nuis C, Kurland LT (1966): Amyotrophic lateral sclerosis and parkinsonism-dementia complex of Guam. Neurological reevaluation. *Arch Neurol* 14:356–368

Gajdusek DC (1982): Foci of motor neuron disease in high incidence in isolated populations of East Asia and the Western Pacific. In: *Human Motor Neuron Disease*, Rowland LP, ed. *Advances in Neurology* 36:363–393 New York: Raven Press

Garruto RM, Yanagihara R, Gajdusek DC (1985): Disappearance of high-incidence amyotrophic lateral sclerosis and parkinsonism-dementia on Guam. *Neurology* 35:193–198

Gibbs CJ Jr, Gajdusek DC (1982): An update on longterm in vivo and in vitro studies designed to identify a virus as a cause of amyotrophic lateral sclerosis, parkinsonism-dementia and Parkinson disease. In: *Human Motor Neuron Disease*, Rowland LP, ed. *Advances in Neurology* 36:343–351 New York: Raven Press

Hirano A, Arumugasamy N, Zimmerman HM (1967): Amyotrophic lateral sclerosis. A comparison of Guam and classical cases. *Arch Neurol* 16:357–363

Hirano A, Kurland LIT, Krooth RS, Lessell S (1961a): Parkinsonism-dementia complex, an endemic disease on the island of Guam. I. Clinical features. *Brain* 84:642–661

Hirano A, Malamud N, Kurland LIT (1961b): Parkinsonism-dementia complex, an endemic disease on the island of Guam. II. Pathological features. *Brain* 84:662–679

Hudson AJ, Rice GP (1990): Similarities of guamanian ALS/PD to post-encephalitic parkinsonism/ALS: possible viral cause. *Can J Neurol Sci* 17:427–433

Kurland LT, Mulder DW (1954): Epidemiologic investigations of amyotrophic lateral sclerosis. 1. Preliminary report on geographic distribution, with special reference to the Mariana Islands, including clinical and pathological observations. *Neurology* 4:355–378; 438–448

Malamud N, Hirano A, Kurland LT (1961): Pathoanatomic changes in amyotrophic lateral sclerosis on Guam. *Neurology* 5:401–414

Mulder DW, Espinosa RE (1969): Amyotrophic lateral sclerosis: comparison of the clinical syndrome in Guam and the United States. In: *Motor Neuron Diseases: Research on Amyotrophic Lateral Sclerosis and Related Disorders*, Norris JH Jr, Kurland LT, eds. New York: Grune & Stratton

Oppenheimer DR, Esiri MM (1992): Diseases of the basal ganglia,cerebellum and motor neurons. In: *Greenfield's Neuropathology* 5th Ed., Adams JH, Duchen LW, eds. New York: Oxford University Press

Parkinson J (1817): An essay on the shaking palsy. London: Reproduced in *James Parkinson*, Critchley M, ed. London: McMillan, 1955

Reed D, Labarthe D, Chen KM, Stallones R (1987): A cohort study of amyotrophic lateral sclerosis and parkinsonism-dementia on Guam and Rota. *Am J Epidemiol* 125:92–100

Reed D, Plato C, Elizan T, Kurland LT (1966): The amyotrophic lateral sclerosis/ parkinsonism-dementia complex: a ten-year follow-up on Guam. I. Epidemiological studies. *Am J Epidemiol* 83:54–73

Rodgers-Johnson P, Garruto RM, Yanagihara R, Chen K-M, Gajdusek DC, Gibbs CJ Jr (1986): Amyotrophic lateral sclerosis and parkinsonism-dementia on Guam: a 30-year evaluation of clinical and neuropathologic trends. *Neurology* 36:7–13

Snow BJ, Peppard RF, Guttman M, Okada J, Martin WR, Steele J, Eisen A, Carr G, Schoenberg B, Calne D (1990): Positron emission tomographic scanning demonstrates a presynaptic dopaminergic lesion in Lytico-Bodig. The amyotrophic lateral sclerosis-parkinsonism-dementia complex of Guam. *Arch Neurol* 47:870–874

Torvik A, Meen D (1966): Distribution of the brain stem lesions in postencephalitic parkinsonism. *Acta Neurol Scand* 42:415–425

20

Discussion: Session 5 – 8 P.M. – 9 February 1993

RECORDED BY DONALD B. CALNE

Reichmann: After Reichmann's paper, Beal asked whether the problem of differences in tissue collection, tissue preparation, and analytic technique might provide a possible explanation for the disparity in the results of mitochondrial enzyme studies reported from various laboratories. While these factors might contribute to the results, it was hard to imagine that they could provide a complete explanation.

McGeer raised the next issue which was the problem of interpreting changes in the substantia nigra when a large number of neurons were lost and a large number of immunologically activated glia were gained. It was agreed that this might be a significant flaw in the interpretation of some findings. Because of this difficulty, immunohistochemical observations were particularly important, since here the cell types could be identified.

McGeer also asked Reichmann whether all the mitochondrial diseases were inherited maternally. The answer was most, but not all.

Snow suggested that differences in the level of muscle activity might contribute to some of the variation in the reported findings. Reichmann thought it unlikely that muscle activity could be a major factor determining the diversity of the results.

Youdim stated that in the brain, histochemical techniques only revealed complex I in the neurons, yet the neurons represented less than 5% of the cells. Mizuno stated that the glia and the neurophil could be shown, by immunostaining, to contain complex I, but the staining was weak. In fact, he considered that the histological and biochemical data were in agreement; in Parkinson's disease there was a reduction of complex I by some 30% in the substantia nigra. Youdim then asked if the weak staining for complex I in the glia and neurophil was about the same in patients with Parkinson's disease and controls. Reichmann said it was.

Mizuno commented that he considered that changes in complex I in

Parkinson's disease were more likely to represent a secondary phenomenon rather than a primary one. Nevertheless, Mizuno explained, a secondary depletion of complex I could be important. Certainly, it would be worthwhile to seek the cause of the 30% reduction of nigral complex I. He pointed out that similar changes in complex I seemed to be part of the normal aging process. He suggested that in Parkinson's disease there was localized accelerated aging of the substantia nigra, but what could cause this? He considered the best current explanation was a combination of high oxidative metabolism and a high level of neurophysiological activity.

Tsui then asked whether the magnitude of the postmortem reduction of nigral complex I was related to the duration of Parkinson's disease or to the cumulative exposure to levodopa. Reichmann replied that there was insufficient evidence, at this time, to provide an answer.

Olanow suggested that the difference between the levels of complex I in nigral neurons and muscle might derive from the fact that muscle cells can replicate, while nigral neurons cannot. Reichmann did not believe that this provided a satisfactory explanation.

Youdim returned to the issue of disease progression. He said that as Parkinson's disease advances he found an increase in iron and a decrease in glutathione, in keeping with the oxidative stress hypothesis.

Baimbridge asked if the analytical techniques employed for measuring complex I would reveal the presence of a possible neurotoxin. Reichmann thought this would be most unlikely.

Nagatsu asked if complex I had been measured in the locus ceruleus. Reichmann said it had not.

Oertel: Following Oertel's paper, Calne asked about the relationship between gangliosides and growth factors. Oertel said that gangliosides had no place in treating human disease, because in Europe three cases of Guillain–Barré syndrome had now been attributed to them. Oertel suggested that subfractions of gangliosides should be explored instead.

Gajdusek: After Gajdusek's paper, Calne asked why there was not a better correlation between amyloid deposition and clinical deficits in Alzheimer's disease, if amyloid was neurotoxic. Gajdusek replied that the clinical consequence would depend primarily on the intellectual expertise achieved by the Alzheimer patients before their illness. The variations in the level of premorbid intelligence were more important than the extent of amyloid deposition in determining the clinical outcome.

Perl: Following Perl's paper, Gajdusek and Baimbridge discussed the possible role of mineral intoxication in Guamanian neurodegeneration. They stressed the importance of a low intake of calcium being combined with a high level of aluminum exposure. The absorption of aluminum is substantially increased by the adjustments that take place to enhance calcium intake in a setting of low dietary content.

Olanow asked why there was selective distribution of metals to certain regions of the central nervous system. Gajdusek pointed out that characteristic patterns of distribution also occurred with viruses. He said that the same virus underwent totally different distribution, in the brain, in different species. Perl argued that the way the various minerals were distributed in characteristics patterns in the central nervous system made him wonder if they might be spread along anatomical neuronal pathways.

Erratum

The publisher wishes to apologize for an error that was made in *Advances in Research in Neurodegeneration, Volume I: Definitions, Clinical Features and Morphology*. On page 69 of Chapter 7, "The Biology of Toxic Events in Parkinson's Disease," by M.B.H. Youdim, the wrong figure was shown as Figure 1. The correct Figure 1 is shown below.

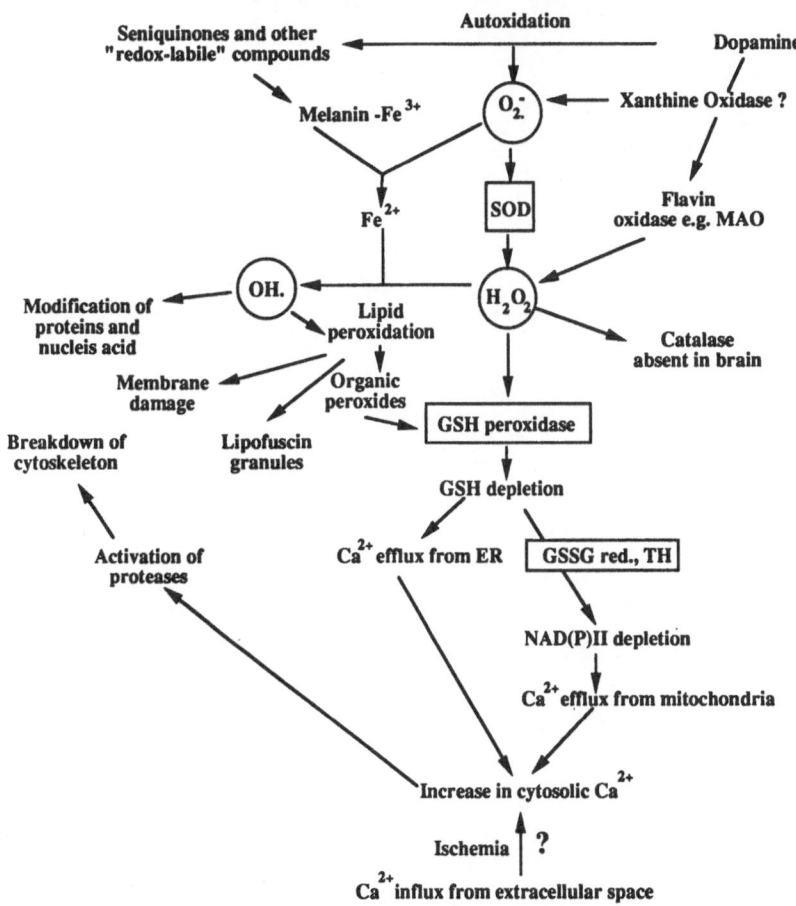

Figure 1. Metabolism of dopamine in the human brain substantia nigra via oxidative deamination by MAO-B and autooxidation, with the generation of hydrogen peroxide. In the absence of gluthathione peroxidase activity or reduced gluthathione or excess decompartmentalized iron, an interaction between hydrogen peroxide and Fe^{2+} (Fenton reaction) is envisaged. This can lead to the formation of cytotoxic hydroxyl radical (OH·) (Fenton reaction) and membrane lipid peroxidation via oxidation reduction of iron by hydrogen peroxide and melanin, respectively. The consequence of increased nigral iron (siderosis) can be tissue-oxidative stress (Youdim et al., 1989; Ben-Shachar et al., 1991b).